Please remember that this is a library book,
and that it belongs only temporarily to each
person who uses it. Be considerate. Do
not write in this, or any, library book.

Anna Metteri, MSocSc
Teppo Kröger, PhD
Anneli Pohjola, PhD
Pirkko-Liisa Rauhala, PhD
Editors

Social Work Visions from Around the Globe: Citizens, Methods, and Approaches

Social Work Visions from Around the Globe: Citizens, Methods, and Approaches has been co-published simultaneously as *Social Work in Health Care*, Volume 39, Numbers 1/2 and

Pre-publication REVIEWS, COMMENTARIES, EVALUATIONS . . .

"IMPORTANT. . . . AN EXTRA-ORDINARY CONTRIBUTION TO THE SOCIAL WORK LITERATURE. This collection brings the world of social work from five different continents into the classroom as well as into everyday practice. Chapters from around the world bring a refreshing new light to social work practice and understanding. With each chapter, the reader is introduced to challenging concepts and methods of practice that reflect the cultures and histories of diverse communities."

Robert Blundo, PhD, LCSW
Associate Professor
Department of Social Work
University of North Carolina at Wilmington

The Haworth Social Work Practice Press
An Imprint of The Haworth Press, Inc.

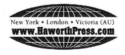

New York • London • Victoria (AU)
www.HaworthPress.com

Social Work Visions from Around the Globe: Citizens, Methods, and Approaches

Social Work Visions from Around the Globe: Citizens, Methods, and Approaches has been co-published simultaneously as *Social Work in Health Care*, Volume 39, Numbers 1/2 and 3/4 2004.

The *Social Work in Health Care*™ Monographic "Separates"

Series Editors: Gary Rosenberg, PhD, Editor, *Social Work in Health Care*, and Andrew Weissman, PhD, Managing Editor, *Social Work in Health Care*, Mount Sinai School of Medicine, The Mount Sinai Medical Center, New York, NY

Below is a list of "separates," which in serials librarianship means a special issue simultaneously published as a special journal issue or double-issue *and* as a "separate" hardbound monograph. (This is a format which we also call a "DocuSerial.")

"Separates" are published because specialized libraries or professionals may wish to purchase a specific thematic issue by itself in a format which can be separately cataloged and shelved, as opposed to purchasing the journal on an on-going basis. Faculty members may also more easily consider a "separate" for classroom adoption.

"Separates" are carefully classified separately with the major book jobbers so that the journal tie-in can be noted on new book order slips to avoid duplicate purchasing.

You may wish to visit Haworth's website at . . .

http://www.HaworthPress.com

. . . to search our online catalog for complete tables of contents of these separates and related publications.

You may also call 1-800-HAWORTH (outside US/Canada: 607-722-5857), or Fax 1-800-895-0582 (outside US/Canada: 607-771-0012), or e-mail at:

docdelivery@haworthpress.com

Social Work Visions from Around the Globe: Citizens, Methods, and Approaches, edited by Anna Metteri, MSoc et al. (Vol. 39, No. 1/2 and 3/4, 2004). *"VALUABLE to practitioners in health and mental health. . . . Shows in a practical way how citizenship can be an inclusive practice related to social justice, rather than a way of excluding people from opportunities and resources in our societies." (Heather D'Cruz, PhD, MSW, Senior Lecturer in Social Work, School of Health and Social Development, Faculty of Health and Behavioural Sciences, Deakin University, Geelong, Victoria, Australia)*

Social Work Health and Mental Health: Practice, Research and Programs, edited by Alun C. Jackson, PhD, and Steven P. Segal, PhD (Vol. 34, No. 1/2 and 3/4, 2001, and Vol. 35, No. 1/2, 2002). *Explores international perspectives on social work practice in health and mental health.*

Clinical Data-Mining in Practice-Based Research: Social Work in Hospital Settings, edited by Irwin Epstein, PhD, and Susan Blumenfield, DSW, (Vol. 33, No. 3/4, 2001). *"Challenging and illuminating. . . . This remarkable collection of exemplary studies provides inspiration and support to social workers. This book will be valuable not only as a guide to practitioners, but also is an important addition to the teaching materials for courses in social work in health care and in social research methodology." (Kay V. Davidson, DSW, Dean and Professor, University of Connecticut School of Social Work, West Hartford)*

Behavioral and Social Sciences in 21st Century Health Care: Contributions and Opportunities, edited by Gary Rosenberg, PhD, and Andrew Weissman, PhD (Vol. 33, No. 1, 2001). *"Stimulating and provocative. . . . The range of topics covered makes this book an ideal reader for health care practice courses with a combined health/mental health focus." (Goldie Kadushin, PhD, Associate Professor, School of Social Welfare, University of Wisconsin-Milaukee)*

Seventh Doris Siegel Memorial Colloquium: Behavioral Health Care Practice in the 21st Century, edited by Gary Rosenberg, PhD, and Andrew Weissman, PhD (Vol. 31, No. 2, 2000). *"A valuable group of research studies examining important and pertinent issues. . . . Offers a fresh perspective on critical problems encountered by health care institutions, providers, patients, and families. Excellent." (Mildred D. Mailick, DSW, Professor Emerita, Hunter College School of Social Work, City University of New York)*

Social Work in Mental Health: Trends and Issues, edited by Uri Aviram (Vol. 25, No. 3, 1997). *"Suggests ways to maintain social work values in a time that emphasizes cost containment and legal requirements that may result in practices and policies that are antithetical to the*

profession." (Phyllis Solomon, PhD, Professor, School of Social Work, University of Pennsylvania)

International Perspectives on Social Work in Health Care: Past, Present and Future, edited by Gail K. Auslander, DSW (Vol. 25, No. 1/2, 1997). *"The authors explore the need for new theoretical and practice models, in addition to developments in health and social work research and administration."* (Council on Social Work and Education)

Fundamentals of Perinatal Social Work: A Guide for Clinical Practice with Women, Infants, and Families, edited by Regina Furlong Lind, MSW, LCSW, and Debra Honig Bachman, MSW, LCSW (Vol. 24, No. 3/4, 1997). *"A knowledge summation of the essence of perinatal social work that is long overdue. It is a must for any beginning perinatal social worker to own one!"* (Charlotte Collins Bursi, MSSW, Perinatal Social Worker, University of Tennessee Newborn Center; Founding President, National Association of Perinatal Social Workers)

Professional Social Work Education and Health Care: Challenges for the Future, edited by Mildred D. Mailick, DSW, and Phyllis Caroff, DSW (Vol. 24, No. 1/2, 1996). *Responds to critical concerns about the educational preparation of social workers within the rapidly changing health care environment.*

Social Work in Pediatrics, edited by Ruth B. Smith, PhD, MSW, and Helen G. Clinton, MSW (Vol. 21, No. 1, 1995). *"It presents models of service delivery and clinical practice that offer responses to the challenges of today's health care system."* (Journal of Social Work Education)

Social Work Leadership in Healthcare: Directors' Perspectives, edited by Gary Rosenberg, PhD, and Andrew Weissman, DSW (Vol. 20, No. 4, 1995). *Social work managers describe their work and work environment, detailing what qualities and traits are needed to be effective and successful now and in the future.*

Social Work in Ambulatory Care: New Implications for Health and Social Services, edited by Gary Rosenberg, PhD, and Andrew Weissman, DSW (Vol. 20, No. 1, 1994). *"A most timely book dealing with issues related to the current shift in health care delivery to ambulatory care and social work's need to position itself in this health care arena."* (Barbara Berkman, DSW, Director of Research and Quality Assessment, Massachusetts General Hospital; Associate Director, Harvard Upper New England Geriatric Education Center, Harvard Medical School)

Women's Health and Social Work: Feminist Perspectives, edited by Miriam Meltzer Olson, DSW (Vol. 19, No. 3/4, 1994). *"[Chapters] explore how social workers can better understand and address women's health, including such conditions as breast cancer, menopause, and depression. They also discuss health care centers and African–American women and AIDS."* (Reference & Research Book News)

The Changing Context of Social Health Care: Its Implications for Providers and Consumers, edited by Helen Rehr, DSW, and Gary Rosenberg, PhD (Vol. 15, No. 4, 1991). *"Required reading for every student and practitioner with a vision of improving our health care delivery system."* (Candyce S. Berger, PhD, MSW, Director of Social Work, University of Washington Medical Center; Associate Professor, School of Social Work, University of Washington)

Social Workers in Health Care Management: The Move to Leadership, edited by Gary Rosenberg, PhD, and Sylvia S. Clarke, MSc, ACSW (Vol. 12, No. 3, 1988). *"Social workers interested in hospital social work management and the potential for advancement within the health care field will find the book interesting and challenging as well as helpful."* (Social Thought)

Social Work and Genetics: A Guide to Practice, edited by Sylvia Schild, DSW, and Rita Beck Black, DSW (Supp #1, 1984). *"Precisely defines the responsibilities of social work in the expanding field of medical genetics and presents a clear, comprehensive overview of basic genetic principles and issues."* (Health and Social Work)

Advancing Social Work Practice in the Health Care Field: Emerging Issues and New Perspectives, edited by Gary Rosenberg, PhD, and Helen Rehr, DSW (Vol. 8, No. 3, 1983). *"Excellent articles, useful bibliographies, and additional reading lists."* (Australian Social Work)

Published by

The Haworth Social Work Practice Press, 10 Alice Street, Binghamton, NY 13904-1580 USA

The Haworth Social Work Practice Press is an imprint of The Haworth Press, Inc., 10 Alice Street, Binghamton, NY 13904-1580 USA.

Social Work Visions from Around the Globe: Citizens, Methods, and Approaches has been co-published simultaneously as *Social Work in Health Care,* Volume 39, Numbers 1/2 and 3/4 2004.

The development, preparation, and publication of this work has been undertaken with great care. However, the publisher, employees, editors, and agents of The Haworth Press and all imprints of The Haworth Press, Inc., including The Haworth Medical Press® and The Pharmaceutical Products Press®, are not responsible for any errors contained herein or for consequences that may ensue from use of materials or information contained in this work. Opinions expressed by the author(s) are not necessarily those of The Haworth Press, Inc.

Cover design by Kerry E. Mack

Library of Congress Cataloging-in-Publication Data

International Conference on Social Work in Health and Mental Health Care (3rd: 2001 : Tampere, Finland)
Social work visions from around the globe: citizens, methods, and approaches/ Anna Metteri, . . [et al.], editors.
      p. cm.– (The social work in health care series)
    "Co-published simultaneously as Social work in health care, volume 39, numbers 1/2, and 3/4 2004"
    Revised versions of selected papers first presented at the 3rd International Conference on Social Work in Health and Mental Health that was organised in July 2001 in Tampere.
    Includes bibliographical references and index.
    ISBN 0-7890-2366-0 (hard cover : alk. paper)–ISBN 0-7890-2367-9 (soft cover : alk. paper)
    1. Medical social work–Congresses. 2. Psychiatric social work–Congresses. 3. Social work with minorities–Congresses. 4. Ethnic groups–Services for Congresses. I. Metteri, Anna. II. Title. III. Series.
HV687.I565 2001
362.1′0425–dc22
                                            2004011706

Social Work Visions from Around the Globe: Citizens, Methods, and Approaches

Anna Metteri, MSocSc
Teppo Kröger, PhD
Anneli Pohjola, PhD
Pirkko-Liisa Rauhala, PhD
Editors

Gary Rosenberg, PhD
Andrew Weissman, PhD
Series Editors

Social Work Visions from Around the Globe: Citizens, Methods, and Approaches has been co-published simultaneously as *Social Work in Health Care*, Volume 39, Numbers 1/2 and 3/4 2004.

The Haworth Social Work Practice Press
An Imprint of The Haworth Press, Inc.

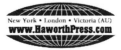

New York • London • Victoria (AU)
www.HaworthPress.com

Indexing, Abstracting & Website/Internet Coverage

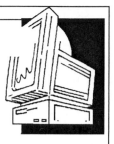

This section provides you with a list of major indexing & abstracting services. That is to say, each service began covering this periodical during the year noted in the right column. Most Websites which are listed below have indicated that they will either post, disseminate, compile, archive, cite or alert their own Website users with research-based content from this work. (This list is as current as the copyright date of this publication.)

(continued)

(continued)

(continued)

*Special Bibliographic Notes related to special journal issues
(separates) and indexing/abstracting:*

- indexing/abstracting services in this list will also cover material in any "separate" that is co-published simultaneously with Haworth's special thematic journal issue or DocuSerial. Indexing/abstracting usually covers material at the article/chapter level.
- monographic co-editions are intended for either non-subscribers or libraries which intend to purchase a second copy for their circulating collections.
- monographic co-editions are reported to all jobbers/wholesalers/approval plans. The source journal is listed as the "series" to assist the prevention of duplicate purchasing in the same manner utilized for books-in-series.
- to facilitate user/access services all indexing/abstracting services are encouraged to utilize the co-indexing entry note indicated at the bottom of the first page of each article/chapter/contribution.
- this is intended to assist a library user of any reference tool (whether print, electronic, online, or CD-ROM) to locate the monographic version if the library has purchased this version but not a subscription to the source journal.
- individual articles/chapters in any Haworth publication are also available through the Haworth Document Delivery Service (HDDS).

Social Work Visions from Around the Globe: Citizens, Methods, and Approaches

CONTENTS

PART II: SOCIAL WORK METHODS IN HEALTH
AND MENTAL HEALTH

ABOUT THE EDITORS

Anna Metteri, MSocSc, is Associate Professor in Social Work at the Department of Social Policy and Social Work at the University of Tampere in Finland, where she is finalizing her doctoral studies. She worked as a social work practitioner in health and mental health for 12 years before returning to school. She was nominated as Social Worker of the Year in 1993 in Finland. Ms. Metteri is a former member of the Nordic Committee of the Schools of Social Work from 1999-2003 and has been a member of the Executive Committee of the European Association of Schools of Social Work since 2003. She was Chair of two international social work conferences held in Tampere: the 3rd International Conference on Social Work in Health and Mental Health "Visions from Around the Globe" (July 2001) and the 4th International Conference on Evaluation for Practice (July 2002). She was the leader and teacher in charge of six professional postgraduate programmes in social work in health and mental health and empowering social work at the University of Tampere's Centre for Extension Studies. She is the author of many scientific and professional publications, which include six edited books, one co-authored book, numerous journal articles, book chapters, and conference proceedings.

Teppo Kröger, PhD, is Lecturer of Social Work in the Department of Social Sciences and Philosophy at the University of Jyväskylä in Finland, and Docent of Social Work in the Department of Social Policy and Social Work at the University of Tampere in Finland. He is a member of the Nordic Committee of Schools of Social Work. He was a member of the local organizing committee of the 3rd International Conference on Health and Mental Health in Tampere in July of 2001. He has lectured widely on issues connected to social care. In addition to his publications in Finnish, Dr. Kröger has published articles in English in the *Scandinavian Journal of Social Welfare*, the *Journal of Social Policy*, the *Nordic Journal of Social Work*, and in several edited books. In 2001, the European Commission published his book "Comparative Research on Social

Care: The State of the Art." Recently, he has coordinated a large comparative research project on combining the use of formal and informal care with participation in paid employment, funded by the European Commission.

Anneli Pohjola, PhD, is Academy Researcher in the Academy of Finland and works at the University of Lapland in Rovaniemi, Finland, where she previously served as a lecturer and research in social work. She has worked for Finland's Ministry of Education as a project administrator for social work education. She is a member of an expert group in the EC Phare Consensus Program "Training of Social Workers in Lithuania" and is one of three experts called upon by the Estonian Higher Education Accreditation Centre to evaluate social work education in Estonia. At the national level, she has held many confidential posts at the ministry of Social Affairs and Health, such as a member of the research section of the Consultative Committee for Equality, a member of the Consultative Committee of Social Work, and a member of the management group of Networking Special Services.

Pirkko-Liisa K. Rauhala, PhD, is University Lecturer of Social Work at the University of Helsinki in Finland, and Visiting Professor of Social Policy and Social Work at the University of Tartu in Estonia. She is an expert member of the Welfare Research Financing Committee of the Nordic Council of Ministers and has served as a scientific advisor to the UNFPA/Expert Group on Population Ageing and Development. She is a member of the European Social Policy Research Group at the Europaeische Akademie in Germany and a member of the Finnish Literature Society.

PART I

CITIZENS' NEEDS AND PARTICIPATION IN HEALTH AND MENTAL HEALTH

Introduction:
Women's and Men's Needs
as a Challenge
for Gender-Sensitive Services

Teppo Kröger, PhD
Anna Metteri, MSocSc, PhD
Anneli Pohjola, PhD
Pirkko-Liisa Rauhala, PhD

In our hands, we have here a rare collection of articles discussing key issues in social work in health and mental health. What is most significant is the fact that these papers come from five different continents. The collection is a result of a long process. First versions of these papers were presented in the 3rd International Conference on Social Work in Health and Mental Health that was organised in July 2001 in Tampere, Finland. From the 433 papers and posters that were presented in this conference, 96 were submitted to be considered for publication. During the following years, these papers have been developed by their authors, supported by several review rounds by external reviewers and the editors of this collection. The language of the papers has been checked by translators in different parts of the world and polished in a final phase by the publisher.

[Haworth co-indexing entry note]: "Introduction: Women's and Men's Needs as a Challenge for Gender-Sensitive Services." Kröger, Teppo et al. Co-published simultaneously in *Social Work in Health Care* (The Haworth Social Work Practice Press, an imprint of The Haworth Press, Inc.) Vol. 39, No. 1/2, 2004, pp. 3-5; and: *Social Work Visions from Around the Globe: Citizens, Methods, and Approaches* (ed: Anna Metteri et al.) The Haworth Social Work Practice Press, an imprint of The Haworth Press, Inc., 2004, pp. 3-5. Single or multiple copies of this article are available for a fee from The Haworth Document Delivery Service [1-800-HAWORTH, 9:00 a.m. - 5:00 p.m. (EST). E-mail address: docdelivery@haworthpress.com].

Digital Object Identifier: 10.1300/J010v39n01_01

Finally, we are proud to present a collection of all together 35 articles that come from Australia, Botswana, Canada, Finland, Germany, India, Ireland, Israel, Lithuania, South Africa, Taiwan, Ukraine, the UK and the US. In all, the themes of these papers range from early historical roots of social work in health to doing social work with men who face capital punishment, from the self-help organisations of parents of disabled children to collective management structures in hospital social work. The commentary to the year 2000 definition of social work by the International Federation of Social Workers says that "social work interventions range from primarily person-focused psychosocial processes to involvement in social policy, planning and development," and this is reflected in the sphere of the papers of this collection. Nonetheless, each article touches upon fundamental principles and dilemmas of social work with people whose health is under threat.

The articles have been organised into two parts, but this has not been done according to the geographical location of the authors. Neither have the papers been divided into two topics: those discussing social work in health and those focusing on social work in mental health. Even though the national and local health and mental health care systems do provide the basic context where social work will have to function and even though the organisational and social contexts of these articles could hardly be more remote from each other, we have been struck by the many similarities in people's experiences all over the world. People from diverse parts of the globe seem to be more similar than different in their needs and problems. Though there are huge geographical disparities in the quantity of human suffering, its basic quality is the same everywhere. Consequently, social work with people with illness or disability faces the same basic challenges everywhere. Even people's difficulties in encounters with the health care system have many features in common: a feeling of being bypassed even when your own life is concerned, facing inequalities in accessing services, seeing that still today health care is often dominated more by professional hierarchies and administrational boundaries than by actual needs of people.

Therefore, instead of a geographical categorisation, the papers are organised theoretically into two thematical parts. The first part discusses the position of women, men and children as users of health and mental health care services. The second part focuses on the methods of social work in health and mental health.

Thus, in this first part of the collection, the health and mental health care systems are looked at from a bottom-up perspective. Examples come from around the globe, but the basic theme in all of these articles is about access to care services that are responsive to one's needs. In countries like India, the lack of services is evident but even in welfare states like Finland or Canada, people have difficulties in obtaining services.

The first three papers concentrate particularly on the situation of women and it is showed clearly that health care systems easily overlook their needs. Even deep suffering does not always bring forward service provisions addressing women's fundamental health needs. Male-dominated structures and cultural practices are to blame for many of these deficiencies but, however, the fourth paper shows that even individual men's actions and mental health are constrained by the same cultural barriers and social structures. Social work has a lot of work to do in empowering both women and men to bring their needs and preferences out to the public, calling for changes in prevailing gender-blind policies and practices.

Another group of four papers focuses on those families with children where one member has become ill or disabled. Whether it is a child or a parent who is personally met by illness or disability, the situation always affects the whole family. Health professionals often concentrate their attention solely to the person who is diagnosed ill, ignoring the needs of other family members. However, for example, it is not only children having cancer who need help, their siblings and parents need formal and informal support as well. In promoting support from public and private providers, extended families and social networks, social workers can have a significant role.

A third group of three articles addresses the general issues of citizenship and participation of service users. Dimensions of citizenship are prescribed by the principles and practices of the service systems: how much participation from people in need of services is allowed and encouraged. An issue requiring particular attention is to ensure that services are culturally sensitive to the values of ethnic minorities, responding to health and mental health views of aboriginal as well as migrant populations.

Opening Remarks, 1 July 2001, Tampere

Jorma Sipilä

Ladies and gentlemen,

I am delighted to be here to welcome you to the University of Tampere. I think that our university and the City of Tampere in July offer a fine setting to discuss the subjects of this conference.

Our university is one of the larger universities in Finland (large in this case means 14,000 students) with an emphasis on the social sciences and their applications. The university has a 75-year history in which social welfare, social work, and social policy have been the main disciplines since the beginning. In the 1970s a medical faculty was established with a specialisation in public health care. Collaboration between social work and health sciences is becoming more important all the time, and we want to promote this cooperation. However, we are also aware of the risks inherent in this process. The aims of social work and medical care are not entirely the same, nor do they define situations in the same way. Social work has its own understanding of the human condition, and it needs considerable autonomy to respond to human needs in its own way.

The title of this conference refers to globalisation. Globalisation is a concept which, at the moment, is highly significant for governments and international business. Globalisation is the frame of reference they use when advocating certain policies that they regard as essential. For governments and multinational enterprises globalisation primarily means

[Haworth co-indexing entry note]: "Opening Remarks, 1 July 2001, Tampere." Sipilä, Jorma. Co-published simultaneously in *Social Work in Health Care* (The Haworth Social Work Practice Press, an imprint of The Haworth Press, Inc.) Vol. 39, No. 1/2, 2004, pp. 7-10; and: *Social Work Visions from Around the Globe: Citizens, Methods, and Approaches* (ed: Anna Metteri et al.) The Haworth Social Work Practice Press, an imprint of The Haworth Press, Inc., 2004, pp. 7-10. Single or multiple copies of this article are available for a fee from The Haworth Document Delivery Service [1-800-HAWORTH. 9:00 a.m. - 5:00 p.m. (EST). E-mail address: docdelivery@haworthpress.com].

competetion. The problem is not only that they understand the purpose of human existence in terms of competition but also that their time perspective is becoming shorter and shorter.

For instance, the world of business can no longer wait for yearly reports. Quarterly business reports have become indispensable and so have monthly statistics, not to speak of the daily stock indexes. On the political side too we can see a similar development. Elections are too rare to measure success in politics. The media defines the biggest party on the basis of almost weekly opinion polls. This shortening of the time perspective seems to mean that no important organisations care about what our world will look like after ten years. Even universities are included in this short-term thinking. Twenty years ago they were still allowed to be institutions preparing students for their lives and discussing the future alternatives of the world–today governments ask them to concentrate on their yearly output numbers.

Perhaps today more than ever, the powerful organisations of all the world speak in the same voice. Globalisation and competition, those are the topics of our time. There are no alternatives, we are told. We have to cut social benefits and public services to be competitive and to make savings for future recessions.

The big questions are never asked by powerful organisations, although there are many difficult world-wide issues seen to be without alternatives. We have to save for the future because of the ageing population. But nobody asks why the population is ageing so fast. Why are birth rates so low that these wonderful cultures cannot reproduce themselves? Has it something to do with the fact that long-term investments in children are not compatible with economic efficiency, nor does the stiff economic competition leave much space for unconstrained family life? And there is an endless list of other serious questions:

- Why are children's social problems growing fast although we have so few children?
- Why do young people behave in such a destructive way against the power elites who insist that there is no alternative?
- Why are so many adult working people always tired and say that they never have time for anything important that they used to do before?
- Why do so many people toy with the idea of getting out of the so-called rat race?

The conditions for human reproduction have become drastically weaker during the last decades in the Western world. More and more people feel that they have no reasonable ways to influence social development. After a hundred years of shortening, the working day is getting longer again and so are travel times. People are tired after work; we do not have strength enough to be politically active during our free time. All we need is entertainment.

When researchers ask ordinary people what is most important in their lives, they get quite similar answers every place and every time. What is most important in the world is birth and death, love and care, friendship and solidarity, health and wisdom, safety and peace. These are the basic issues. But what is their status in political discourses?

The media do not give too much support to discussing the fundamental issues of life. The news is dominated with daily competition between the power elites of the economic and political field. The slightest movements on the market are described in detail. There is no daily index for children dying from starvation. The topics people consider essential are pushed aside into soap operas, non-action movies, and novels. And it is not only the media that have assumed the role of promoting short-term competition. Education is expected to give its full support to this game. Ministers speak of skills and qualifications; we seldom hear the word "understanding" as an aim of education.

However, globalisation as a word does not only mean the promotion of narrow, short-term interests. The use of the word "globalisation" also means that all we have, after all, is this lonely planet and that our future depends on its fate. As human beings we are infinitely dependent on each other. All the social structures that repress people and all the political processes with no alternative are human constructions, based on decisions among human beings. Globalisation has taken the direction that people have given to it. We are here to prove that globalisation does not always mean competition or protection of short-term interests.

We are interested in visions from around the globe. Your presence and the reasons for it show that there are visions that offer alternatives. Globalisation, in itself, is not a negative phenomenon but a process that also opens up enormous chances to improve the human condition all around the world. This global conference, for instance, did not exist ten years ago.

On behalf of the University of Tampere I thank all the organisers for the tremendous work they have done, and I wish you exciting talks in the auditoria, during the breaks and in the evenings, all that a good conference may offer. You are cordially welcome!

Understanding the Interconnections Between Ethnicity, Gender, Social Class and Health: Experiences of Minority Ethnic Women in Britain

Ravinder Barn, PhD
Kalwant Sidhu, MSW

SUMMARY. This paper presents the findings of a qualitative study about the impact of ethnicity, gender, and socio-economic status upon health, and use and access to appropriate service provision. A total of 54 interviews were carried out with women who identified themselves as Muslim and Bangladeshi. Health and social care professionals were also interviewed. However, the focus of this paper is upon the ways in which women conceptualised their health and social care needs and concerns. Our findings indicate that individual characteristics serve to mediate the influence of gender and ethnicity on health, but for the women in our study, socio-economic status represents the most potent factor in adversely affecting their health status and access to health care. *[Article copies available for a fee from The Haworth Document Delivery Service: 1-800-HAWORTH. E-mail address: <docdelivery@haworthpress.com> Website: <http://www.HaworthPress.com> © 2004 by The Haworth Press, Inc. All rights reserved.]*

Ravinder Barn is Reader, Department of Health and Social Care, Royal Holloway, University of London, Egham, Surrey, TW20 OEX, UK (E-mail: r.barn@rhul.ac.uk). Kalwant Sidhu is Senior Lecturer, School of Social Work and Health Care, South Bank University, United Kingdom.

[Haworth co-indexing entry note]: "Understanding the Interconnections Between Ethnicity, Gender, Social Class and Health: Experiences of Minority Ethnic Women in Britain." Barn, Ravinder, and Kalwant Sidhu. Co-published simultaneously in *Social Work in Health Care* (The Haworth Social Work Practice Press, an imprint of The Haworth Press, Inc.) Vol. 39, No. 1/2, 2004, pp. 11-27; and: *Social Work Visions from Around the Globe: Citizens, Methods, and Approaches* (ed: Anna Metteri et al.) The Haworth Social Work Practice Press, an imprint of The Haworth Press, Inc., 2004, pp. 11-27. Single or multiple copies of this article are available for a fee from The Haworth Document Delivery Service [1-800-HAWORTH, 9:00 a.m. - 5:00 p.m. (EST). E-mail address: docdelivery@haworthpress.com].

KEYWORDS. Ethnicity, gender, health, culture, mental health, social class, Bangladeshi

INTRODUCTION

Research studies exploring the lives of minority ethnic women in Britain have tended to emphasise 'race,' culture, and gender in a highly parochial and fragmented fashion preventing an understanding of the interrelationship between these variables (Bowes and Domokos 1996). Moreover, the class relationship has been inadequately conceptualised to understand the impact of poverty, poor housing, low income, and unemployment upon health.

This paper presents the findings of a qualitative study examining how ethnicity, gender, and socio-economic status combine to impact upon health and access to service provision, as experienced by Bangladeshi women living in East London (Barn and Sidhu 2000). In-depth semi-structured and focus group interviews were carried out with 54 women who identified themselves as Muslim and Bangladeshi. Findings arising from our interviews with health and social care professionals are discussed elsewhere (Barn and Sidhu 2002).

BANGLADESHIS IN BRITAIN

The Bangladeshi community is one of the most disadvantaged in Britain. As recent migrants, the Bangladeshis face much disadvantage and discrimination in the areas of housing, employment, education, and social services. Moreover, the Bangladeshi community in Tower Hamlets could be regarded to be one of the most 'over-researched' without any notable improvements in health services (Hillier and Rahman 1996). Indeed it is a concern that minority groups simply become a focus of research, and in the accompanying rhetoric the reality of their existence becomes lost.

The Bangladeshi community in Britain has been described to have a number of distinct characteristics including its rapid and continuing growth; the high number of children and young people (43% of the population is under the age of 18, according to the 2001 census figures), dependence on social housing, high rates of social and economic deprivation, high unemployment amongst men, and low levels of female employment in the formal sector (Eade, Vamplew and Peach 1996). The contextual reality of a studied population should be an essential pre-requisite in the design and conduct of any research study. Our study was mindful about the lived reality of our respondents and the importance of this in understanding women's conceptualisation of needs and concerns (Humphries and Truman 1993).

THE STUDY

The study aimed to identify Bangladeshi women's constructions of their health and social care needs, and the barriers they perceived to exist in accessing and using health and social care services. The data collection involved demographic profile questionnaires (subjected to SPSS analysis) and semi-structured interviews and focus groups. The interview and focus group schedules were designed to incorporate themes and issues identified by previous research and current literature and were initially piloted with Bangladeshi women and health and social care professionals outside of the London borough of Tower Hamlets.

The inclusion criteria were identified as Bangladeshi women (self assigned ethnicity) aged between 18-55 with dependent children, residing in Tower Hamlets (n = 54). All the respondents were Muslim. Purposeful sampling was employed to draw our sample from a range of voluntary community organisations. This initial contact then snowballed into access with informal networks. The strengths of this approach were that it provided a sample of women who were already engaged with some kind of health and social care intervention and could provide a useful reflection upon their experiences. This also helped to facilitate an easier dialogue with the women, which may not have been possible with a purely randomly selected sample. Importantly, the intention was not to produce a definitive account of the needs of Bangladeshi women, which would be a futile exercise in any case given the dynamism of the different facets of health, but to ground these experiences within a specific context.

CONCEPTUALISING PHYSICAL AND MENTAL HEALTH

In analysing our findings, we sought to identify how gender, ethnicity, and socio-economic status affected physical and mental health needs. Whilst it is recognised that gender, ethnicity, and socio-economic status all impact upon health status (Acheson 1999), what is difficult to substantiate is the relative influence of each. In common with their construction of health, the women in our study did not describe clear and concise parameters to their identity.

A composite picture emerged which presented the complexity of the women's lives and health needs. The experience of gender and ethnicity upon health differed according to the problem or need being discussed, but socio-economic status emerged as a key underlying issue in the problems experienced. The women employed a holistic perspective of health, which was not merely confined to the absence of illness or disease. Significantly, the majority of women did not perceive themselves to be ill but equally did not perceive themselves to be in good health either. They experienced a diverse range of chronic health problems, including gastric ulcers, headaches, and backaches. Although the majority of the interviews were conducted in Sylheti, when describing their poor health women used these exact terms rather than Bengali words. Good health was perceived as enabling the women to fulfil their different roles, particularly in relation to childcare and domestic tasks. It was perceived, however, that these chronic health problems affected their ability to undertake these roles with any satisfaction.

Gender Roles and Health

The vast majority of women in our study were not involved in any paid employment outside of the home. The majority of the women were also married, and all the women had dependent children. The key roles undertaken by the women were that of mother, wife, and housewife. The experiences of these roles were problematic for a variety of reasons, but the majority of women attributed their difficulties to the socio-economic context within which their roles were undertaken rather than the construction of these. Many of the women expressed their fears about the 'westernisation' of their children and the loss and continuity of Bangladeshi culture and traditions (see Barn 2002).

In describing their circumstances and the different roles they undertook, for married women, the husband was predominantly absent from this. In part this was attributable to the type of employment in which men were involved, for example, catering work which demanded long hours. Also, some men were said to be in Bangladesh for long periods of time. Most of the women felt unable or unwilling to share their concerns with their husbands or other family members. Thus, although positioning themselves within a family context, the women conveyed a sense of being isolated with their difficulties. These included worries about their own health, practical difficulties around domestic tasks, and concerns about their children's welfare. The demarcation between male and female roles described by the women meant that they did not wish to burden their husbands with their own or their children's health and social welfare.

Although women identified their socio-economic context as affecting their health, our findings would suggest this was influenced by the gender roles they undertook, and how these were specifically conceptualised with their own families. In terms of family, the husband and mother-in-law were influential in a range of health related needs. The difficulties emerging from this interface, and their impact upon health, for example family conflict, childcare concerns, domestic violence, and mental health distress, were experienced in isolation. Belliappe (1991) reported that Asian women identified distress as emanating from dissatisfaction around their roles with family members. For the majority of the women in our studies, it could be argued that the role of mother and spouse were their significant roles.

Ethnicity and Health

In considering the relationship between ethnicity and health, external sources of stress arising out of socio-economic difficulties, such as housing, unemployment, and shared experiences of racial discrimination, afforded a common identity around being Muslim Bangladeshi women. However, women do not constitute a homogenous group, but gender roles were defined through this identity. All the women identified themselves as part of the Bangladeshi community, which was grounded in a shared religion and tradition and experiences of migration. It was also founded in their experiences of living in East London. For example, from our focus groups, experiences of racial abuse and the hostility from their urban environment met with great consensus, which conferred a greater sense of kinship. Significantly, although all women could be defined as British in nationality, the majority still referred to England as a 'foreign' place. Thus many women would make references to 'back home' or 'going home.' Significantly, all the women in our study were born in Bangladesh, which would seem influential in their construction of a Bangladeshi identity.

However, given this perception of community, it was interesting that one of the key problems identified by the women was about isolation and a lack of support. The main source of support identified by the women in our study was their religion. Whilst this brought great solace and comfort, many women predominantly maintained their faith through solitary activity, such as praying in their own home, rather than attending a mosque. In line with other studies, which have looked at the experiences of Muslim women, religion was an important strategy for coping positively with difficulties (Currer 1984, Westwood, Couloute, Desai, Mathew, and Piper 1989; Belliappe 1991). Although religion was a shared identity and perceived to be an important part of being Bangladeshi, the issue of women not attending a mosque for prayer was founded in tradition, encompassing social and political factors, and child care responsibilities rather than emanating from Islam. Given the importance of religion to women, having this as a mechanism to facilitate both support and social contact could be an important strategy.

The experience of being Bangladeshi was perceived to be different for men and women. From our findings this would seem to be attributable to the distinct roles men and women were required to undertake within their family and community. The women in our study also indicated that men were more likely to be English speaking which afforded greater respect, independence, and accessibility to a range of facilities. Interestingly, Bowler (1988) documented the negative attitude of midwives towards Asian women who did not speak English. It was found that midwives perceived these Asian women as incompetent, lacking in maternal instincts, and did not feel obligated to help. The gender roles were also significant in terms of how women articulated their identity, but the nature of these roles was bound up and dictated by religious, cultural, and traditional beliefs encapsulated in the term Bangladeshi.

The correlation between health and ethnicity is often made in the literature. For the women in our study, it was specifically in relation to mental health needs where the women made explicit reference to Bangladeshi culture or tradition. The women referred to possession within the context of Jinn (spirits), Shaitan (satan/satanic beings), and Farishta (angels). However, whilst this was described as affecting an individual's behaviour and health, in terms of seeking health care, women identified traditional healers and imams as the main source of support. Thus religion was also an important facet in explaining and treating possession as illustrated by the following quotes:

> *I know a woman whose daughter has seen death. If that happens you should get a holy man to say special prayers and get rid of the bad spirits.*

In this country the jinn got my child once. She used to run out through the door at night outside. It happened after she came back from the park where she was wearing red clothes, other things she used to do was to grab me and hit me.

However, the majority of women in our study conceptualised these experiences as distinct from mental ill-health problems. Instead problems affecting their emotional or psychological health were conceived, as part of their general health needs, rather than being compartmentalised as specific mental health problems. For example, isolation was identified as a particular problem, and in part this was a reflection of their role as homemaker. The following quotes illustrate the experience of isolation:

Some people who live on their own start to become crazy from being alone. Socialising with other people, and keeping yourself busy keeps you sane.

I can't walk too much. I get depression–sometimes it's too much–I feel like crazy. I need help with shopping–you know with Muslim food. I need big onion boree (bag), rice boree; I have to carry it myself.

I suffer from migraines very frequently and I constantly get muscular aches and pains. Sometimes I feel I cannot cope with the pressures of family life. It's never ending–the cooking and cleaning . . .

It's not our age that affects our health; it's the stress and problems we have to deal with in our daily lives.

The women described their worries through physical symptoms, but this was not perceived to convey a lack of understanding about emotional or psychological needs, rather that the mind was not separated from the body. The issue of somatisation is an interesting one because it implies that an individual is unable to articulate their emotional needs, and this concept has been employed to explain the under-representation of Asian groups in mental health services (Rack 1982). However, such an interpretation fails to acknowledge that the notion of somatisation actually reflects a western construction of the normal mode of presentation for depression (Fernando 1996; Douki and Tabbane 1996). Equally, conditions such as anxiety do have a recognised physical dimension to them, and depression will have an effect on an individual's functioning (Gelder, Lopez-Ibor and Andreasen 2000). Current research on the prevalence of mental health problems suggests that Pakistani and Bangladeshi women are currently under-represented (Cochrane and Sashidharan 1996). However, qualitative research, which has examined the mental health needs of Asian groups, has challenged this (Currer 1984, Fenton and Sadiq 1993, Avan 1991). Beliappe (1991) reported that both Asian men and women (which included Bangladeshis) did recognise that their emotional problems affected their physical health, but the emotional needs were not viewed as pathological. She suggested that the differences in prevalence rates could be attributed to differences in defining mental health problems. Given this non-compartmentalised understanding of mental health needs, the issue becomes one of appropriate service provision. The fact that traditional mental health services are inadequate for meeting the needs of minority ethnic groups is well-established (Fernando 1996; Nazroo 1997b). Current policy regarding the modernisation of mental health services is aimed at ensuring that the mental health needs of local populations are assessed and met together with a better network of assertive outreach care (DOH 1998). Our findings suggested that to date this has not been the experience of Bangladeshi women. The majority of the women in our study perceived of improvements in their general health as being rated to a range of activities, which fall outside of traditional notions of mental health care. Thus greater attention needs to be given to groups and activities which provide social contact, support, and purposeful activity which does not pathologize the experience of being Bangladeshi.

These problems were not perceived as shared concerns with other Bangladeshi or with the Bangladeshi community but experienced in isolation. The majority of the women felt they had very little help or support. The need for a more sophisticated understanding of ethnicity and culture is illustrated by a study by Khanum (1994). She undertook interviews with 140 Bangladeshi women in a British city. She identified that class differences as defined by belonging to either 'choto lok' (poor people) or 'bhoro lok' (rich/high status people) were influential in women's perception of health status and access to services. Thus both 'cultural norms' around 'choto or bhoro lok' within the Bangladeshi community, as well as the experience of racism from outside the Bangladeshi, were significant. In discussing the issue of service provision with the women in our study, perception of gender roles was also cited as significant. The perception of 'women only' services were said to be considered by some Bangladeshis men as a threat to the family rather than a source of support for the woman. For some women, services failed to recognise their responsibilities for childcare. In this sense women cannot be empowered in isolation since this removes them from their family context. The difficulty is that relationships within the family may be perpetuating the problem. Notwithstanding the heterogeneity of Bangladeshi women, Bangladeshi women as opposed to the Bangladeshi community must be enabled to advocate for themselves regarding their health needs.

Socio-Economic Status and Health

Although the women regarded gender and ethnicity as being influential in terms of how they defined their health needs and their ability to access services, socio-economic status was identified as the most potent factor in adversely affecting their health. Importantly, this was not seen as being synonymous with their ethnicity. However, the experience of being Bangladeshi was an important factor in their ability to access health and social care needs.

In his comprehensive analysis of the health status of Britain's ethnic minorities, Nazroo (1997a) identified that the Bangladeshi and Pakistani groups reported the poorest health, which was perceived to be related to their socio-economic context. Benezeval et al. (1997) assert that as our understanding about the multiple determinants of health increase, the fact that health cannot be divorced from the social and economic environment becomes more fixed.

In describing health, each woman referred to her social context and described this as inextricably linked to her health status. In particular the majority of women experienced problems with housing and poverty. Almost all lived in local authority or housing association accommodations. The average household size was consistent with the census data on Bangladeshi families, that is, 5.3 persons per household. Poor living conditions and problems of over-crowding were reported by almost all of the women. The experiences of racial harassment and racial attacks were described as particular difficulties.

> *Some people are not healthy because they've got problems with housing, overcrowding–and the children are giving you a hard time. The children have nowhere to do their homework. My daughter's got asthma. She has to share the room with another three family members, because I've only got a two bedroom flat. Four people in one bedroom. There's nothing you can do. Overcrowding is causing health problems.*

I live in a two bedroom flat, which is damp and horrible. My handi-capped son will not share with his brother. Since his racial attack he suffers from terrible nightmares and wants a room for himself. I have to share a bedroom with my 18 year old son. I wish the coun-cil will re-house me. We are so congested that it feels as if the four walls will eat me.

Women described their poor housing situation and the negative im-pact of that on themselves and their family. They expressed anger and dissatisfaction at a system, which turned a blind eye to their needs and concerns. The system was perceived to be racially discriminatory which was reflected by housing decisions that saw Bangladeshi families being placed in high rise tower blocks with little or no consideration being given to the needs of children, or disabled or elderly members within the family.

Yuval-Davis (1997) highlights the fact that the home is a central ex-pression of culture and source of kinship, but also that women are un-derstood to have the responsibility for maintaining the home. This is an important point, since women expressed dissatisfaction with their role of homemaker, and this difficulty was largely related to problems with their housing. The women also conveyed a great sense of responsibility for the problems experienced by their children in relation to health and education because of damp conditions and inadequate space. It would appear therefore that the women, because of the roles they assumed, ex-perienced the effects of poor housing and poverty more acutely. The following quotes illustrate these tensions:

How am I going to survive with the children on income support? They are growing up fast, and we need lots of school material for them. My middle child is going on a school trip; I am worried I have to find money for that trip. I don't know how we're going to do that.

Well there's a mother and father, the mother takes care of everything in the house and the father can take the outside role, but when you're on your own, you have to do everything even if your health is not good.

The concern to resolve this problem was identified as a priority for the women, and the fact that it remains a longstanding unmet need evoked a great deal of distress. The problem with housing would thus be more accurately defined as an issue about having a home. A house represents a shelter which is not only a determinant to an individual's health status (Dahlgren and Whitehead 1991), but also a means to establishing a sense of security and well-being (Maslow 1970), upon which other needs can be more successfully attained.

TOWARDS A HOLISTIC PERSPECTIVE

In determining the health needs of Bangladeshi women and appropriate and relevant service provision, gender, ethnicity, and socio-economic status are all important facets to the equation. In order to determine their relative merit, factors such as age, marital status, children and the role within the family, and the influence of religion must be considered as part of this equation. An understanding and acknowledgement of this dynamic and complex picture means that at a fundamental level, Bangladeshi women need to be able to advocate for themselves as individuals without the constraints imposed on them by perceptions of their culture or ethnicity. In defining their needs, whilst notwithstanding this complexity, the women were able to convey what they prioritised to be as their key need against a backdrop of deprivation, poverty, and insecurity. However, the problem with poor housing has remained a longstanding unmet need which has been also widely documented (CRE 1988, Phillips 1986, Hyndman 1990, Collard 1995, Holmans 1997), together with problems of racial harassment and hostility.

The desire to attain the user perspective and for service provision to be needs led is a prevalent theme in current British health and social care policy (DOH 1997). However, the experiences of the women in this study suggest that whilst the women present a holistic perspective of their health needs, these become compartmentalised by service providers, and in so doing, the problem becomes re-defined into one which fits with service delivery. The problem with housing provides a striking example of this. We found that whilst the women presented their poor health as a consequence of poor housing, the intervention was perceived to be focusing on the symptoms and not addressing the cause. It is interesting that in his description of Bangladeshis for 'The Ethnic Health Handbook—A Fact File for Health Care Professionals,' Karmi (1996) asserts the following as a specific health issue:

Many Bangladeshis suffer from anxiety and depression as a result of poor housing conditions, unemployment, culture shock and racial harassment.

This begs the question that whilst health and social care professionals seem to recognise and assess from a holistic perspective, does their intervention fall short of actually meeting the individual's defined health needs? Correspondingly, in espousing the empowerment of Bangladeshi women, or any given minority ethnic community, in order for this to be meaningful, empowerment must encompass and accommodate an interpretation which reflects their experience of the intersection and influence of gender, ethnicity, and socio-economic factors and its relationship to health.

Current policy emphasises the need for health and social care practice to be underpinned by sound reasoning and research (DOH 1997). We would argue that given the dynamic nature of culture and its interface with other variables, it is impossible and futile to attain a definitive understanding of Bangladeshi culture. Instead, all health and social care professionals need to critically examine how culture impacts upon each individual's health and social care needs. Culture is a dimension in how health and social need is conceptualised (Helman 1994; Fernando 1993). The difficulty lies in what is assigned as a cultural issue and the consequence of this in terms of where the onus of change is cited, within the culture or service providers (Ahmad 1993; Ahmad 1996; Kelleher 1996). In determining this, practice should be based on credible knowledge rather than assumption. Where differences are perceived, the notion of what is normal needs to be carefully examined, and specifically practitioners need to establish what the evidence is for a 'normal' presentation. The difficulties in mental health practice in terms of how need is defined and met illustrates powerfully that how ill-health may manifest itself is bounded by social and cultural norms, and these are not shared by everyone. However, it is more problematic that need is judged from a baseline which reflects western norms, and this should be open to some critical debate and discussion. More generally, the health needs of minority ethnic groups and the related discourse about ethnicity and 'race' needs to be examined within the context of evidence based health and social care. In line with this, what is accepted as evidence needs to be scrutinised as well as the source from where the evidence is attained.

The current impetus towards an integrated policy of social care and the development of health action zones should aim to address the socio-economic factors affecting health (Jacabson and Yen 1998). However, in order to ensure these changes are meaningful and relevant, the service providers need to seriously reflect upon Bangladeshi women's definitions and experiences of health and social care. Moreover, service planning and delivery requires an understanding of the interconnections between gender, social class, ethnicity, and health. A compartmentalised understanding and misplaced targets serve not only to perpetuate disadvantage but also lead to greater social and economic costs in the long run.

REFERENCES

Acheson, D. (1999) Independent Inquiry into Inequalities in Health. Stationary Office.

Ahmad, W. and Atkin, K. (1996) Race and Community Care, Buckinghamshire: Open University Press.

Ahmad, W. I. U. (1993) Race and Health in Contemporary Britain, Open University Press.

Ahmad, I. U. (1996) The Trouble with culture. In: Kelleher D. and Hillier S. (1996). Research Cultural differences in Health, London: Routledge.

Atkins, K. and Rollings, J. (1993) Community Care in a multi-racial Britain: A critical review of literature, London: HMSO.

Avan, G. (1995) Perceived Health Needs of Black and Ethnic Minority Women: An Exploratory Study, Glasgow Healthy City Project.

Balarajan, R. and Soni Raleigh, V. (1992) The ethnic populations of England and Wales: The 1991 census, Health Trends. 24 113-116.

Balarajan, R. and Soni Raleigh, V. (1993) Ethnicity and Health. A Guide for the NHS, Department of Health, London.

Balarajan, R. and Raleigh, S. V. (1997) Patterns of Mortality among Bangladeshis in England and Wales, Ethnicity and health. 2(1/2): 5-12.

Balarajan, R. (1995) Ethnicity and variations in the nation's health, Health Trends, vol 27 no 4. 114-9.

Barn, R. (1998) Race and Racism: Can Minority Ethnic Groups Benefit from Social Work, in Discourse on Inequality in France and Britain, (eds), Edwards, J. and Revauger, J. P., Ashgate, Gower House.

Barn, R. (2001) Black Youth on the Margins, York: Joseph Rowntree Foundation.

Barn, R. and Sidhu, K. (2000) Health and Social Care: A Study of Bangladeshi Women in Tower Hamlets, London: Department of Health.

Barn, R. (2002) Parenting in a 'foreign' climate: The experiences of Bangladeshi mothers in multi-racial Britain, in Social Work in Europe, 9(3), 28-38.

Barn, R. and Sidhu, K. (2002) Dealing with Difference: Professional Conceptualisations of Health and Social Care Needs of Bangladeshi women in London, Journal of Social Work Research and Evaluation, 3(2), 145-158.

Barn, R., Sinclair, R. and Ferdinand, D. (1997) Acting on Principle: An Examination of Race and Ethnicity in Social Services Provision for Children and Families, London: BAAF.

Barot, R., Bradley, H. and Fenton, S. (1999) Ethnicity, Gender and Social Change. London: Macmillian Press Ltd.

Belliappe, J. (1991) Illness or Distress: Alternative models of mental health, Confederation of Indian Organisations (UK).

Bhopal, R. and Senior, P. A. (1994) Ethnicity as a variable in epidemiological research, BMJ vol 309:327-30.

Bowes, A. M. and Domokos, T. M. (1993) South Asian Women and Health Services: A Study in Glasgow, in New Community, 19(4), 611-626.

Bowes, A. M. and Domokos, T. M. (1995) 'South Asian Women and their GPs: Some Issues of Communication, in Social Sciences in Health, 1, 1:22-33.

Bowler, I. (1988 or 93) 'They're Not the Same as us,' Midwives Stereotypes of South Asians Maternity Patients, Sociology of Health and illness, 15(2).

Brah, A. (1992) Women of South Asian Origin in Britain: Issues and Concerns, in Braham, P., Rattansi, A. and Skellington, R., (eds) Racism and Anti-Racism: Inequalities, Opportunities and Policies, London: Sage, 64-78.

Butt, J. and Mirza, K. (1996) Social Care and Black Communities, London: HMSO.

Clare, A. (1983) Psychiatry in Descent (2nd ed), Tavistock Publications Ltd.

Cochrane, R. (1996) Women's Experiences of Antenatal Care in Tower Hamlets, in L. Mckie (ed), Researching Women's Health, Methods and Process, Wiltshire: Quay Books, 151-175.

Collard, A. (1995) Homing In. Providing for the Health and Resettlement Needs of Rehoused Homeless Families. Summary Report of The Health for Rehoused Families Project (HERFA), A Joint City and East London FHSA and Tower Hamlets health Strategy Group Venture.

Cooper, H., Smaje, C. and Arber, S. (1998) Use of Health Services by Children and Young People According to Ethnicity and Social Class; A Secondary Analysis of a National Survey, British Medical Journal, v317 n7165 p1047(5).

CRE (1988) Homelessness and Discrimination, London: Commission for Racial Equality.

Currer, C. (1984) Pathan women in Bradford–Factors affecting mental health with particular reference to effects of racism, International Journal of Social Psychiatry. Vol 30:72-76.

Department of Health (1992) The Health of the Nation–A Strategy for Health in England, London: HMSO.

Department of Health (1998) Modernising Mental Health Services, London: HMSO.

Department of Health (1997) The First Class Service: Quality in the New NHS, London: HMSO.

Douki, S. and Tabbane, K. (1996) Culture and Depression, World Health v49, n2 p22(2).

Eade, J., Vamplew, T. and Peach, C. (1996) The Bangladeshis: The Encapsulated Community, in C. Peach (ed) Ethnicity in the 1991 Census, vol.2, London: HMSO.

East London and The City Health Authority (1997) Health in the East End. Annual Public Health Report 1996/7. EL and CHA.

Erikson, E. (1968) Identity: Youth and Crisis, New York: W W Norton.

Fenton, S. and Sadiq, A. (1993) The sorrow in my Heart, London: Commission for Racial Equality.

Fernando, S. (1991) Mental Health, Race and Culture, Macmillan in Association with MIND.

Fernando, S. (1996) Mental Health in a Multi-Ethnic Society, Macmillian Press.

Gelder, M. G., Lopez-Ibor, Jr. and Andreasen, N. C. (2000) New Oxford Textbook of Psychiatry, Oxford University Press.

Greenhalgh, T., Helman, C. and Chowdhury, A. M. (1998) Health Beliefs and Folk Models of Diabetes in British Bangladeshis; A Qualitative Study, British Medical Journal v 316 n7136 p978.

Helman, C. (1994). Culture, Health and Illness. An Introduction for Health Professionals (3rd ed), Oxford: Butterworth-Heinmann.

Higginbottom, G. (1998) Breastfeeding and black women: A UK investigation. Health Visitor, Vol 71, no1, 12-15.

Hillier, S. and Rahman, S. (1996) Childhood development and behavioural and emotional problems as perceived by Bangladeshi parents in East London, In Kelleher D. and Hillier S. (eds) (1996) Researching Cultural Differences in Health. London: Routledge.

Hopkins, A. and Bahl, V. (1993) (eds) Access to Health Care for People from Black and Ethnic Minorities, London: Royal College of Physicians of London, RCP.

Humphries, B. and Truman, C. (1994) (eds) Re-thinking Social Research, Avebury.

Hyndman, S. J. (1990) 'Housing and Health Amongst British Bengalis in Tower Hamlets, Research Paper No. 3, Department of Geography, Queen Mary and Westfield College, London.

Jacabson, B. and Yen, L. (1998) Health Action Zones, British Medical Journal. V316 n7126 p1641(1).

Karmi, G. (1996) The Ethnic Handbook. A Factfile for Health Care Professionals. Blackwell Science.

Kelleher, D. (1996) In defence of the use of terms 'ethnicity' and 'culture.' In: Kelleher, D. and Hillier, S. (1996) Research Cultural differences in Health. London: Routledge.

Kelleher, D. and Islam, S. (1996) How Should I live? Bangladeshi People and non-insulin dependent diabetes. 220:237, In Kelleher D. and Hillier S. (eds) (1996) Researching Cultural Differences in Health, London: Routledge.

Kelleher, D. and Hillier, S. (eds) (1996) Researching Cultural Differences in Health, London: Routledge.

Khanum, S. M. (1994) 'We Just Buy Illness in Exchange for Hunger': Experience of Health Care, Health and Illness Among Bangladeshi Women in Britain. Unpublished PhD Thesis, University of Keele.

Madood, T. et al. (1997) Ethnic minorities in Britain; Diversity and Disadvantage, London: Policy Studies Institute.

Mandlestam, M. and Schwehr, B. (1995) Community Care Practice and the Law, London: Jessica Kingsley.

Maslow, A. H. (1970) Motivation and Personality, Harpers and Row Publishers Inc.

McAvoy, B. R. and Raza, R. (1988) Asian Women: (I) Contraceptive Knowledge, Attitudes and Usage (ii) Contraceptive Services and Cervical Cytology, Health Trends, 20, 11-17.

McAvoy, B. R. and Raza, R. (1991) Can Health Education Increase Uptake of Cervical Smear Testing Amongst Asian Women?, British Medical Journal, 302, 833-6.

McKeigue, P. M., Marmot, M. G., Syndercombe Court, Y. D., Cottier, D. E., Rahman, S. and Riemersma, R. A. (1988) Diabetes, Hyperinsulinaemia and Coronary Risk Factors in Bangladeshis in East London, British Heart Journal. 60(5):390-396.

McKeigue, P. and Chaterved, N. (1996) Epidemiology and Control of Cardiovascular Disease in South Asians and Afro-Caribbeans, NHS Centre for Reviews and Dissemination, University of York.

McKenzie, K. J. and Crowford, S. (1994) Race, ethnicity, culture, and science; researchers should understanding and justify their use of ethnic groupings (Editorial), EMJ July 30, v309 n6950 p286(2).

McNaught, A. C. (1988) Race and Health Policy, London: Croom Helm.

Nazroo, J. Y. (1997a) The Health of Britain's Ethnic Minorities, London: PSI.

Nazroo, J. (1997b) Ethnicity and Mental Health, London: Policy Studies Institute.

Nazroo, J. Y. (1998) Genetic, cultural, or socio-economic vulnerabilty? Explaining ethnic inequalities in health, Sociology of health and illness. Vol 20 no 5: 710-730.

Pearson, M. (1986) Racist Notions of Ethnicity and Culture in Health Education in Rodmell, S. and Watt, S. (Eds.) The Politics of Health Education: Raising the Issues, London: Routledge and Kegan Paul, 38-56.

Philips, D. (1986) What price equality? Report on the allocation of GLC Housing in Tower Hamlets, London: Greater London Council.

Rack, P. (1982) Rack, Culture and Mental Disorder, Tavistock Publications Ltd.

Rehman, H. and Walker, E. (1995) Researching Black and Minority Ethnic Groups, Health Education Journal, 54, 489-500.

Robertson, C. and Goddard, D. (1997) Monitoring the quality of breastfeeding advice. Health Visitor, 70, 11:422-424.

Rocheron, Y. (1988) The Asian Mother and Baby Campaign: The Construction of Ethnic Minorities Health Needs', Critical Social Policy, 22: 4-23.

Rudat, K. (1994) Black and Minority Ethnic Groups in England: Health and Lifestyles, London: Health Education Authority.

Smaje, C. (1995) Health 'Race' and Ethnicity: Making sense of the Evidence, King's Fund Institute/Share, London.

Smaje, C. (1996) The ethnic patterning of health; new directions for theory and research. Sociology of health and illness, Vol 18 no 2: 139-171.

Stanfield, J. H. and Routledge, M. D. (eds) (1993) Race and Ethnicity in Research Methods, Sage Publications Ltd.

Thompson, D. (1993) Mental Illness. The Fundamental Factors, The Mental Health Foundation.

Tower Hamlets Health Strategy Group (1994) Primary Care Users' Information Project: Project Report.

Wallis, S. (1981) Bengali Families in Camden, in J. Cheetham et al. (eds) Social and Community Work in a Multi-racial Society, London: Harper and Row.

Watson, E. (1984) Health of Infants and Use of Health Services by Mothers of Different Ethnic Groups in East London, Community Medicine, 6, 127-35.

Westwood, S., Couloute, J., Desai, S., Mathew, P. and Piper, A. Sadness in my Heart: Racism and Mental Health. Leicester Black Mental Health Group, University of Leicester 1989.

Williams, D. R. (1996) Race/ethnicity and socio-economic status: Measurement and methodological issues, International Journal of Health Services. Vol 26 no 3:483-505.

Williams D. R. (1997) Race and Health: Basic questions, emerging directions, Annuals of Epidemiology, Vol 17 no 5:322-333.

Woolett, A., Marshall, H., Nicolson, P. and Dosanjh, N. (1994) Asian Women's Ethnic Identity: The Impact of Gender and Context in the Accounts of Women Bringing up Children in East London, in Feminism and Psychology, 4(1), 119-132.

Yuval-Davis, N. (1997) Gender and Nation, London: Sage.

Psychosocial Problems and Coping Patterns of HIV Seropositive Wives of Men with HIV/AIDS

Elizabeth Betcy Joseph, MSW, MPhil
Ranbir S. Bhatti, MA, DPSW, PhD

SUMMARY. The sociocultural milieu provides HIV positive women with fewer resources and more role responsibilities. The present research aimed at studying the psychosocial problems encountered in living, post HIV infection, and the coping patterns adopted by HIV seropositive wives of men with HIV/AIDS. In the background of an exploratory research design, thirty (n = 30) HIV positive women, attending Counseling Clinics in Bangalore (South India), selected through purposive sampling, were assessed using an interview schedule and a standardized coping scale. Majority of the respondents were the primary caregivers for their infected spouse and/or children. Content analysis of the problems revealed increased financial difficulties; problems in child care and support; compromised help-seeking due to stigma; problems in sexual interactions and communication in their marital relationship; role

Elizabeth Betcy Joseph is Social Worker, St. Barnabas Hospital, 183rd Street, 3rd Avenue, Bronx, NY 10457 USA (E-mail: betcyjoseph@yahoo.com or betcyjoseph@rediff.com). Ranbir S. Bhatti is Professor, Department of Psychiatric Social Work, National Institute of Mental Health and Neuro Sciences (NIMHANS), Bangalore 560 029, India (E-mail: ranbirbhatti@yahoo.com or bhatti@nimhans.kar.nic.in).

[Haworth co-indexing entry note]: "Psychosocial Problems and Coping Patterns of HIV Seropositive Wives of Men with HIV/AIDS." Joseph, Elizabeth Betcy, and Ranbir S. Bhatti. Co-published simultaneously in *Social Work in Health Care* (The Haworth Social Work Practice Press, an imprint of The Haworth Press, Inc.) Vol. 39, No. 1/2, 2004, pp. 29-47; and: *Social Work Visions from Around the Globe: Citizens, Methods, and Approaches* (ed: Anna Metteri et al.) The Haworth Social Work Practice Press, an imprint of The Haworth Press, Inc., 2004, pp. 29-47. Single or multiple copies of this article are available for a fee from The Haworth Document Delivery Service [1-800-HAWORTH, 9:00 a.m. - 5:00 p.m. (EST). E-mail address: docdelivery@haworthpress.com].

Digital Object Identifier: 10.1300/J010v39n01_04

strain in caregiving; gender discriminatory and inadequate care; and increased concerns about parenting efficacy, post HIV infection. Escape avoidance was the most preferred coping strategy adopted by them. Situating the illness in a socio-familial context is indicated, and implications for social work and mental health practice follow from the findings. *[Article copies available for a fee from The Haworth Document Delivery Service: 1-800-HAWORTH. E-mail address: <docdelivery@haworthpress.com> Website: <http://www.HaworthPress.com> © 2004 by The Haworth Press, Inc. All rights reserved.]*

KEYWORDS. HIV seropositive wives, men with HIV/AIDS, attending counseling clinics, purposive sampling, help seeking, psychosocial problems, primary care givers, coping scale, escape avoidance, stigma

A diagnosis of HIV seropositivity is the beginning of a long road of challenging life events and extraordinary personal changes, which can overwhelm even the most psychologically well-adjusted individual. Though HIV made a relatively delayed entry into India as compared to the rest of the world, the current Indian scenario is a frightening scene postulating fatal projections. There has been an alarming and steep rise in seropositivity rates from 11.2 per thousand (March, 1992) to 25.84 per thousand (December 2000). Although India's adult prevalence rate is only 0.82%, an estimated 4.1 million Indians were living with HIV at the end of 1999 (UNAIDS, 2000), making India the country with the largest number of HIV infected people in the world.

With increasing evidence of heterosexual transmission being the predominant mode for the spread of the HIV infection in India, more and more women are getting infected, and the predictions of the possibility of equal numbers of both men and women infected with HIV are proving true. In some areas the sex ratio is changing from 1: 1 to 1:1.4 to the detriment of women. Rising HIV infection rate in women of reproductive age, with their high birth rate, has led to increased incidence of pediatric AIDS. The infant and child mortality has risen by 10-15%. As per the Centers for Disease Control (CDC), globally, nearly 6-8 million were infected with the virus (Malhotra, 1998). A study conducted by Gangakhedkar et al. (1997) on the spread of HIV infection among married monogamous women in India revealed that HIV infection among women who are not sex workers was increasing in India, and the likely mode of transmission was from these women's husbands. The researchers had noted that the infection rate among non-sex workers was "disturbingly high" considering their relatively low-risk behavioral profile. In addition, the spread of HIV infection from urban to the rural areas is a serious threat that has just recently been recognized (UNAIDS, 1999). While the psychosocial sequela of HIV infections are reasonably well documented for men, the unique experiences of women with HIV illness have been the focus of recent research efforts. Such information is imperative, given the fact that the incidence of AIDS has increased at a faster rate for women than for any other subgroups. Moreover, the disease dramatically impacts women and children, and globally HIV/AIDS has a ripple effect on families.

WHAT DOES RESEARCH SAY?

Although cases of HIV/AIDS in women were reported as early as 1981, it was not until late 1990 that women were routinely included in clinical studies and attention was focussed on gender-specific HIV issues (Nakajima and Rubin, 1991). Women with HIV infection are often faced with multifarious predicaments, which compound their adaptation to the illness. They are faced with socioeconomic stressors that exacerbate the negative consequences of HIV for physical and mental well being (Cochran and Mays, 1989; Osmond et al., 1993; Quinn, 1993).

The investigations on the psychosocial concerns of women infected with HIV have found that women generally had fewer resources, more role responsibilities, and fewer social and community supports than the men (Kneisll, 1993). Gillman and Newman (1996) found that when women with HIV rank ordered their psychosocial concerns, after HIV diagnosis, financial issues (46%) topped the list followed by concerns about housing (41%), HIV related health issues (38%), issues related to death and dying (37%), and concerns for their children with HIV (32%).

Women who shared their HIV or AIDS diagnosis with family or friends risked stigmatization and isolation and subsequently lost their self-esteem through the process of self-blame (Hackl et al., 1997). Other issues raised by the HIV positive women were their children's future (Chung and Magraw, 1992; Gillman and Newman, 1996), child care arrangements when sick (Chung and Magraw, 1992), guilt and self blame for their inability to care for the children (Gillman and Newman, 1996), and protecting children from crisis and stigma (Hackl et al., 1997).

HIV infection often complicated the traditional family caregiving responsibilities of the women. As women living with the infection, they struggle to continue with caregiving responsibilities and also wrestle with the grief and loss issues that accompany their own terminal illness. Anger and frustration about future goals, mourning of the loss of a long life, and the risk of losing custody of the children as a result of their HIV status were identified as common bereavement issues among HIV infected women (Sherr et al., 1993).

A study on household and community responses to HIV/AIDS, on a gender dimension by Bharat (1996) in Mumbai (former Bombay, India) revealed that the household responses to HIV/AIDS in the case of women with HIV/AIDS was not as supportive. And the situation of the seropositive wives and widows was even more precarious. While they were the major caregivers for their male sex partners, they were not assured of care to the same extent. Widows invariably found themselves faced with problems of shelter, economic maintenance, children's welfare, and their own health care. The HIV positive wives were burdened with caring for a sick and dying partner, and with the burden of planning for the future. Returning to their own parental home was not always an easy choice due to stigma, isolation due to fear of transmission through non-sexual contact, societal labeling of being promiscuous, and sometimes marrying the 'wrong' person without parental consent.

The array of physiological, sociocultural, economical, and psychological stressors faced by HIV positive women almost invariably triggered major stress responses and coping strategies, which have been the context of various research efforts as well. Seeking information, peers were prominent among the coping strategies utilized by a diverse group of HIV positive women in Australia (Lawless et al., 1996). HIV positive young mothers had used confrontive coping most frequently and found it to be significantly related to physical quality of life (Rose and Clark-Alexander, 1996). Hackl et al. (1996) identified that the primary coping strategies most often employed by HIV positive women had been denial, concealment of their health status from others, isolating oneself and crying.

Moore et al. (1996), on assessing the depressive symptoms and coping strategies among HIV infected women, found high rates of depressive symptomatology and utilization of the coping style of disengagement, positive cognitive or behavioral coping, and seeking social support for emotional expression. Positive coping strategies had been associated with fewer depressive symptoms.

Somlai et al. (1998) noted that following the diagnosis of HIV positive women had invested on spiritual coping strategies and had believed that there had been a divine intercession renewing their spiritual growth and connectedness with others. Tolliver (2001) cited that positive women who provided care called upon their spirituality to deal with existential issues related to their HIV status and identified cognitive coping and immersion in the issue as a coping resource to deal with the stress of HIV/AIDS in their lives.

Discrepant research findings concerning the psychological distress levels of women with HIV infection also suggest that coping success was related to a number of factors including circumstances surrounding test result feedback, presence or absence of current illness symptoms, general stress coping style and other competing life stressors, adequacy of effective social supports, access to health care, and hope or pessimism concerning the effectiveness of available treatment regimens. It is likely that distress and successful coping patterns are fluid and changing over time due to multiple factors–psychological, social, physical, economic, and medical (Rose and Clark-Alexander, 1996; Solomon et al., 1993; Hertz, 1996; Fleishman et al., 1996; Lawless et al., 1996; Hackl et al., 1996; Pinel, 1996; Moore et al., 1996; Romano et al., 1996; Siegal et al., 1997; Pederson and Elkitt, 1998).

In spite of the critical role of Indian women as natural nurturers and primary caregivers, there has been little that has been written about their problems post HIV infection as wives, mothers, and daughters. And the family context of the epidemic, especially the havoc it brings on intimate relationships like couple behavior, child care, social supports, and sense of future, have been largely ignored. The purpose of this discovery oriented investigation had been to fill in the informational gaps and to extend the research efforts for service intervention. The sample in the present study is composed of the women whose husbands were infected with HIV/AIDS; therefore these women considered it to be "man's disease."

METHOD

The present study sought to identify the psychosocial problems in living post HIV diagnosis and the coping patterns adopted by the HIV positive women. A purposive sampling technique was chosen for selection of respondents, and the respondents who met the criteria of being HIV seropositive wives of men infected with HIV/AIDS (whether living or deceased) formed the sample. Those positive women who suffered from any other kind of terminal illness, had a diagnosed psychiatric illness, or those women whose husbands had been diagnosed with any other kind of terminal illness were excluded from the study. The final sample thus included thirty (n = 30) HIV seropositive women, who had contacted the three study sites (counseling clinics) chosen for the study, which again had been chosen on the basis of proximity and grant of permission to the researcher for the purpose of data collection.

A semi-structured socio-demographic data sheet designed for the purpose of the study solicited information about the demographic and illness variables. An interview schedule, which consisted of a series of open-ended probe questions on the psychosocial problems and the women's experiences in the domains of childcare, finances, marital interactions, social support, disclosure, and emotional reactions, was developed. The responses were audio recorded by the researcher with the written consent of the participants. The audiotapes were then transcribed and qualitatively analyzed for predominant concerns and themes. In addition to the semi-structured interview, the coping patterns of the respondents were assessed using the modified version of the Coping Scale developed by Lazarus and Folkman (1984). The scale consisted of 50 items in eight subscales, having a response format of a four-point Likert scale. The subscales assessed the following patterns of coping–Confrontive, Distancing, Self-Control, Seeking Social Support, Accepting Responsibilities, Escape Avoidance, Planful Problem Solving, and Positive Reappraisal.

The items were arranged in a chronological order and not as subscales, in order to avoid personal bias, and were ranked from 0-3, representing strategies not used or not applicable, to strategies that they used a great deal.

The actual procedure of data collection from a respondent was carried in a one-to-one situation, in the privacy of an interview room, and alternate arrangements were made for the supervision of the small children of the respondents. On average an interview required 60-75 minutes with each respondent. The data were collected over a period of six months in the year 2000.

SAMPLE CHARACTERISTICS

The age of the respondents ranged from 18 to 40 years, with the majority being in their early twenties. The mean age of the respondents was 21.57 years. The highest level of education attained by the majority of the respondents was upper-primary education (36.7%). On the whole, the highest educational qualification among the respondents was pre-university education, and only 6.2% of the respondents had achieved that feat. The majority of the respondents were unemployed and were housewives (63.3%), and those who were working were employed in the unorganized sector as unskilled laborers. The income of these employed women ranged from three hundred and fifty Rupees (Rs. 350) per month to seven thousand five hundred Rupees (Rs. 7500) per month. The mean income of the respondents was 1363 Rupees per month. Forty-three percent (43%) of the respondents hailed from a rural background and 56.7% hailed from an urban background. Health status varied between the respondents. Twelve women (40%) had been aware of their HIV positive status for less than two months, nine (30%) had been aware for a period of 3-9 months, and another nine (30%) for more than 10 months. Only 11 respondents (36.66%) did not report any symptoms post HIV testing, but the rest of the 19 respondents reported varied HIV related symptoms that consisted of opportunistic infections and disturbed biological functioning. Nine women (30%) whose husbands were alive reported a poor health status in them.

FINDINGS

Psychosocial Problems

The psychosocial problems experienced by HIV seropositive wives of men with HIV/AIDS that emerged are described below in the domains of finance, children, marital relationship, disclosure, social support and stigma, caregiving and receiving, quality of life, and emotions.

Finances

The majority of the women (n = 25, 83.33%) had experienced financial problems following the diagnosis of HIV/AIDS in their families. The women experienced increased financial difficulties due to decreased income following the loss of jobs of their husbands and/or themselves. In few instances financial problems arose due to the spouse's death or HIV disease related limitations. The women were burdened financially because they were either engaged in low paid jobs themselves, ill equipped to start working, or unable to sustain a job full-time, due to care taking responsibilities that they had to adopt, due to an infected spouse and/or child.

The women reported financial strain due to an increased expenditure that they had to incur in health care and in costs of treatment, for their husbands, for self and children, or the entire family unit. This had affected their living standards in return and had forced the women to dip into savings, incur debts for sustenance, and in some instances take up the breadwinner role, either completely or partially. A few women (n = 3, 10%) reported of their children taking up the earning responsibility to meet the financial demands on the family. Another respondent reported that

> *my husband is dead, I am ill and so are my two children . . . My family won't support me and neither can I do anything . . . my mother-in-law is 70 years old, has started working in a quarry . . . we have to live somehow, and without money, we won't be alive for long. (Mrs. S., 33 years)*

Children

The children had been a main source of concern for the respondents. The majority of women had children (n = 24, 80%), and seven of them had HIV positive children (29.16%). Two women (6.66%) were in the life cycle stage of their first pregnancy. Four women (13.33%) had been childless.

The women perceived a decrease in their parenting efficacy and experienced a problem in the fulfillment of the role of a mother and nurturer for their children. Following HIV seropositivity in them and suffering from a compromised health status, along with fears of infecting their children through non-sexual contact, caregiving burden and financial constraints led the women to have decreased interaction with their children. They were unable to concentrate on their education and feared the possibility of a discontinued education for their children. Several women reported an increase in behavioral problems in their children, which they attributed to their inconsistent disciplining and the altered status of being a single parent post HIV infection.

Another source of concern for the women was the physical separation from their children (n = 7, 23.33%), which had been largely situational owing to a compromised health status, increased burden in caregiving, and also their fear of transmission. One respondent reported restrictions imposed on her interacting with her non-positive children by her in-laws, due to the stigma attached to the illness and the lack of awareness regarding transmission of the infection *they (in-laws) don't let me go anywhere near my children . . . my baby will run to hug me, but they scream at me if I let the child do that . . . (Mrs. G., 38 years)*

The women who had positive children experienced problems in disclosing the HIV status of the children to them and adequately reassuring the children about the inexplicable health problems that they had to face at a very young age. Another problem reported by the women in the study had been the paucity of childcare facilities and respite care for their children. The pregnant women lived with the fear of giving birth to a positive child and felt guilty for being the reason for it. The women feared the premature death and isolation of their positive children, due to associated stigma in society and the absence of care takers for the children in the future, especially when the women were no longer capable or alive to do so. One respondent expressed that

today I am there . . . but for how long . . .? what will happen after that . . . who will see to their care . . . there are so many things that need to be taken care of when you have children . . . after me who . . .? (Mrs. T., 29 years)

A sizable number of the respondents (n = 11) were more concerned about the care of their daughters in the future and feared restricted marriage alliances for them due to parental HIV positivity. Several women also feared desertion of their married daughters by the son-in-laws following disclosure of HIV infection in the family. Four women perceived denial of biological motherhood to them as a problem, and they faced the constant pressure to conceive from family members, particularly from in-laws, who were unaware about the HIV status of their sons and daughters-in-law.

Marital Relationship

Eight respondents (26.66%) in the study had been widowed, following the death of their husbands from AIDS. One respondent had separated from her husband following her HIV status confirmation, and another one had been deserted by her spouse. The majority of the respondents reported a qualitative change in their marital interaction following HIV diagnosis. The marital relationship was characterized by problems in sexual interaction with the spouse, and a loss of sexual intimacy.

The women reported a decreased desire for sex (5%) and a reduction in the frequency of sexual activity (10%), sometimes to the point of celibacy (65%). Few women (20%) reported of being forced to have unprotected sex by their husbands, despite being aware of their mutual HIV positivity. These women cited difficulty in negotiating condom use and safer sex practices with their husbands

> *. . . I know that we should be careful . . . even he knows it, but he doesn't listen to me . . . the doctor also asked us to use 'nirodh' (condom) . . . if I tell him, he gets angry at me . . . what can a woman do . . .? (Mrs. R., 22 years)*

The women also cited communication problems in their marital relationship. Following HIV infection, the spousal communication pattern was characterized by need-based communication (50%), a decrease in dyadic communication (15%), and higher noise levels, due to frequent quarrels following increase in negative affective responses such as anger, frustration, fear, mutual blame, and sadness. In some instances the women reported the absence of any discussion about the threat posed by the infection and planning for the future with their husbands, which was sought by them but avoided by their husbands. One respondent reported that

> *I can't talk anything with him . . . he is so ill that he doesn't even recognize me, his wife . . . what can I possibly do . . . he doesn't comprehend anything. (Mrs. V., 40 years)*

Widowhood with the concomitant stress of single parenthood, forced earning responsibility, loneliness, and unfulfilled support needs were reported as problems by the women who had lost their husbands to the illness.

Disclosure and Social Support Stigma

The stigmatizing nature of HIV/AIDS was a major concern for the women who participated in the study. The women reported the ever-present undercurrent of stigma and shame. Disclosure about their HIV status was a feared process. A sizable number of women (n = 25, 83.33%) reported that their HIV status was known to 'others' such as parents, in-laws, siblings, other relatives, neighbors, and heads of religious institutions. The women reported that voluntary disclosure to family members had been a highly selective process. A few women experienced a problem when their HIV status was disclosed to their family members without their consent by health professionals and at times faced stigma following the intelligent speculations of the people in their social network. Some women reported that

> *I have just stopped meeting people . . . I used to get stared at . . . as if in a zoo . . . (Mrs. K., 30 years)*

> *. . . everyone knows that I have it (HIV) . . . my husband used to go to all 'those' women . . . now even I'm considered a bad woman . . . (Mrs. M., 34 years)*

Following disclosure the women experienced difficulty in maintaining the social network that had existed prior to it. Their social supports dwindled, and the women reported decreased social interactions, maintenance of physical distance by others while interacting, and in extreme instances a complete severance of social ties with them. Nine respondents (31%) reported discrimination in their households as a couple, post HIV serostatus disclosure, wherein their interactions were characterized by social discrimination. They would be excluded from family gatherings or social functions. In the household, the relatives covered their face and mouth while speaking to them and gave them utensils and other articles for daily use separately.

Another problem reported by the women was compromised help seeking that they had to face following disclosure, which was mainly due to the stigma attached to the illness. The women felt hesitant to seek support as sometimes they had been outrightly refused any help. In other times the women reported feelings of shame, which influenced hesitation in seeking help. Two respondents had married without parental consent, and following seropositivity, their help seeking was even more compromised.

Caregiving and Receiving

Despite their HIV infection, the women were perceived as caretakers of others, especially their husbands and children whose infections had reached a stage of severity. Nine women (30%) had been the primary and only identified caregivers for their husbands and children. The women cared for and supported their husbands directly through actual caregiving tasks related to personal care and medical treatment. In some instances the women cited the assumption of additional family roles and responsibilities, including earning, following their husband's inability to be gainfully employed and in some instances due to an absent husband, for reasons of separation, desertion, or death. The women reported role strain and an increase in caregiving burden which was often compounded by HIV disease-related health limitations, financial constraints, minimized support networks, negative feelings of anger, fear, sadness and betrayal, and in few instances, pregnancy.

The problems that the women experienced in receiving care centered on inadequate care provisions from primary and secondary social support networks. Eight women (26.66%) had no one to care for them. The women also cited actual instances of stigma and discrimination within the household, which were largely gender discriminatory, in receiving care. The women faced these situations in their husband's house from the in-laws. The women attributed discriminatory care to their status of being a daughter-in-law and to the blame that they had infected their husbands, when the reality had been quite the opposite. The care and maintenance had shifted to the families of origin for a few women.

Quality of Life

All the respondents in the study reported a disruption in their normal pattern of living following the diagnosis of HIV in their families. Their activities of daily functioning became restricted to health related concerns and preoccupations about the future. Their leisure time activities were characterized by an increase in religious activities and self-imposed restrictions in social interactions due to shame, fear of stigma, and negative perception of the physical attractability of self. The spouse's illness, the children's debilitation, and their own disease progression curtailed a normal family interaction. Frequent hospitalization became the norm in their life. To top it all the women also experienced difficulty in accessing a non-discriminatory, non-stigmatizing public health care system, all of which increased their burden in coping with the HIV infection.

Emotions

The concerns described by the women had been replete with a myriad of emotions. The women had been in different stages of HIV seropositivity and disease progression, and they faced an emotional roller coaster. The predominant emotion expressed by the women was that of fear. The women reported constant thoughts of death and dying and feared being left alone in the terminal stages of their illness. Some women feared discovery of their HIV status in their social repertoire. Several women identified shock and anger when the dual life led by their husbands was revealed to them. The women reported of an erosion of trust in their spousal relationship and felt cheated. Some women cited an emergence of a negative perception of men in general, which they identified as a fallout of the jeopardies their own 'men' (husbands) had wrought in their lives. They viewed HIV as a shatterer of their dreams in having a fulfilling life experience. Especially poignant were the expressions of sadness and the feelings of helplessness that the women experienced. Strong feelings of guilt and concern for their innocently infected children led some women to question the justice of the 'Supreme Being' in their sufferings.

Coping Patterns

The commonly adopted coping pattern by the respondents in the study was that of escape avoidance. Following that they preferred seeking social support, self-control, distancing, positive reappraisal, planful problem solving, confrontive coping, and accepted responsibilities to cope with the problems following HIV diagnosis.

Differences tested (t-tests) between the urban and rural respondents on the adoption of coping patterns revealed a preference for confrontive ($t = -2.892$; $p = 0.007$) and positive reappraisal ($t = -2.035$; $p = 0.051$) coping by the urban women than the rural ones, which was statistically significant ($p = < 0.05$).

Analysis of variance (ANOVA) results for coping patterns among the seropositive women on the duration of awareness of HIV seropositivity revealed the adoption of the coping patterns of positive reappraisal ($F = 12.774$; $p = 0.000$), planful problem solving ($F = 5.851$; $p = 0.008$), seeking social support ($F = 4.094$; $p = 0.024$), confrontive coping ($F = 4.094$; $p = 0.028$), and self-control ($F = 4.179$; $p = 0.026$) by those women who had been aware of their seropositive status for a longer duration (i.e., 10 months or more), which had been statistically significant ($p = < 0.05$).

DISCUSSION

The findings from this study highlighted that most HIV infected women had been of child-bearing age and had been in the productive age group, which was a pointer to the increasing evidence of changing sex ratios in the AIDS epidemic in India. It is also a predictor in the rise of pediatric cases of HIV/AIDS. The predominance of lower levels of education, presence of an unemployed or underemployed occupational status, and lower income brackets revealed that the respondents had been from an economically disadvantaged background with limited resources.

Lower incomes exacerbate the familial difficulties following HIV infection, especially during the rising health problems that warrant pharmacotherapeutic interventions, which can be extremely expensive. A higher representation of urban women (n = 17) revealed the increased prevalence of HIV infection in urban adults. Interestingly, the presence of 13 rural women was an indicator of the spread of HIV infection even to rural India. Due to the erosion of the joint family structure in the society, the women experienced depletion in their social support resources, and that had been cited as a concern in their post-HIV living experience.

The women in this study were a representative population of the increasing heterosexual transmission of HIV infection in India when they pointed to the spouses as the predominantly identifiable source of infection. The women in this study had discounted high-risk behavior in them. It also gives an insight into the sexual ethos of the society, particularly to the existence of a normative social presumption for men to have multiple sexual partners and to the covert contract that women could not question the sexual behavior of their men. Another finding that indicated interventions aimed at women was the presence of a higher proportion of women who had not requested for testing themselves but had been tested due to their husbands or children. This highlights the sociocultural canvas of lowered prioritization by women to their own health needs in the households. It could also be assumed that the women had a lowered perception of personalization of risk which was due to their lack of knowledge, wherein they did not relate their partners' sexual behaviors to risk of HIV and STDs in themselves.

Glimpses of reality and poignant experiences were contained in the HIV seropositive women's citations regarding their problems. Loss of jobs and unstable incomes in the family unit, compounded by a pre-existing lower socioeconomic status, resulted in financial limitations that influenced decisions about health care needs and access to social support networks. Health care being an expensive affair placed the women in a state of double jeopardy. Parentification of adolescent children and assumption of breadwinner roles in a compromised health state characterized the plight of these women and their children. Childcare concerns permeated many of the women's responses.

The women perceived a threat to parenting efficacy, care of children in the future and separation from them, as a resultant effect of their HIV seropositivity. This tenor indicated the felt need of the women to maintain their parental role and to protect their children from any distress. Increased concerns for their female children could be attributed to the sociocultural factors that often influenced the lives of the girl children, in terms of low economic and educational status, threats to physical safety and the linkage of women's status to marriage and motherhood. A good number of women had received support in the care of their children, which could be possibly explained by the flexible cohesiveness of the families in India, where children and the aged still find compassionate care.

The erosion of intimacy and the emergence of a minimal-interactive spousal sub-system characterized the marital relationship of these women. Though negative affective cognitions underlay their mutual exchanges, the expressions of it were often suppressed when concerns about the spouse's health status took precedence over all other emotions and the women subscribed to their nurturing role, despite requiring care themselves.

The HIV positive women experienced significant levels of stigma and discrimination following disclosure of their HIV status, and it severely affected their help seeking roles. These discriminations are indicative of wide spread misconceptions about non-sexual transmission modes of HIV infection that exist in the communities and the fear of the unknown that accompanies it.

A feminization of care and support was observed in the context of HIV where the caregiving burden was on these women. They had to cope with the effects of it in a non-supportive, gender discriminatory, and inadequate care-recipient state. In doing so the women underwent intense physical strain and emotional stress.

The women in the study had been at different stages in their experiences with HIV infection. The most preferred coping pattern by them had been that of escape avoidance, wherein they wishfully thought that the situation would go away, hoped that a miracle would happen, and had fantasies about how things might have turned out. These women tried to make themselves better by eating and taking medications; they avoided people in general and slept more than usual. Even though their multifarious problems demanded a full-thronged and more proactive approach to coping with them, the HIV positive women in this study preferred escaping or avoiding the situation.

Seeking social support in terms of efforts to seek information about the illness and talking to someone about one's feelings had also been adopted by the women to cope with the situation but it had not been in the same intensity or frequency of wishing the situation away. This could be attributed to the overwhelming burden that HIV had imposed on these women. Thus, not confronting the issue seemed a better alternative even though it was dysfunctional.

A go-getting urban ethos can be contrasted with the more fatalistic approach that had colored the adoption of the coping patterns of confrontive coping and escape avoidance among the urban and the rural respondents.

The adoption of the strategies of confrontive coping, seeking social support, planful problem solving, and self control by respondents, who had been aware of their HIV status for a longer period, was indicative of the presence of more active strategies in coping, as the women perceived the limited time dimension and the importance of the same in their unpredictable life span. It could also be assumed that these women might have worked through their anger. They may had reached the 'acceptance' stage, wherein it was not a happy stage but rather void of feelings with the set realization that life goes on though different from the old life.

RECOMMENDATIONS AND CONCLUSION

Responses to the needs of women with HIV should be culturally sensitive in terms of gender specificity. Services need to be family oriented, community based, with the utilization of existing formal and informal resources, for holistic health care. Given the predominant theme about children and child care concerns by the women, the interventions should assist them in planning for their children's future by activating their social support networks, addressing parenting skills, and enhancing their perceptions of parenting self-efficacy, thereby working through their guilt of infecting their children. Services need to be garnered to improve the emotional and mental health of the women through the provision of support groups and individual therapy sessions, which should be routinely made available to all women with HIV. These services would enable women to address and resolve issues in relationships, childcare, life choices and handle emotions of anger and grief reactions. Cognitive behavioral therapies, with a psychoeducational approach on safer sex practices, skills-building training to manage high-risk situations, assertiveness training to negotiate safer sexual interactions, and relaxation instructions for stress management need to be part of the intervention repertoire in the development of effective coping strategies by the HIV positive women.

Given the centrality of the family in the women's needs, the interventions should also provide supportive services to their family units through augmenting primary support systems, facilitating increased HIV/AIDS knowledge, providing information on medical and social services, and provision of family-focused therapies to address disclosure, so as to help destigmatize HIV within the family unit. Policy and program actions targeting the socio-economic determinants of women's risk of HIV infection need to be activated. On a broader policy level, it is essential that efforts be made to improve women's economic status through appropriate measures including access to credit, skills training, flexible employment, sheltered workshops, and provisions of primary and secondary education. It is also indicated that the existing community-based organizations improve and expand their existing services to rural areas as well, rather than being polarized in urban cities. There is a definite need to start a socioeconomic intervention package programme towards providing economic relief and improving the social networks. Subsidized medical care and a responsive health care delivery system need to be the order. There is a strong need to widen NGO services to include shelter and care for HIV positive children with networks to initiate foster care and adoption services. As the children of HIV positive parents grow, they will also require age appropriate counseling to help them cope with the knowledge of their parents HIV status and at times their own compromised state.

The limitations of this study centered on the non-random small group of women and in the reliance on subjective responses by them. A longitudinal study designed to detect important changes in social, psychological and spiritual spheres, throughout women's experiences of HIV disease as well as the factors influencing these changes, would be very valuable to service providers, professionals, and ultimately to growing numbers of women with HIV/AIDS.

REFERENCES

Bharat, S. (1996). *Facing the challenge: Household and community responses to HIV/AIDS in Mumbai*. Tata Institute of Social Sciences, Mumbai, India.

Chung, J.Y. & Magraw, M.M. (1992). A group approach to psychosocial issues faced by HIV-positive women. *Hospital and Community Psychiatry*, 43 (9), 891-894.

Cochran, S.D., & Mays, V.M. (1989). Women and AIDS-related concerns, roles for psychologists in helping the worried well. *American Psychologist*, 44(3), 529-535.

Fleishman, J., Sherbaine, C.D., Crystal, S., Marshall, G., Kelly, M., Grant, I., Collins, R., & Hays, R. (1996). Social support and coping factor structures and associations with psychological distress. *Abstracts XI International Conference on AIDS*. Vancouver, Canada.

Gangakhedkar, R.R., Bentley, M.E., & Divekar, A.D. (1994). Spread of HIV infection in married monogamous married women in India. *Journal of American Medical Association*, 278 (23), 2090.

Gillman, R.R., & Newman, B.S. (1996). Psychosocial concerns and strengths of women with HIV infection: An empirical study. *Families in Society: The Journal of Contemporary Human Services*, 3, 131-141.

Hackl, K.L., Somlai, A.M., Kelly, J.A., & Kalichman, S.C. (1996). Women living with HIV/AIDS: The dual challenges of being medical patient and a primary family caregiver. *Abstracts XI International Conference on AIDS*. Vancouver, Canada.

Hertz, E. (1996). Social support and coping–Defining the relationship. *Abstracts XI International Conference on AIDS*. Vancouver, Canada.

Kneisl, C.R. (1993). Psychosocial and economic concerns of women affected with HIV infection. In F.L. Cohen & J.D. Durham (Eds.), *Women, Children and HIV/AIDS*. New York: Springer.

Lawless, S., Greet, B., & Vivienne, M. (1996). 'Seriously Seeking': The experiences and coping strategies of two Australian states. *Abstracts XI International Conference on AIDS*. Vancouver, Canada.

Lazarus, R.S., & Folkman, S. (1984). *Stress, appraisal and coping*. New York: Springer.

Malhotra, S. (1998). AIDS and women: AIDS–ABC to XYZ. 3rd Edition. Chandigarh: Tagore Medical Publishers.

Moore, J., Solomon, L., Schoebaum, E., Schuman, P., Boland, B., & Smith, D. (1996). Depressive symptoms and coping strategies among HIV-infected and HIV uninfected women in four urban cities. *Abstracts XI International Conference on AIDS*. Vancouver, Canada.

Nakajima, G., & Rubin, H. (1991). Lack of racial, gender, and behavior risk diversity in psychiatric research on AIDS/HIV in the United States [Poster M.B 2044]. *Proceedings of the Seventh International Conference on AIDS*, 1, 193.

Osmond, M.W., Wambach, K.G., Harrison, D.F., Byers, J., Levine, P., Immershein, A., & Quadagno, D.M. (1993). The multiple jeopardy of race, class, and gender of AIDS risk among women. *Gender and Society*, 7, 99-120.

Pederson, S.S., & Elkitt, A. (1998). Traumatization, psychological defense style, coping, symptomatology and social support in HIV positives: A pilot study. *Scandinavian Journal of Psychology*, 39(2), 55-60.

Pinel, A. (1996). Personal dynamics of women who risk unprotected sex with HIV-infected partners. *Abstracts XI International Conference on AIDS*. Vancouver, Canada.

Quinn, S. (1993). AIDS and African American women: The triple burden of race, class and gender. *Health Education Quarterly*, 20, 305-320.

Regan-Kubinsky, M.J., & Sharts-Hopko, N. (1995). Illness cognitions of HIV-infected mothers. *Issues in Mental Health Nursing*, 16, 327-344.

Romano, E.M., Aplasca, M.R., & Monzon, O.T. (1996). Coping mechanisms of families/households of HIV-infection AIDS Patients. *Abstracts XI International Conference on AIDS*. Vancouver, Canada.

Rose, M.A., & Clark-Alexander, B. (1996). Quality of life and coping styles of HIV positive women with children. *Journal of the Association of Nurses in AIDS Care*, 7(2), 28.

Sherr, L., Petrak, J., Melvin, D., Davet, T., Glover, L., & Hedge, B. (1993). Psychological trauma associated with AIDS and HIV infection in women. *Counselling Psychology Quarterly*, 6, 99-108.

Siegel, K., Gluhoski, V.L., & Karus, D. (1997). Coping and mood in HIV positive women. *Psychological Reports*, 81(2), 435-442.

Solomon, G., Kemeny, M., & Tomoshok, L. (1991). Psychoneuroimmunologic aspects of HIV infection. In R. Ader, D. Felten, & N. Cohen (Eds.), *Psychoneuroimmunology* (2nd ed., 1081-1114). San Diego, CA: Academic Press.

Somlai, A.M., Heckman, T.G., Hackl, K., Morgan, M., & Welsh, D. (1998). Developmental stages and spiritual coping among economically impoverished women living with HIV disease. *Journal of Pastoral Care*, 52 (3), 227-240.

Tolliver, D.E. (2001). African-American female caregivers of family members living with HIV/AIDS. *Families in Society: The Journal of Contemporary Human Services*, 82(2), 145-156.

UNAIDS (1999). Breakup of HIV/AIDS. *www.unaids.org.in*

UNAIDS (2000). Current update of HIV/AIDS. *www.unaids.org.in*

Rehabilitation
of the Wandering Seriously Mentally Ill
(WSMI) Women:
The Banyan Experience

P. Nalini Rao, MA, MPhil, PGDHRM

SUMMARY. Started in 1993, in a small way, by a social worker as a response to the growing destitution of mentally ill women and with the objective of giving shelter, treatment and mainstreaming them, The Banyan has so far given 'Adaikalam' (refuge) to 413 women, of whom 252 have been rehabilitated. The entire care process starts from the time the women are picked from the streets in a disheveled and deranged state and brought to the home after much difficulty. On arrival they are spruced up and clinically assessed by a psychiatrist and put on medication. Slowly and steadily they return to the world of reality. Simultaneously, the inmates are put through various therapies like individual counseling, music, art, yoga, and vocational training. Finally, the address of the inmates is traced, and a team from The Banyan accompanies them, and they are rehabilitated. The family is enlightened about the illness, the woman's stay at The Banyan, need for continuous medication. The Banyan is a lifetime service provider of medicines, keeping track by regular follow up and above all a friend to whom they can seek any help

P. Nalini Rao is Lecturer, Madras School of Social Work, Chennai, India.

[Haworth co-indexing entry note]: "Rehabilitation of the Wandering Seriously Mentally Ill (WSMI) Women: The Banyan Experience." Rao, P. Nalini. Co-published simultaneously in *Social Work in Health Care* (The Haworth Social Work Practice Press, an imprint of The Haworth Press, Inc.) Vol. 39, No. 1/2, 2004, pp. 49-65; and: *Social Work Visions from Around the Globe: Citizens, Methods, and Approaches* (ed: Anna Metteri et al.) The Haworth Social Work Practice Press, an imprint of The Haworth Press, Inc., 2004, pp. 49-65. Single or multiple copies of this article are available for a fee from The Haworth Document Delivery Service [1-800-HAWORTH, 9:00 a.m. - 5:00 p.m. (EST). E-mail address: docdelivery@haworthpress.com].

at any time. The role played by the social workers is so vital that the success of the programme hinges on their repertoire of skill and commitment. *[Article copies available for a fee from The Haworth Document Delivery Service: 1-800-HAWORTH. E-mail address: <docdelivery@haworthpress.com> Website: <http://www.HaworthPress.com> © 2004 by The Haworth Press, Inc. All rights reserved.]*

KEYWORDS. The Banyan, women, mentally ill, destitutes, rehabilitation, Nalini Rao, India

INDEX

Banyan: A huge tree with widespread branches supported by lateral roots. This tree is found in India and often finds mention in religious scripts as a benevolent tree giving succor and fulfilling the wishes of the devotee.

Adaikalam: A place where a person takes refuge.

India, the largest country in the Asian sub-continent, has inherited a rich civilization grounded in religion and philosophy. She has nurtured the cultural diversity of her vast landscape, which is reflected in her teeming millions. But, this hoary past has not ensured a comfortable present. Population explosion, poverty, illiteracy, new economic policy focusing on structural adjustments, the growing digital divide, and migration of people from rural to urban centers have initiated rapid social change. This has torn asunder the conventional social support configurations like value systems, the joint family norm, and neighborhood networks, making survival far from a pleasurable experience. These subsequently have had a deleterious effect on the psyche of the common man and much more, as explained below, on the women.

SHIFTING PARADIGMS–THE DOUBLE EDGED SWORD

When we look into the concepts of culture, gender, and health, it is indeed amazing to see the linkages between them, so intricately intermeshed and interdependent. Culture is a broad domain wherefrom constructs of gender and mental health draw their origin and sustenance. This is obvious and beyond debate. Gender does not merely indicate biological differences but is an essential part of the socio-cultural paradigm that has been painstakingly constructed and preserved over the centuries. The Indian society follows the patriarchal system of governance, where men are endowed with a lot of rights and privileges both legally and socially. Preference for sons, female feticide, girl-child marriage, and multiple pregnancies (resulting in fetal wastages and high maternal mortality rates) have resulted in low health status for women. Although there are several legal enactments since independence, focusing on enhancing the status of women in areas of inheritance, marriage, and education, how far they have been successfully implemented is questionable. Limited rights to property and education, battering, sexual exploitation and bride burning has had a cumulative toll on women.

The current globalization era not only symbolizes economic and technological development but also reflects a philosophy of life, de-layering the old for the new at every step. The merging geographical boundaries have unleashed change at an exponential rate. Women are not only major players in maintaining biodiversity and ecological balance; they are also the preservers of herbal medicine and seed conservation,[9] but given the current context they are not able to live up to this critical role. Technological development has dismantled the village crafts. Mechanization of agriculture and other forms of production have raised the demand for skilled labour, thereby pushing women out of gainful employment, resulting in feminization of poverty, increase of women headed households due to desertion/widowhood, or migration of male population to cities.[7] The modern women that we see in the media as informed, educated, decisive, assertive, and totally in control is an antithesis of the prevailing reality.

Although the relationship between globalization, mental distress, and high levels of vulnerability of women as a spillover of transition[3] has been established, whether this has resulted in greater neglect and subsequent wandering away of the mentally ill women is yet to empirically established. "Increases in incidence of health and mental health problems, and of social disintegration within the families and communities, are anticipated results."[1] Nevertheless the growing number of vagrant mentally women has become a social issue and a public hazard.

MENTAL ILLNESS–THE BIG PICTURE

There has been no national mental health survey to date. But there have been several epidemiological studies conducted in different parts of the country at different points of time. Hence, the following data are the result of an extrapolation exercise. Conservative estimates place the national prevalence rate of mental illness at 73/1000 people (Urban rate at 73 and rural at 70.5–a difference of 2.5). Prevalence rate for all mental disorders in India is higher than Sri Lanka, but lesser than West Asian and African countries. The Indian urban rate is four times more than the median Asian rate. Schizophrenia occurrence is placed at 3.6 rural and 2.5 urban per 1000, and MDP at 37.4 and 33.7 (includes both psychotic and neurotic depression), respectively. Females have higher rates than males on an average of 1.5 times at the all India level. Women belong to the high-risk group. The vulnerable among them are the housewives with a prevalence rate of 104/1000, and among them, the married are even more susceptible, followed by widows. Statewise break down of urban prevalence rate of mental disorders shows Tamil Nadu, with an alarmingly high rate of 83/1000, 14% higher than the national figure and MDP at 43.3/1000, and schizophrenia at 2.5.

There are variations in a woman's experience of mental illness/distress as she moves across different stages of her life cycle; it peaks during reproductive years, as demands on her are many, in terms of adjustment to her new roles and status as a wife, daughter-in-law, and mother (anger, disappointment and frustration that she may experience during this time find no avenues for release in a culturally approved manner) and tapers off during subsequent age periods. Although the prevalence rate is almost the same for both the sexes as far as severe mental disorders are concerned, there is a preponderance of male patients in terms of hospital admissions. This high percentage is due to 'unconscious' neglect of women based on feudal cultural values.[3] Psychosocial factors pre-empt mentally ill women from accessing medical help. They are normally routed either to religious faith healers or are deserted/abandoned. But some do reach the level of GP consultation, and a few even access psychiatric help (mostly by default).

The current situation here is so typical of Ogburn's 'cultural lag' theory, wherein he observes that material culture accumulates and religion, law, art, and custom replace rather than build on one another. He further asserts that material culture grows faster than adaptive culture, and hence modern society suffers from a great burden of unresolved social problems.[6] Although there is legislation pertaining to mental health and National Institutes established with sophisticated treatment modalities, and societal attitudes, poverty, and family breakdown nullify all efforts. The Banyan, through its efforts, to a certain extent tries to bridge this lag.

THE ROOTS

The complex social issues are a spillover of rapid and haphazard economic development. Although the state emerged as a major service provider in the nineties, it was realized that the government was not competent enough, given its political and procedural constraints, to address the issue single-handedly. The adoption of the structural adjustment programmes saw declining investment in the health sector.[5] When physical health is getting such a cursory treatment, mental health is not even mentioned in the overall health policy.

The National Mental Health Programme is limited in its implementation and out of focus. Both in the erstwhile Indian Lunacy Act (1912) and the more recent Mental Health Act (1987), there are provisions for the mentally ill persons who wander about without ostensible means of support (dubbed wandering lunatics by the 1912 Act), to be picked up by the police and produced before the nearest judicial court to receive orders for rehabilitation in the government and other approved hospitals. But the provision is only on paper. The police by and large ignore the deranged person on the street unless she proves to be a threat to the public. The need gap is to a certain extent taken care of by the non-governmental organizations (NGOs). These have the support of the local community, and they are more a response to the emerging needs of the people and have greater accountability and transparency.[4] In this context 'The Banyan' is emerging more than a mere caretaker for WSMI (wandering seriously mentally ill) women in India.

THE ORIGIN

A deranged, half-naked woman living in her own world of delusions and hallucinations soon became an object of public taunts and ridicule and caught the attention of two young professionals: Vandana Gopikumar (Founder Trustee), a professionally qualified social worker; and Vaishnavi Jayakumar (Founder Trustee), a management student. They took her to established hospitals and welfare centers to admit her, but no one would admit her, as legal hurdles were quoted as an escape route. The burning desire to be of help to these women saw the beginnings of The Banyan–the roots were struck. That was in August 1993, seven years ago, and slowly the numbers grew, and the tiny sapling has now grown into a huge banyan tree–giving succor to hundreds of destitute mentally ill women in a home called Adaikalam, meaning refuge.

Starting a home for women who are suffering from an illness that is highly stigmatized is no mean task. The first step was to scout for premises to house these patients. People were contacted and after some search a house was finally selected, and the rent was borne by some well-wishers. This was just the beginning. There was lot of protests from the neighbors; it took some time to pacify them. Financial implications were high–mounting medical bills, transport costs, food, electricity charges, etc., meant more lobbying for funds from philanthropists and the general public and also for the cause of The Banyan.

PROFILE OF THE REHABILITATED WOMEN

Records as of 30-05-2001 show that, of the total number of 473 beneficiaries that have taken refuge in the home since its inception, 112 are currently residents. A total of 38 beneficiaries have been referred to other organizations, over a period of time, as these women were mainly non-psychiatric destitute women picked from the streets, and 34 have expired due to secondary complications–in most cases, these women were long standing street wanderers who were not only mentally ill but were also afflicted with severe malnutrition/TB/diarrhoea/fever, etc. Those who escaped constitute the 37 and are grouped under 'failures.' 252 women have since been rehabilitated (see Figure 1).

Geographic Spread

A look at the map (see Figure 2) indicates the fact that the women have come from all parts of the country, even from distant states of Rajasthan and Punjab. But the majority of them (63 percent) seem to come from within the state of Tamil Nadu, where The Banyan is situated, followed by the neighboring state of Andhra Pradesh (12 percent). The rest have their origin from different states.

Area

Distribution of the residents indicates that most of the inmates come from the rural areas, followed by cities and towns. Of the total of 252, those who trace their origin to villages are 175, and 62 are from urban centers, and the remaining are from towns. There is a group labeled as

'Not Known,' a category referring to residents whose hometowns are yet to be identified. A multiplicity of factors, like high illiteracy rates, low nutritional status, less employment opportunities, and conservative norms of a village society make women from rural sectors more vulnerable to stress, as they find it difficult to overcome economic and psychological distress in a culturally determined context. Severe social control coupled with poverty pushes the women into the twilight zone of insanity, leading them away to strange lands and peoples.

Age

Figure 3 reflects the age distribution of the residents. Nearly 70% of the women belong to the 20-40 years age group, a critical and established age for the precipitation of psychotic disorders, especially for schizophrenia and manic depressive psychosis, a fact well established by earlier research findings the world over, when onset during these

FIGURE 1. Distribution of Residents

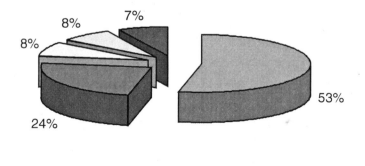

rehabilitated current residents referred escaped died

FIGURE 2. Geographic Spread of the Rehabilitated Women

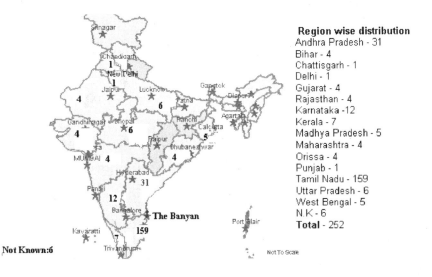

Region wise distribution
Andhra Pradesh - 31
Bihar - 4
Chattisgarh - 1
Delhi - 1
Gujarat - 4
Rajasthan - 4
Karnataka -12
Kerala - 7
Madhya Pradesh - 5
Maharashtra - 4
Orissa - 4
Punjab - 1
Tamil Nadu - 159
Uttar Pradesh - 6
West Bengal - 5
N.K - 6
Total - 252

prime years leaves both the individual and the family totally devastated.

Marital Status

Married women succumb to various pressures. As already quoted earlier, married women also belong to the 20-40 years age group, when vulnerability to the illness is at the highest, as marriage entails adjustment to a stranger of a husband (most of the marriages in India are arranged by the elders in the family based on factors like caste, economic status, dowry–and compatibility between the two individuals does not find a place at all as a consideration for marriage), harassment by in-laws, physical and sexual abuse, pregnancies in quick succession, demand for a male child, deteriorating health, desertion by husband, polygamy, and low social status all have a cumulative effect on the mental health of the women. Of the total number of residents, 179 are married and 73 are either single or have been since deserted by their husbands.

Educational Status

Literacy levels are low; almost 50% of the rehabilitated are illiterate. Some of them have had school education up to primary level, and few of

FIGURE 3. Distribution of Rehabilitated Women–Age Wise

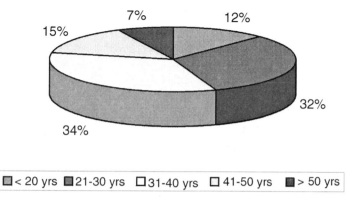

☐ < 20 yrs ■ 21-30 yrs ☐ 31-40 yrs ☐ 41-50 yrs ■ > 50 yrs

them have gone up to the secondary level. Three of them are post-graduates. The rest of them are illiterate, hailing mostly from the rural areas where educating girls is still looked upon as a luxury both in terms of financial implications and sparing a hand from farm labor/sibling responsibility.

Economic Status

All of the women, except for a handful, come from families who belong to low economic strata, having incomes on an average less than Rs 3000 or $60 per month. Most of them hail from agrarian families, which are large in size. Fragmentation of land holdings, failure of monsoons, drought conditions, and heavy debt burden put these families within the vicious grip of poverty for generations to come. Even in the urban areas, most of them live off daily wages/petty business having irregular flow of finances, and computing income for a month is based on conjecture. Dohrenwend and Dohrenwend (1980) found that psychopathology was two and half times more in the lower classes than the upper class.[8] This general pattern suggests that mental disorders are most likely to occur in disadvantaged sectors of society. However, the cause may be due to cumulative effects of environmental adversity or to selection process, or to some combination of social causation and selection. There is very little systematic information on the effectiveness of early outreach and treatment of childhood-onset or adolescent-onset disorder.[2]

Poverty and mental illness seem to act jointly to erase the ill-fated women's self-identity and somehow make them undertake a random voyage to far-away places (for example, the distance from Rajasthan to Chennai is nearly 2000 miles). Such wanderings (impelled by some kind of accession of wanderlust which may be a part of the syndrome) seem to continue until they are stopped by a powerful, beneficial social force such as The Banyan, which seeks to reconstruct their past, their personality, and individuality and arranges for their return journey to their original abode.

Duration of Stay

The duration of stay at The Banyan varies from less than three months to more than three years. Although it is heartening to note that 40% of the inmates stayed less than three months, it is even more distressing that an equal percentage have stayed from six months to two years. Only 9% of the patients' stay stretched beyond three years.

For long standing psychotics who stayed away from home for a lengthy period of time, tracing their families becomes a very challenging and arduous task. The younger the inmate, the shorter the stay. Nearly 87% of the less than 20 years age group was rehabilitated within six months. As the age increases, the residents' stay spreads over a longer period. Although, of the 21-30 years age group, 50% successfully move out, nearly 44% stay on for nearly a year or two. The same applies to the subsequent two age groups ranging from 31-50 years. The duration of stay of inmates is even higher for those above 50 years (see Table 1).

Table 2 indicates that the marital status of the individual does seem to influence the duration of stay. The married ones seem to stay on longer. There is the usual argument as to who should take the woman back. In many instances, it is between the husband who absolves himself of responsibility of taking care of her (unless there are grown up children in the family, who insist that they want their mother back) and the women's natal family. The resolution of the tussle takes a while

REHABILITATION–THE QUALITATIVE PROCESS

The residents of The Banyan are literally picked up from the streets. Someone calls up or comes personally to inform about a 'mad woman' in their area, and immediately a social worker, along with one of the staff members, goes and after much cajoling and help from the members of the public brings her to Adaikalam. Simultaneously, the social worker informs in writing to the police officers on duty that the patient is being taken to The Banyan, and anyone seeking her can be directed to

TABLE 1. Age and Duration of Stay

Age (Years)	Duration of Stay (Months)						Total
	< 3	4-6	7-12	13-24	25-36	> 36	
< 20	16 51.6%	8 25.8%		3 9.7%	4 13%		31 100%
21-30	33 40.7%	5 6.1%	25 30.8%	17 29%		1 1.2%	81 100%
31-40	22 25.8%	15 17.6%	17 20%	18 21.1%	8 9.4%	5 5.8%	85 100%
41-50	10 27%	5 13.5%	10 27%	8 21.6%		4 10.8%	37 100%
> 50	8 44.4%		4 22.2%			6 33.3%	18 100%
TOTAL	89 35.3%	33 13%	56 22.2%	46 18.2%	12 4.7%	16 6.3%	252 100%

the home. Other legal formalities (though cumbersome) like procuring the reception order from the magistrate, a statutory requirement of the Mental Health Act, is also taken care of. Bringing her to the home is a herculean task by itself.

When she makes her first entry she is in a totally disheveled and deranged state with her body covered by grime and in a pitiable condition. At first her head is shaved carefully (lest the sores on the scalp bleed), as the unkempt hair is matted and infested with lice, then she is given a bath, dressed in a clean a set of clothes, fed, and examined by a consultant psychiatrist, diagnosed and put on medication, which usually comprises antipsychotic drugs, antidepressants, tranquilizers, and other supportive medication. They are also de-wormed, and tested for sexually transmitted diseases. Other secondary infections/diseases are also treated. Some of these women are pregnant when they arrive and are totally unaware of their delicate status. The team consists of a doctor, professional social worker, voluntary workers, and resident caretakers for each inmate for monitoring purposes.

The role of the social worker starts from bringing the patient home, informing the doctor, subsequent supervision, medication management, documenting the progress of the resident, and planning the rehabilitation strategy and accompanying them on their journey of reintegration. After due assessment of their psychosocial functioning and residual capabilities, all residents are put in any one of the following four groups.

TABLE 2. Marital Status and Duration of Stay

Marital status	Stay at The Banyan (in Months)						TOTAL
	< 3	4-6	7-12	13-24	25-36	> 36	
Married	72	19	35	37	6	10	179
	39.70%	10.70%	19.10%	20.60%	3.10%	6.90%	100%
Single	31	6	18	16	1	1	73
	41.20%	8.80%	23.50%	20.60%	3.0%	3.0%	100%
Total	103	25	53	53	7	11	252
	40.00%	10.30%	20.00%	20.60%	3.0%	6.10%	100%

Group 4

This is meant for new entrants, for whom warmth, food, clothing, medicines, love, and affection become vital inputs to put them on the road to recovery. The social worker, with her professional zeal to help, is constantly in association with the patient and slowly but steadily establishes a rapport and a bonding that has a therapeutic effect on them. In the meantime medicines also do their wonderwork. Sometimes the patients are so violent and unpredictable, more so at this stage than others, that there are instances when the social workers and caretakers have been at the receiving end.

Group 3

This is for manageable and improving patients. During their stay at the home, which may range from one week to four years, the inmates are put through a series of psychosocial therapeutic techniques comprising individual and group counseling sessions. Once the inmates become oriented to reality, and they are able to establish some meaningful communication, they are able to relate better, and some crucial information is obtained from them. Everything gets recorded in their respective case files. The number of counseling sessions is determined by the chronicity of the illness, rate of recovery, personality of the inmate, education level, nativity, and other factors.

Group 2

The inmates progress. Slowly and steadily, the patients improve, drug dosages are altered accordingly, individual sessions continue, and the social worker becomes a pivotal and important person in the life of the inmate. Group sessions are planned and carried out by the social worker in the form of ADL (activities of daily living), exercises, yoga, aerobics, music and dance therapy. This helps them to develop interpersonal skills, and they form group affinity after several sessions.

Group 1

This group of residents is almost ready to return to their homes. They are now taught some vocational skills through workshops on candle making, greeting cards, block printing on napkins, table linen, basket making, threading flowers and making bouquets, etc. This acts both as a therapeutic exercise and also as a viable means of sustenance later on. They are entrusted with some housekeeping duties and also to take care of other residents. They are given an opportunity to attend meetings for a limited audience, to speak for their cause of inclusion.

Recreation includes outings to the beach, movies, celebrating festivals and sports, all of which, along with regular medication, love, and care, put these inmates slowly but surely on the road to recovery. Cultural differences of the residents are respected and maintained. Above all the dignity of the individual is upheld and nurtured.

THIS IS ONLY THE BEGINNING

Eliciting of information and tracing the address of the resident are both a rewarding and frustrating experience. Illiteracy, strange local dialects (residents come from all over India), inability to recall, and loss of contact with home makes case history construction an arduous and long drawn out process. Over several sessions, the social worker puts the bits and pieces of the puzzle together and finally a blurred picture emerges–life incidents, family constellation, name of hometown, and disjointed address. With this the search begins. Letters are sent out to the local post office/police station/school, depending on the clues given, and when there is a positive response from the other side then half the battle is won. Sometimes a member of the family comes to take her back resulting in a happy reunion.

Many a time there is no response. Efforts are then made to take the residents to their native place. The rehabilitative team led by the social worker selects a few of them, forming a homogenous group, those belonging to the same state or neighboring states based on certain reference points, like name, language, food habits, and way of dressing that they take to after improvement, and the vague address and landmarks that the resident often quotes, are grouped together. The date of journey is decided, and the team along with the residents leaves. It may be a month or more before the team returns.

They traverse thousands of miles by train/bus and even walk if it is to a remote village with just a single street and cannot be accessed by road. Sometimes the homes are traced without much difficulty, and the women are reunited. The family is educated about the illness, inmate's stay, need for continuous medication and with an assurance that The Banyan is there for any other help if need be. Once the women are successfully reintegrated with their families, medicines are dispatched every month, and local doctors are identified and contacted for periodic review of the beneficiary.

There are instances when after a period of time the drug parcels return unaccepted either because the family has moved away to another town or village leaving no forwarding address, or the woman has wandered away/expired. There are also instances when the family brings back the woman as she has had a relapse or societal stigma is so high that they would rather not have her at home. In all these cases the Banyan once again takes them back into its fold . . . *The role of The Banyan as not a mere transit home* . . . but a lifetime service provider of medicines, follow up and above all a friend to whom they can seek any help at any time.

At times, for the other residents, after the long and arduous journey, the resident's family is not traceable or there is a complete rejection of her and in a few such cases, there are instances when a local NGO, or a benevolent school teacher or the police came forward voluntarily as caretakers. At times, it turns out that it is not the resident's hometown after all. In such situations, she is brought back once again to The Banyan, and she is helped to come out of her trauma of rejection/not finding her family. Specific skills are taught to her based on her interests, and she is sent for work in the neighborhood as a maid/flower seller/fruit vendor or in a small shop that stocks sweets, biscuits, pencils, stationery items, etc., so that she becomes economically independent. This process of mainstreaming is an essential part of The Banyan's activities.

The Banyan's useful endeavors give sociological significance under ecological perspectives theorized by Hauser and Duncan. This theoreti-

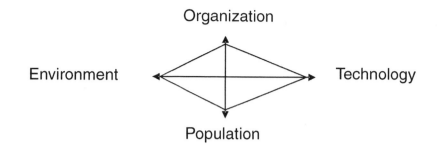

cal framework interrelates four aspects of the ecological complex, as illustrated below:
"The four sets of variables are in reciprocal relationship and the lines in the presentation above are meant to suggest the idea of functional interdependence." Hauser and Duncan called it and 'equilibrium-seeking' system.

In the Banyan context, the population would be the composition of its inmates and the outside people it tries to reach out to; the organization would refer to the family and other institutions that at times fail to take care of the mentally ill, and as a result, consciously or unconsciously seek relief from the environment. They wander away from their original habitat and make their get-away in different directions. The technology that comes in handy for them is in the shape of transport–a long distance running train; overloaded with its passengers, it helps these women to remain unidentified and unnoticed. Here ecology of space meshes into the technology of transport.

The Banyan's efforts become the equilibrium-seeking mechanism. Family's failure and that of government agencies in providing relief to the destitute mental patients is made good by NGOs like The Banyan. The restoration of equilibrium is almost complete (a) when the government recognized and cooperated with The Banyan in setting up an office in its premises to give the official seal of approval for admission of inmates as per the act, and (b) when these women are reunited with their families.

It is ecological incongruity–a half naked woman in front of a prestigious educational institution in an upscale neighborhood–that sparked the starting of The Banyan, and it has over the years taken on the role of an ecological leveler.

It is almost ten years now since The Banyan was started, a long and tough journey, with miles still to go. But nevertheless there have been several bright spots that have brought cheer to the Banyan team. Several programmes are on the anvil, like starting a research wing, adopting neighborhood for community mental health programmes, and to identify like-minded individuals to start similar organizations in different parts of the country. But at the end of the day, the social work profession needs to gear up to the challenging demands of a society in transformation.

LANDMARKS IN THE HISTORY OF THE BANYAN– CELEBRATING LIFE

- August 1993–The Beginning.
- New Year–The first resident enters–Ms. Chellamal.*
- October 1994–Ms. Leela the first inmate to be rehabilitated
- End 1994–Media recognition–since then it has played a vital role in championing the cause of mental health and the Banyan.
- February 1995–Fund raising programmes a whooping success, the first of the series to follow.
- Mid 1995–Inauguration of community awareness programmes, followed by several over the years–talk shows, debates, contests, awareness walks.
- August 1996–Government grants six grounds of land to build a center.
- 1997–Formation of the Alliance for the mentally ill–volunteers of the Banyan, who help out from caring the residents, vocational training, fund-raising, rehabilitation, administration, etc.
- October 2000–Outreach programme is started to cover the neighboring rural village to spread awareness of mental illness and related issues.
- April 2001–Moving to a newly constructed three-floor center from small cramped house after a massive fund-raising drive, with contributions from the public, corporate houses, film stars, etc.

Names of the residents mentioned are real.

BIBLIOGRAPHY

1. *All Our Futures, Principles & Resources For Social Work Practice in a Global Era.* Chathapuram S. Ramanathan & Rosemary J. Link. Wadsworth Publishing Company, USA. 1999.
2. *Bulletin of the World Health Organization*, 200, 78(4), WHO International, 2000, Geneva.

3. *Mental Health of Women, a Feminist Agenda*. Bhargavi V. Davar, Sage Publications, New Delhi, 1999.
4. *NGOs in The Changing Scenario*. Meher C. Nanavatty, D. Kulkarni, Uppal Publishing House, New Delhi. 1998.
5. *Social Impact of Social Reforms in India*, P. R. Panchamukhi, Economic and Political Weekly, March 4, 2000.
6. *Sociology an Introduction,* Neil J. Smelser, Wiley Eastern Pvt. Ltd, New Delhi, 1970.
7. *Women-Headed households. Coping with caste, class, and gender hierarchies.* L. Lingam, Economic and Political Weekly, XXIX (12), 19 March.
8. *World Health Organization-Report,* Geneva, 1993.
9. *Staying Alive, Women Ecology and Survival in India,* V. Shiva, 2000.
10. *Epidemiological Findings on Prevalence of Mental Disorders in India.* H.C. Ganguli, 2000.

Time to Father

Natalie Bolzan, PhD
Fran Gale, PhD
Michael Dudley, PhD

SUMMARY. This paper reports the qualitative findings from 40 couples involved in a study exploring men's post-natal mental health. Interviews were conducted with individuals soon after the birth of their first child. Findings suggest that new fathers want to be more involved in the direct care and nurturing of their children than their fathers were with them. Discourses which construct fathers and inform social structures have not kept pace with men's changed attitudes and role expectations limiting the options available to men as fathers. In particular men's employment circumstances figure in their experience of adjusting to life as a father. Those fathers having least flexibility and autonomy in their work report experiencing, since the birth of their child, more unhappiness, anxiety, and generally higher levels of stress. These findings sug-

Natalie Bolzan is Senior Lecturer, School of Applied Social and Human Sciences, University of Western Sydney, Bankstown Campus, Locked Bag 1797, Penrith South Distribution Centre, NSW 1797, Australia (E-mail: n.bolzan@uws.edu.au). Fran Gale is Lecturer, School of Applied Social and Human Sciences, University of Western Sydney, Bankstown Campus, Locked Bag 1797, Penrith South Distribution Centre, NSW 1797, Australia (E-mail: fw.gale@uws.edu.au). Michael Dudley is affiliated with Prince of Wales Hospital, University of New South Wales, Sydney, NSW 2520, Australia (E-mail: m.dudley@unsw.edu.au).

[Haworth co-indexing entry note]: "Time to Father." Bolzan, Natalie, Fran Gale, and Michael Dudley. Co-published simultaneously in *Social Work in Health Care* (The Haworth Social Work Practice Press, an imprint of The Haworth Press, Inc.) Vol. 39, No. 1/2, 2004, pp. 67-88; and: *Social Work Visions from Around the Globe: Citizens, Methods, and Approaches* (ed: Anna Metteri et al.) The Haworth Social Work Practice Press, an imprint of The Haworth Press, Inc., 2004, pp. 67-88. Single or multiple copies of this article are available for a fee from The Haworth Document Delivery Service [1-800-HAWORTH, 9:00 a.m. - 5:00 p.m. (EST). E-mail address: docdelivery@haworthpress.com].

gest increasing workplace flexibility and provisions such as parental leave are important for men's post-natal mental health. *[Article copies available for a fee from The Haworth Document Delivery Service: 1-800-HAWORTH. E-mail address: <docdelivery@haworthpress.com> Website: <http://www.HaworthPress.com> © 2004 by The Haworth Press, Inc. All rights reserved.]*

KEYWORDS. Fatherhood, discourse, social construction

Fatherhood has not generally been regarded as a life-transforming event for men in the same way that motherhood has for women (Eggebeen and Knoester, 2001). In Western societies fatherhood for most of the 20th century came to be equated with increased financial responsibility and the expanded role of breadwinner for 'a family.' Men's contribution in terms of moral leadership and gender-role modeling were also acknowledged but not framed as requiring any great transformation in men's lives. Men's experience of fatherhood was generally seen in instrumental rather than in personally transformative terms. Until the closing decades of the 20th century, very little scholarly exploration or examination was concerned with the changes which accompanied men's transition to fatherhood. The meaning of fatherhood to men and the sense men make of fatherhood are areas that are just beginning to be explored.

Emerging evidence suggests that fatherhood may require more than a mere adjustment for men, that it may in fact have a much greater impact than previously acknowledged. Research which investigates fatherhood suggests that there is an impact on men of fatherhood in terms of: psychological distress (Barnett, Marshall and Pleck, 1992; Grove and Mongione, 1983); personal growth (Parke, 1981; Russell, 1982); involvement in religious activities (Chaves, 1991; Ploch and Hastings, 1998); and social relationships with family and kin (Eggebeen and Hogan, 1990). The weight of this evidence suggests that fatherhood is associated with substantial changes in men's daily activity and with the way in which they experience or relate to the world. Fatherhood may well be a life-transforming event for men. Whilst society is prepared for this impact on women and acknowledges through various programs, structures, debates, and discourses the shift which occurs when a woman becomes a mother, it appears less prepared for the impact of the transition from man to father. Indeed, fathers' mental health problems have been comparatively absent from psychiatric literature which has predominantly focussed on mothers' postnatal depression (Dudley, Roy, Kelk, and Bernard, in press). Similarly whilst social workers are alert to the strains, demands, and insecurities women have about motherhood, they are less attuned to these aspects of men's transition to fatherhood.

The current paper briefly reviews the dominant discourses constructing fatherhood in Australia at the beginning of the 21st century and identifies the presence of these discourses in public policies affecting fathers. Results of interviews with first time fathers are then presented that suggests men are negotiating fatherhoods which, to varying degrees, accept or challenge the constructions offered them by the dominant discourses of fatherhood and consequent policies.

DISCOURSES CONSTRUCTING FATHERS IN AUSTRALIA

Use of Discourse

Fairclough states 'discourse is in an active relation to reality . . . language signifies reality in the sense of constructing meanings for it' (Fairclough 1992:42).

The discourses that are available at any point in time serve to construct the ways in which we think, talk about, or understand certain experiences or situations. Thus knowing the social discourses around fatherhood provides some insight into the ways society expects men to be when they are fathers. The types of fatherhoods which men have available to them are at worst restricted to, and at least influenced by, the discourses available at any time in society. Academic and policy literatures provide two sites in which we come to know discourses constructing fathers in Australia today.

Four main themes emerge from the literature concerned with fathering.

Men as Ill-Equipped to Parent

Psychologists from the developmental school emphasised the role of the maternal-child bond and the primacy of such a bond for healthy emotional and psychological development. A focus on the naturalness of the mother-child relationship tended to relegate fathers to the periphery of intimate parenthood. This 'excluded' status was reinforced by research which tended to focus on problematic situations in which a 'deficit model of men' (Doherty, 1997) or a 'role-inadequacy perspective' of fathering was exposed (see Hawkins and Dollahite, 1997). The literature that constructed men in this way informed discourses such as 'deadbeat dads' or referred to absent fathers. Much of the more recent writing in this area focussed on fathers, who after separation from their partner, would slowly withdraw from their children's lives as well (see Doherty, 1997, for a discussion of this). Such literature focused on men's connection to fatherhood as, at best, conditional.

In Australia a range of programs appear to have emerged in response to this 'incompetent fathers' discourse. Parenting and fathering programs that are either fully or partially funded by the state to enhance the contribution men can make to the family are provided in a variety of venues. Such programs acknowledge the support men need in the transition to fatherhood and are also beginning to accommodate the varying needs men have as they make this transition. There is an apparent increasing commitment from the state to develop and fund services, which recognise men's needs in terms of learning how to father.

Men's Contribution as Fathers

In contrast to the 'incompetent father' discourse is research which considered the cognitive manifestations of father's involvement (see, for example, Palkovitz, 1997).

This approach began to place value on what it was that men did as fathers, and focussed on interaction, accessibility, and responsibility (Lamb, 1997). In this way an alternate construction of men as fathers was proposed. The contribution of fathers has also been explored through notions of generativity (Hawkins and Dollahite, 1997). This approach emphasises the contributions fathers make to their child's development through their active involvement and participation in fathering.

In Australia, the Child Support Scheme, administered by the Department of Social Security and the Child Support Agency, exists to encourage biological fathers to be responsible for children's financial support rather than the state support these children. Similar to recent moves in the United States, the Australian government has moved responsibility for the well-being of children (including low-income, high-risk children) from the state back to the biological parents (Fox and Bruce, 2001).

Fathers as Located in a Social Context

Another set of academic writing attempts to locate men in either the context of the family or the wider society. A systemic ecological approach

(Doherty, Kouneski and Erickson, 1998) sites fathering within a set of individual, interpersonal, and social factors which have a specific influence on fathering and underscore the contextual nature of fathering. In exploring the literature which locates fatherhood in a larger social context, a range of articles emerged which described 'responsible' fathering. Responsible fathering construes fathers as 'not only financial providers but also as affective companions and caregivers' (Curran and Abrams, 2000:669). Research which investigates the impact of parenting programs on children's behaviour (Dishion, McCord and Poulin, 1999) and that which talks about generative or 'involved fathering' (Palkovitz, 1997) places men in a web of relationships and networks which can have an impact over time. Such literature often details programs and policy premised upon the belief that 'involved, nurturing fathers are a key component in raising competent, healthy and responsible children' (*Dads Make a Difference*, University of Minnesota, 1998).

It is interesting to note that despite an apparent commitment to actively engaging men as fathers as suggested by the programs described above, there are limits to this involvement which the state sets. Involvement should not come at the cost of smooth labour force activity. Thus only tentative forays into the arena of policy making which have any real impact on changing structures such as the work force participation are evident in Australia. A reluctance to affect major changes on employment conditions reflects an underlying assumption that men are, and possibly should be, the key breadwinners in the family.

Fatherhood as Fluid and Negotiated

A further emergent approach to understanding fatherhood is concerned with the fluid and changing nature of men's experience of fatherhood. In this literature men are seen as making a commitment in varying degrees to fatherhood (Fox and Bruce, 2001), as acknowledging the growing diversity of life course and residency patterns for men and children (Marsiglio, 1998), and to how men perceived and construct their identities as fathers in diverse situations (Amato and Rezac, 1994). The way in which men are negotiating a construction of fatherhood in response to the various discourses is also dealt with in this literature (Lupton and Barclay, 1997).

Most recently identity theory (Daly, 1995; Marsiglio, 1998) has been used to accommodate the many diverse situations, family arrangements and cultural situations in which men locate themselves and a diversity of ways in which men construct themselves as fathers.

The discourse of men as occupying a diversity of fatherhoods which are negotiated as the result of individual life circumstances and relationships is not apparent in Australian social policy. Such policy would need to be cognizant of the many fatherhoods which exist, but this is not the case. A recent report into fatherhood in Australia, 'Fitting Fathers into Families' (Department of Family and Community Services, 1999), revealed that policy makers and practitioners did not embrace a genuine belief that both fathers and mothers had a shared responsibility for children. The report argued that policies and programs in Australia, whilst beginning to emphasise the needs and contribution of fathers, are largely premised on a belief that the mother has the primary responsibility for the children and that fathers are neither interested nor competent in being parents.

Within these competing discourses and constructions of fatherhood, and in the context of public discourses which appear to restrict the fatherhoods available, how do first time fathers construct and give meaning to their experience? Our research suggests that men's mental health is affected by the intersecting discourses which construct fatherhood and that men are finding a tension exists from these intersecting discourses.

METHODOLOGY

In the current project the stories or narratives of 40 men who have become fathers for the first time are examined to provide some insight into the ways in which new fathers are negotiating their changed status.

Narratives are a response to a limited set of public and private stories that guide our thoughts and actions in certain ways and not others (Somers and Gibson, 1994). Narratives can be much broader than this; however, because ontological narratives are used to define who we are and are a precondition for knowing how to behave (Somers and Gibson, 1994), we used them to help explore the construction men have of themselves as fathers.

In acknowledgment of the contribution of the mother of the child to the repertoire of narratives available to men, we also gained information about the expectations of mothers around fatherhood. The data gathered from the women were used to triangulate information around particular behaviours such as drug and alcohol use, but was also used to provide some insight into one set of negotiations in which the men were involved, that is mothers' expectations around fathers.

Sample: The sample comprised of fathers and mothers in the Eastern Suburbs of Sydney, Australia, attending several nearby early childhood centres. The early childhood centres see most new mothers from the immediate geographic catchment area in the post-natal period. The eastern suburbs geographic area is socio-economically diverse, and a wide variety of social and occupational groups were represented. The sample collection was opportunistic, and each family of a newborn attending the clinic during the data collection phase was invited to participate.

A structured interview was conducted by one member of the research team, and a set of questionnaires was administered and completed by both parents independently. Mothers were interviewed as soon as possible after attending the early childhood centre. Fathers were interviewed as soon after the mother's interview as possible. Interviews were conducted face-to-face where possible but otherwise were conducted over the telephone. The qualitative data obtained in interviews form the basis of this paper. The quantitative data have been and are still being analysed and will be presented at a later date.

A total sample of 150 couples participated in the research. Interviews from the first 40 men and women selected from the larger study are reported here.

WHAT WE FOUND

The first thing to note in the findings is the very high proportion of men who state they wish to father differently from their own fathers. Fully 29 fathers out of 40 (72.5%) made comments such as

I am doing things differently from my father.

My experience is completely different from my father, my father was more old fashioned, he was mainly about 'bringing in the money.'

My father worked 18 hour days—I didn't get the chance to be close to him.

He (my father) spent too long at work.

This group of new fathers are re-working images of 'father' and articulating a desire to be different to their own fathers, whether that be in terms of less time at work, or having a closer relationship, or just doing things differently. For many the image they have carried of 'father' is an image they increasingly are unable or unwilling to relate to.

These new fathers recognised that their own fathers provided some of their most powerful models of fatherhood with all the restrictions of those models. Some expressed regret for their own father: *'my father had to work hard, he was denied the chance for any education and for being involved with his children.'* Many commented that they saw their father as caring towards them, recognised a continuity with their own fathering and did not completely reject their father's legacy, but clearly wanted to transform aspects of it.

One of the ways many of the fathers in this group distinguished their fathering from their own fathers' (fathering) was around expression of feelings:

> *My father didn't say much or express feelings much to us, I'm more talkative and express my feelings more.*

> *I'm very different from my own father, I'm more affectionate to my child, I don't find it a problem to show affection.*

For others 'hands on' involvement is also an important difference:

> *My father was more removed, I'm much more hands on, my father sat around and did little, my experience is very different, I change nappies, make milk and get up in the middle of the night.*

> *For my father having children was all about responsibility, for me it is also a privilege, I took an active part in the birth and take a much more active part in rearing our child than he did with us.*

Re-working images of fatherhood involved, for some, 're-assessing' what it means to be 'male':

> *My father wasn't around much when I was growing up, he was a coal miner and had lots of bravado and machismo. Bonding with your child is important I think, you get more in touch with what it really means to be male.*

Another commented:

We don't know how to behave as men and fathers–we have no older male models.

A challenge arose for these men in contesting the familiar images of 'father' which left them as some put it *'open to surprise,' 'waiting and learning how to be involved,' 'fatherhood is important and I'm impatient in learning about it.'* For some there was pleasure in *'being opened to surprise in one's self and one's child.'* This sense of new possibilities and trust in their changing identity was expressed succinctly by one as; *'I'm re-writing the book on fatherhood for myself.'*

The emerging discourse around fatherhood as a fluid and negotiated identity is evident in these findings, the sense of an identity of father as an important and multifaceted person in a child's life.

For ease of discussion in the following section, men's narratives that describe their fathering as being actively and or emotionally involved with their children will be referred to as the 'new fatherhood.' Narratives that refer to fathers as being breadwinners, or less actively engaged with their children will be referred to as 'traditional fatherhoods' or narratives. Whilst we acknowledge that not all 'traditional fathers' were emotionally or physically removed from their children, we nonetheless acknowledge that some men are saying they want something different from their father's approach.

We now come to the second interesting finding from the men's stories. Not only was there an apparent lack of guidance available to these men on how to achieve the new fatherhood, but there were considerable obstacles in the way.

Many fathers explained that they felt marginalised by early childhood services at the very times they felt they most needed help, were doubting their own competence, and wanted sources of support. In the words of one:

I felt shit scared. Having a new baby is a worrying time and I feel I lack a bit of confidence . . . fathers are invisible to some of these facilities–facilities don't take fathers into account.

Another summed it up this way:

Services are prepared for mums but dads aren't in the equation.

For the majority of this group, early childhood institutions, professionals and the systems in which they are embedded maintain traditional narratives:

Professionals focus heavily on the mother and the father is pushed aside.

Society is still sexist. I went to the Royal Women's hospital to-day–there was no toilet there for me–I had to go next door.

They (maternity hospital) were talking to mothers about breast feeding but they didn't talk to us both about breast feeding.

If fathers wished to pursue a different type of fatherhood from those defined in society's dominant discourses, a determined, sustained effort was required to actively challenge the constructions of fatherhood on offer. As one father said,

I had to take the initiative with early childhood services, I had to push to get involved–men have to take more initiative in services, but if they push they get what they want.'

Another commented:

They should make it easier for fathers to stay–I had to insist in the hospital.

Without the support that might facilitate fathers making other choices, services and professionals are 'colluding with and reinforcing social processes' that consign fathers to more traditional narratives such as of the 'disengaged father' or actively excluded father. This invisibility of fathers in early parenting appears as much a by-product of discourses that highlight maternal involvement and ignore a paternal engagement as it is about men choosing not to engage with their baby.

The next set of findings reveal a range of fatherhoods operating in Australian society. Some men were able to negotiate a fatherhood they wanted.

Fathers Who Could Pursue the New Fatherhood

A small group of men (N = 4, 10%) who wanted to be more actively involved in fathering were able to re-organise their lives so that they are able to be active and involved fathers. Three were in the position of being self employed and so re-organised their hours to maximise their time with their child, and the fourth has chosen to work part-time. All worked either a couple of hours a day or two or three days per week. Three saw themselves as their child's primary carer. One, an art dealer, commented

> *My father spent more time at work away from his children than I want to, I spend more time at home and I work more from home because I don't want to miss things with my son. A normal job would be a minus.*

Another father describes his understanding of his new arrangements this way:

> *We are missing fathers in our society. I now work three days a week and my partner (baby's mother) works one day a week. We've bought into a kind of power sharing that distances us from the more traditional family.*

Another describes the recent changes in his life:

> *In our case the baby's mother is going back to work full time and I've decided to finish work to be with the baby. A lot of fathers spend so much time at work. Although we've got some financial worries I'd prefer this than not being with my child. I've always wanted to be with my child. I want to be around for my child in a way my father wasn't for me.*

This group of fathers found that they got vital help in their quest to fashion new forms of fatherhood by being with and talking to other fathers. This entire group reported that talking through their experiences with others in a similar position helped them learn to trust their new identity and the transformations it was bringing about.

> *Fatherhood is a big change for me and the opportunity to share my fathering experiences with others who have children has helped me a lot.*

While these 'small scale solidarities of interpersonal relationships' (Aronson, 2000) were seen as vital, a number also mentioned the importance of literature about fathering. Two fathers commented on how helpful they'd found Steve Biddulph's books (an Australian psychologist who has written several popular books about fathering, particularly fathering boys). Public narratives around the new fatherhood are still slim, and all these fathers commented on their need for more accessible books about fathering.

These men who had re-arranged their lives to give primary emphasis to their fathering reported levels of stress lower than other fathers in the sample. While other groups in the sample self assessed their stress levels as having risen after becoming fathers, this group reported levels of stress similar to those experienced prior to fatherhood. One even commented that since becoming a father he'd felt less stressed and had given up smoking.

Here we see evidence of men negotiating with several systems including the labour market and traditional expectations of fathering to be the type of father they want to be. These men indicated they felt alone until they made contact with other men who were also creating this very engaged type of fatherhood and literature which supported their decision.

Fathers Who Attempted to Combine New Fatherhood and Traditional Narratives

The resources necessary to negotiate a position where a new fatherhood narrative was pre-dominant are not equitably available. The majority of the sample (N = 29, 73%) were in the position of juggling both their desire and their attempts to be more involved with their children with the demands of full-time work and careers. They reported experiencing tension and contradictions between these competing demands on their time.

Such tensions go to the very heart of the issue of men wanting to father in a way which is different to traditional fathering, which is provided for in public discourses and which informs programs and policies. The self rated stress measures reported by these men contrasted quite dramatically with those who could live out their 'new fatherhood narrative.' Those men attempting to combine the traditional and new fatherhood narratives all observed that their stress levels had increased markedly since becoming a father. A number revealed that their smoking and/or alcohol consumption had increased, and some said they were smoking more marijuana than previously.

Comments such as:

I feel emotionally drained.

I'm tired and giddy.

and

I'm more on edge and snappy.

were prevalent.

Most of this group worked hours similar to those they had before the arrival of their baby. Some had adjusted their working hours to maximise their time with their child, but they made up this time working when their baby slept. One, a businessman, commented:

> *I'm having huge difficulty performing across all areas of my life since the baby. I have less sleep, less sexual activity and there's more strain generally. I'm stressed out and drinking too much but the baby has given me an enormous sense of there's more to life than working and having a relationship with one person. Fatherhood amplifies the meaning of life. I've organised my business to take days off during the week to be with the baby but I make it up at night.*

Another, a bookmaker, describes how he *'takes off'* from work to play with his child and look after her, observing:

> *Parenthood interferes with bookmaking. My reason for getting up in the morning is my daughter, but the negative side of fatherhood is my business losses.*

Commented another:

> *I feel more pessimistic at work and have difficulty concentrating. I look forward to coming home more than before we had the baby. Home and work feel like two different worlds now but I'm more snappy at work.*

These fathers who are trying to combine the traditional and new fatherhoods are in a very different position to those who have relinquished the constructions offered in the traditional narrative and created their own construction of father. These men are conflicted. They talk of their social contacts diminishing due to lack of time and energy, and they have become more isolated since the birth of their child. For these fathers their attempts to be the type of father they wish to be is much more private; consequently, their opportunities for help, support and reassurance around developing new identities as fathers are much more limited.

For the men who are attempting to live out both the traditional and new fatherhoods, the time and energy needed to meet both sets of demands meant less time for the ways in which they had traditionally taken care of themselves. As one father said: *'I've given up gym to be with the baby.'* His partner, the baby's mother, commented:

> *He works hard, then comes home, changes nappies, gets up in the middle of the night when the baby cries–he's exhausted all the time–he needs to get out more for himself.*

One father, a doctor, explains:

> *Time is a problem, I'm exhausted and its pretty stressful. I've become socially isolated but the baby delights me, he calls out to people in the street, sings in his cot, shops and highchair. . . that's why I feel proud of him . . . but it's difficult to get out, I used to swim but not now and the bills aren't paid on time.*

Another comments:

> *Being a father has changed me. I'm more aware of the bigger picture. I find fatherhood very satisfying but as the income earner I also find it stressful. I'm more fearful than I used to be–it probably comes down to trying to do everything and lack of sleep. I don't see my squash friends anymore. I'm sacrificing my personal space at present and expect to for some years to come.*

These fathers make a direct link between their increased stress, their mental state, and the pressures and tensions generated negotiating with both the dominant constructions of father and their own construction.

Pervasive dominant discourses of fatherhood do not condone withdrawal from the labour market. It is stressful trying to meet such demands and also attempting to be a new father. For example, one father, a manager of a delicatessen, described this situation in his interview:

> *My baby could be blind. I've lost the desire to be at work. My boss keeps the pressure on me–to a point it's okay but I'm finding it difficult to be positive about being at work now.*

The potential conflict between the competing demands is brought into sharp focus in this father's narrative. All of these fathers, however, expressed worry about being able to manage being both a good provider and a 'hands on' father. They felt a lot of pressure from work and were concerned about work performance dropping.

> *I have to fight to stop work taking over my life. I'm pretty exhausted but I want to be 'hands on' with the baby. I like teaching him, naming, climbing and I'm looking forward to teaching him footy and how ants work. I enjoy time with him but he wears me out with the toys, I feel glad to get away but I'm glad to come back. I'm much more stressed than before and worried because my work performance has dropped.*

> *I'm trying to work less and I find it very positive that the baby needs me. At the same time I feel the extra responsibility and extra pressure, I know I'm drinking more. I'm doing fatherhood differently to my father, I'm not as work orientated and I'm much more involved. I feel an urgency about getting home each day now. I feel more satisfied with the way I'm managing at home than at work.*

> *It's easier to be happy at home. I find it hard being away from the baby.*

> *I often feel detached at work because I feel it's a waste of time not being with the baby.*

> *I get worried about financial pressures. I'm the breadwinner and I'm working very hard at work. I find fatherhood hard but I'm enjoying it, I do everything for the baby when I'm not working.*

> *I do my best to care for her (baby). It's a burden of responsibility that you have for the rest of your life. It's a whole new adventure. Work is stressful. I'm pretty tired all the time. I feel there is pressure at home and at work and feel miserable at times.*

This group appears to be finding the negotiation around fatherhood more problematic than the previous group. For these men the clash between the new fatherhood and the expectation that they not relinquish their obligations in the labour market is causing a great deal of tension. The social context in which these fathers find themselves does not readily accommodate removal from the workforce to forge a new identity as father.

Those Who Engaged with Traditional Fatherhood

A small group of men appeared to accept the construction of traditional fatherhood (N = 3, 7.5%). Having limited choices was a strong theme emerging in the language of this group of fathers. They appeared to believe that they were doing what was expected of them. There was not much sense of 'possibility' generated in relation to fatherhood within this narrative:

> *I work seven days a week. I don't have much choice. I haven't got into fatherhood yet. I expect my experience of it is much the same as my fathers in many ways.*

Statements such as this may reflect the power of the dominant discourse and concomitant structural arrangements that limit new fathers' sense of their possibilities. Certainly notions of choice about fathering do not accord with realities of a system in which there are restricted options and in which power differentials between employers and employees can be large. Scarcity and uncertainty about employment discourages making demands.

> *It's a burden of responsibility you have for the rest of your life. I have more purpose but feel I'm more pressured at work and more irritable and upset. I don't think my experience is very different from my father's.*

There is also another group of men from this sample who did not appear to experience any conflict around their construction of fatherhood.

> *It's difficult with building up a new business (dentistry), but we're managing. I'm feeling pretty depressed and I get worried about the mortgage. We can't have everything at present. I've taken up smoking in the hope it will make me less stressed.*

This man's partner and mother of their child was a scientist who has given up her career to act as his dental secretary in order for them to save money. Both parents feel an increase of tension in their relationship and domestic violence is occurring. This father comments that *'there is a limit to what I can do with the baby'* as *'I need a good nights sleep to deal with my patients.'*

> *I haven't had much time to spend on fatherhood. I finish work when the baby is asleep and I'm always tired from work.*

With these work pressures the dominance of the traditional fatherhood allows fathers to focus only on 'the immediate, the practical, and the surface' with their child (Aronson, 2000:52); this does little to challenge received ideas about fatherhood.

With the exception of one mother who said she had confidence her partner would become more involved as their baby grew up and became more interactive, mothers with partners in this group were also more stressed.

> *I'm always working, there's not enough time in the day to do everything. I don't think fatherhood for me is much different to the way it was for my father. I'm more responsible than I used to be. I used to like going out with my mates but I don't so much now. My wife shouts at me and I put my tail between my legs and run.*

There seems little room in the traditional fatherhood for expressing frustration and anger. We are used to thinking of women as suppressing frustration and anger, yet men can also suppress and deflect anger. The traditional narrative, unlike the 'new fatherhood' narrative, is not a narrative in which men could express feelings and talk things through. Furthermore, whilst these men are contributing as fathers, they are doing so in ways which tend to be instrumental rather than those more aligned with the new fatherhood such as in emotional or active engagement. To varying degrees the men acknowledge changes after becoming fathers, but this is expressed as increased responsibilities, rather than as a transformation in themselves.

Those Who Did Not Appear to Engage with Fatherhood

A further small group of men (N = 3, 7.5%) emerged who did not engage with any constructions of fatherhood. The 'mates' narrative is well publicly rehearsed in the literature and media which is critical of absent fathers. Certainly policies and programs which exist to make fathers accountable are evidence of this disengaged father narrative. For these men this disengagement was apparent through their withdrawal from their baby and partner. One father had withdrawn into work (with no narrative of this being about traditional fatherhood). Two others have withdrawn into drugs and drinking with 'mates.'

One father says of himself: 'Drinking and drugs are my biggest problems.' His partner and mother of their child formulated the problem this way:

> *He's having problems adjusting to being a parent. He avoids me and the baby. I'm lonely with him in the next room drinking. He doesn't want to be here–it's the influence of his friends. He doesn't want to realise there's a third person in our lives.*

Another mother comments about the father of their child:

> *He doesn't get much time with the baby. When he's supposed to be looking after the baby he drops her off at his mother's. When he is around he is abusive and he drinks heavily.*

This withdrawal and lack of attentiveness corresponds most closely, in the literature on fathering, with those fathers characterised as 'dead beat dads' or as having 'deficit parenting.' The discourse of men as ill-equipped and ill-prepared to parent is closely aligned with the men who presented in this cluster.

Interestingly, all the fathers in this last cluster come from groups that are marginalised in Australian society. This suggests an alternate reading to that of the 'deadbeat dad' literature, i.e., members of marginal groups have their choices severely constrained. Members of marginal groups may not easily access the narratives of 'new fatherhood and/or traditional fatherhood.'

What is important for these and all fathers participating in this study is that a range of choices about fathering needs to be opened up and–through supporting policies and structural change–made accessible to all fathers.

CONCLUSION

A dominant discourse of fathers as engaged in the public arena and less involved in the private domain of the family has been around and entrenched for much of the 20th century. This discourse is being challenged by a new fatherhood that is emerging. The narratives of the men in our sample suggest that their lived experience of fatherhood describes a different fatherhood to that offered in the dominant discourses.

For many of the fathers in our research being, as some expressed it, a 'hands on father' is uncharted 'land'; they feel in need of some kind of guide. It also appears that a tension exists between the dominant public discourses of fatherhood and the emerging narratives of fatherhood. Fathers juggling the public and private discourse articulate their exhausting struggle and their pain, they are questioning what is happening. At the same time they look forward to change and some kind of eventual transformation.

Pursuing the type of fatherhood which men want to pursue is by no means an easy path. It is not only the public constructions which limit the choices men have around fatherhood, it is also the social structures which affect the way men can father.

> When . . . men have jobs that allow choice and autonomy, they can base work decisions on how their work enhances or diminishes their ability to be the kind of father they strive to be. Men with a broad orientation to fatherhood but without much autonomy in their work roles may be much more limited in their ability to enact their fathering commitments. (Fox and Bruce, 2001:394)

Fox and Bruce take men's parenting behaviour as reflective of their 'commitments to the fathering role' (Fox and Bruce, 2001:394). We argue that it is not as simple as a commitment to a role, but rather is also dependent on how closely the man's understanding of fathering meshes with the dominant discourse which creates the structures and circumstances that allow or prevent him from realising his expectations. There is some negotiation that can occur between the individual and the social structures, but an inability to reach an adequate resolution or negotiation can result in men experiencing stress and consequent mental health problems.

The reality of the majority of the father's lives is no longer reflected in the dominant discourses. However, to adequately sustain this reality for fathers and their mental health, these fathers' narratives need to inform public discourse. Likewise those working with new fathers will require an ongoing critique of their own positioning among these conflicting 'discourses.' Men's journey to fatherhood needs to be supported by structural change which professionals working with men can facilitate. As Aronson argues, the small scale solidarities in which people or groups come together and support each other can be stimulated and strengthened by public policies (2000:25).

The Department of Family and Community Services Report argues that if parenting and employment options are to increase, a major shift is needed in the attitudes of policy makers: 'This shift must presume mothers and fathers have equal responsibility from conception on-wards' (1999:104). They also argue that there is a general need for greater recognition that men sometimes need support and the opportunity to share their feelings and concerns. Findings from their research indicate that fathers would value from learning more about parenting from media and sharing their experiences with other fathers.

The dominant discourse of the traditional fatherhood is receiving some critique, but professionals striving to assist men to resist the dominant narrative are, often working within social structures which neither acknowledge nor encourage a diversity of fatherhoods, as the fathers participating in this study are, themselves, very aware. Social workers are well positioned to challenge the limited and proscriptive discourses around fatherhood and to assist men in their struggle to construct *themselves* as fathers. Reflexive social work practice requires us to account for our own complicity in engaging in discourses that exclude men or which narrowly construct fathers. Having identified and acknowledged our part in limiting men's choice, we can work to assist men in accessing or developing those tools, resources or structures which will provide them with the opportunity to father as they wish.

The fathers who participated in this research are showing that there are many types of fatherhood, but that choosing amongst them comes at a cost, often in terms of mental health and stress levels. Attention needs to be paid to the transformative impact of fatherhood and that in order to honour this process we need to provide the resources, the commitment, the support, and the time to father.

REFERENCES

Amato, P.R. & Rezac, S. (1994). Contact with non-residential parents, interparental conflict, and children's behaviour. *Journal of Family Issues,* 15, 191-207.

Aronson, J. (2000) Conflicting Images of Older People Receiving Care: Challenges for Reflexive Practice and Research. In Neysmith, S. (Ed) Restructuring Caring Labour Oxford University Press: pp. 47-69.

Barnett, R.C., Marshall, N.L. & Pleck, J.H. (1992). Men's multiple roles and their relationship to men's psychological distress. *Journal of Marriage and the Family,* 54, 358-367.

Chaves, M. (1991). Family structure and Protestant church attendance: The sociological basis of cohort and age-effects. *Journal of the Scientific Study of Religion*, 30, 501-514.

Curran, L. & Abrams, L. (2000). Making men into dads: Fatherhood, the state and welfare reform. *Gender and Society,* Vol 14(5) 662-678.

Daly, K.J. (1995). Reshaping fatherhood: Findings the Models. In Marsiglio W. (Ed), Fatherhood: Contemporary theory, research and social policy. Thousand Oaks: Sage.

Department of Family and Community Services. (1999). Fitting Fathers into Families, Report for the Commonwealth Department of Family and Community Services. Canberra; Media and Publications Unit Department of Family and Community Services

Dishion, T.J., McCord, J. & Poulin, E. (1999). When interventions harm: Peer groups and problem behaviour. *American Psychologist*, (54), 755-764

Doherty, W.J. (1997). The best of times and the worst of times. Fathering as contested arena of academic discourse. In Hawkins, A.J. & Dollahite, D.C. (1997). Generative Fathering: Beyond Deficit Perspectives. Sage Publications: United Kingdom.

Doherty, W.J., Kouneski, E.E., & Erickson, M.F. (1998). Responsible fathering: An overview and conceptual framework. *Journal of Marriage and the Family*, 60, 277-292.

Dudley, M., Roy, K., Kelk, N., & Bernard, D. (In press). Psychological Correlates of Depression in Fathers and Mothers in the First Postnatal Year. Reproductive and Infant Psychology.

Eggebeen, D.J. & Hogan, D.P. (1990). Giving between the generations in American families. *Human Nature*, 1, 211-232.

Eggebeen, D.J. & Knoester, C. (2001). Does fatherhood matter for men? *Journal of Marriage and the Family*, Vol 63(2), 381-392.

Fairclough, N. (1992). Discourse and Social Change. Cambridge, Polity Press.

Fox, G.L. & Bruce, C. (2001). Conditional fatherhood: Identity theory and parental investment theory as alternative sources of explanation of fathering. *Journal of Marriage and the Family*, Vol 63 (2), 394-402.

Grove, W.R. & Mongione, T.W. (1983). Social roles, sex roles and psychological distress: Additive and interactive models of sex differences. *Journal of Health and Social Behaviour*, 24, 300-312.

Hawkins, A.J. & Dollahite, D.C. (1997). Beyond the Role-Inadequacy Perspective of Fathering. In Hawkins, A.J. & Dollahite, D.C. (1997). Generative Fathering: Beyond Deficit Perspectives. Sage Publications: United Kingdom.

Hawkins, A.J. & Dollahite, D.C. (1997). Generative Fathering: Beyond Deficit Perspectives. Sage Publications: United Kingdom.

Lamb, M.E. (1986). The role of father in child development (2nd ed). New York: Wiley.

Lupton, D. & Barclay, L. (1997). Constructing Fatherhood, discourses and experiences. London: Sage Publications.

Marsiglio, W. (1998). Procreative Men. New York: New York University Press.

Palkovitz, R. (1997). Reconstructing "Involvement": Expanding conceptualizations of men's caring in contemporary families. In Hawkins, A.J. & Dollahite, D.C. (1997).

Generative Fathering: Beyond Deficit Perspectives. Sage Publications: United Kingdom.

Parke, R. (1981). Fathers. Cambridge, MA: Harvard University Press.

Ploch, D.R. & Hastings, D.W. (1998). Effects of parental church attendance, current family status, and religious salience on church attendance. Review of Religious Research, 39, 309-320.

Russell, G. (1982). The changing role of fathers. St. Lucia, Australia: University of Queensland Press.

Somers, M.R. & Gibson, G.D. (1994). Reclaiming the Epistemological "other": Narrativity and the Social Construction of Identity. In Calhoun, C. (Ed). (1994) Social Theory and the Politics of Identity. Blackwell: Cambridge.

University of Minnesota. (1998) Dads Make a Difference, Minnesota Impacts, Community Outreach Solutions for people, http://www.extension.umn.edu/mnimpacts/

Disabled Children and Their Families in Ukraine: Health and Mental Health Issues for Families Caring for Their Disabled Child at Home

Gillian Bridge, PhD

SUMMARY. In the Eastern European countries included in the communist system of the USSR, parents of disabled children were encouraged to commit their disabled child to institutional care. There were strict legal regulations excluding them from schools. Medical assessments were used for care decisions. Nevertheless many parents decided to care for their disabled child at home within the family.

Ukraine became an independent country in 1991, when communism was replaced by liberal democracy within a free market system. Western solutions have been sought for many social problems existing, but 'hidden,' under the old regime. For more of the parents of disabled children, this has meant embracing ideas of caring for their disabled children in the community, and providing for their social, educational, and medical

---

Gillian Bridge is Senior Lecturer in Social Policy, Department of Social Policy, LSE, Houghton Street, London, WC2A 2AE, UK (E-mail: g.bridge@lse.ac.uk).

This paper was presented at the 3rd International Conference on Social Work in Health and Mental Health, July, 2001, Tampere, Finland.

[Haworth co-indexing entry note]: "Disabled Children and Their Families in Ukraine: Health and Mental Health Issues for Families Caring for Their Disabled Child at Home." Bridge, Gillian. Co-published simultaneously in *Social Work in Health Care* (The Haworth Social Work Practice Press, an imprint of The Haworth Press, Inc.) Vol. 39, No. 1/2, 2004, pp. 89-105; and: *Social Work Visions from Around the Globe: Citizens, Methods, and Approaches* (ed: Anna Metteri et al.) The Haworth Social Work Practice Press, an imprint of The Haworth Press, Inc., 2004, pp. 89-105. Single or multiple copies of this article are available for a fee from The Haworth Document Delivery Service [1-800-HAWORTH, 9:00 a.m. - 5:00 p.m. (EST). E-mail address: docdelivery@haworthpress.com].

needs, which have previously been denied. The issue of disability is a serious one for Ukraine where the nuclear disaster at Chernobyl in 1986 caused extensive radiation poisoning. This almost certainly led to an increase in the number of disabled children being born and an increase in the incidence of various forms of cancer.

This paper is based on a series of observation visits to some of the many self-help groups established by parents, usually mothers, for their disabled children. It draws attention to the emotional stress experienced both by parents and their disabled children in the process of attempting to come to terms with the disabling conditions, and the denial of the normal rights of childhood resulting from prejudice, poor resources, ignorance, and restrictive legislation. Attempts have been made to identify the possible role and tasks of professional social workers within this context. International comparisons show that many parents and their children do not benefit from the medical model of disability, and that serious consequences include the development of depressive illness among those who find that little help is available from public services. *[Article copies available for a fee from The Haworth Document Delivery Service: 1-800-HAWORTH. E-mail address: <docdelivery@haworthpress.com> Website: <http://www.HaworthPress.com> © 2004 by The Haworth Press, Inc. All rights reserved.]*

KEYWORDS. Disabled, children, families, Ukraine, self-help, communism, transition

INTRODUCTION

On the 20th of October 1999 in the UK, Melody Turnbull murdered her two disabled sons for whom she had cared for 23 years. The story made newspaper headlines, leaving the general public shocked and disbelieving. However, it was probably soon forgotten and replaced by other sensational news events. On the other hand, parents of disabled children and those professionals involved in their treatment and care were probably less shocked, for they were aware of many circumstances where the same thing might have happened. The emotional impact of caring for severely disabled, dependent children is probably too painful for prolonged attention by society.

Throughout the world most disabled children are cared for by their families (Thorburn 1985; Werner 1987; Alur 1987; Bridge 1999). Their quality of life and that of their parents, families, and carers depends on cultural and religious attitudes, medical, educational and social welfare provisions, and on the legal framework that underpins national social policies. Stark contrasts may be found in qualities of care between developing countries, including those in transition from communism, and the Western world. However, the emotional consequences for families are probably very similar. Many parents feel driven by the need to seek treatments and cures for their children, and to find or develop educational opportunities to enable their child to be included in society.

This discussion paper has as its focus community care provided by families for disabled children in Ukraine, one of the largest of the fifteen states to become independent from the Soviet Union in 1991 and to change from communism to a market economy. As the result of these political changes, Ukrainians have turned to Western Europe for aid in developing a liberal democratic welfare system. This has included beginning to identify the role and tasks of professional social workers, and being more open to Western approaches to caring for disabled children.

In addition, Ukraine is of interest in that the number of disabled and sick children has increased considerably since the Chernobyl nuclear disaster in 1986, resulting in the birth of many congenitally disabled children and the diagnosis of many cases of thyroid cancer. The Soviet government deliberately downplayed the gravity of the situation, partly to avoid panic, but largely because the disaster demonstrated to the world the failing of the communist system.

Western aid has been provided to set up hospitals and health care clinics. An example is the US group FOCCUS (friends of Chernobyl), whose group members have been involved in going to Ukraine to provide training and in taking children and staff of centres in Ukraine to the US. The true extent of the disaster and its long-term effects will never be known as the cover-up has been so extensive (Dalton 1999 pp. 25-30).

Through massive publicity in the media, the world has been shocked by the 'subhuman' conditions discovered in Eastern European institutions for disabled children after the transition, particularly those in Romania (UNICEF 1997; Human Rights Watch 1998). However, much less attention has been paid to the many self-help groups, NGOs, and local authority departments of social protection concerned with providing care for disabled children within their families. In common with other Eastern European countries in transition, many social problems in Ukraine, including the plight of disabled children, emerged after having been largely denied and 'hidden' under communism, so that very little definite information exists about the real extent of the problem (Kourktchian 1998).

The material for this paper has been collected during a series of weeklong visits to Ukraine as a consultant to the newly established School of Social Work at the National University, Kiev Mohyla Academy (KMA), funded by Tempus from 1995 (Ramon 2000). Additionally, a similar visit to the Moscow School of Social Sciences provided an opportunity to observe the treatment provisions at the Moscow Centre for Children with Cerebral Palsy in 1998. In order to develop practice placements for the professional social work students from KMA, a series of consultations took place with social welfare agencies, many concerned with providing for disabled children in the community (Bridge 1999). Some interesting themes emerged from these discussions, providing the framework for this article.

Undoubtedly collecting material in this way has many limitations. First and foremost is the problem of not being able to speak Ukrainian or Russian and therefore being dependent on an interpreter. Also, cultural perspectives are very different and require some understanding. For example, Western visitors are always seen as a source of grant aid, so that information is selectively provided with that in mind. Many others involved in developmental projects in Eastern Europe have commented on these difficulties (Monk and Singleton 1995; Solomon 1994). Nevertheless, an emergent theme is about health and mental health issues for families and their disabled children, an aspect of care with global resonance.

DISABILITY IN THE SOVIET UNION DURING COMMUNISM

In order to understand the current situation in Ukraine, it is necessary to consider the historical context for social welfare provision and, in particular, attitudes towards disabled people. Despite obtaining political autonomy, the legacies of communism remain strong; for example, the social security and social welfare systems are based on Soviet legislation, although some responsibility has shifted to the local authorities rather than being primarily work-based. It is crucial, therefore, to examine Soviet attitudes towards the disabled, and the provision of welfare under communism.

Soviet society officially appeared to provide well for the welfare needs of citizens. Full employment was guaranteed and a universal social security system was administered through places of work. Health care, education, and leisure activities were provided free of charge, and vast amounts of affordable public housing were available in pur- pose-built apartment blocks.

In his paper to the First International Conference of Social Work in Paris in 1928, Semachko stated that relief of the needy was the responsi- bility of the State. 'Any worker in need has the right to be assisted by the State in all cases: sickness, infirmity, old age, unemployment, or dis- tress due to any cause whatsoever' (p. 533). While vigorously opposing 'parasitism and begging,' the principle duty of the State was to provide rehabilitation for all those who have found themselves, by chance, 'eliminated from a life of normal work.' For those identified as entitled to assistance, this should be provided in the forms of pensions, institu- tional care, and 'special, vocational re-education' to resume work. So strong was the dual commitment to work and rehabilitation that over- night clinics were set up for workers diagnosed with tuberculosis. After completing the days' work, those diagnosed with tuberculosis would be expected to go to a sanatorium; replace working clothes with hygienic garments, bathe, eat a healthy meal and sleep with windows open to benefit from fresh air. In the morning they would return to work (Semachko 1929).

Thus, this philosophy appears to have provided for those disabled in war and industrial accidents, so long as they were able to resume pro- ductivity. Working people or 'toilers' were actively engaged in 'the he- roic construction of the new society' (White 1999 p. 26). If they did not respond to rehabilitation and retraining programmes, their status was re- duced, and political propaganda sought to deny and hide this evidence of a failing political ideology. Social barriers to inclusion in society ex- isted in the form of poor access to buildings and public transport. Inade- quate provision of wheelchairs and prostheses ensured that disabled people were largely hidden. Abroad the USSR took no part in the Inter- national Year of the Disabled 1981 (White 1999 p. 27).

Those born with disabilities appear to have been even less fortunate. The options were institutional care or being allowed a small pension. Children, assessed as handicapped through stringent medical tests, would usually be admitted to institutions, since legal classification as disabled prevented them from entering mainstream nurseries and schools. Thus, the birth of a disabled child meant that both the mother and child could not be considered as active, valued citizens. While parents or relatives of children less than eight years were considered incapable of gaining a live- lihood by outside work, the expectation was that women as well as men would participate in the labour market. 'Ideally, a woman is expected to have children, be an outstanding worker, take responsibility for the home, and, despite everything, still be beautiful' (Manovona in Slater 1995 p. 77). During the Stalin period, until his death in 1953, collectivist values were promoted. State children's homes were considered to be even better places for the upbringing of healthy children than within families. This policy was discontinued under Khrushchev and Brezhnev (White 1999 p. 31).

Because of this closed system prior to 1991, it is impossible to know how far this political philosophy was implemented over the vast areas of the USSR. There were certainly considerable differences between provisions for urban and rural dwellers, and in different regions. The peasants of Ukraine rural areas were certainly considered to be recalcitrant. The Great famine of 1933 and the severe repressions under Stalin, in order to implement collective farming, had serious effects on the 'rural base of traditional ethnic philanthropy' in Ukraine (Kuts 2002 p. 81). In consequence, it is likely that rural peasants lived in poor conditions with little financial, medical, and educational support for their disabled children. In contrast a large well-equipped rehabilitation centre for children with cerebral palsy existed for wealthy party members in Moscow, staffed by teams of highly trained doctors and physiotherapists.

Accurate figures about the proportions of disabled children within Ukrainian society, and about those cared for in institutions and those in the care of their families, are not available until after 1991 (UNICEF 1997 p. 47). However, according to White (1999), 'despite the totalising aspirations of many party officials and leaders before 1985, Soviet citizens were increasingly forming informal groups and even organisations in an attempt to address some of the unresolved social issues neglected by the official state welfare service' (p. 17). Many of these voluntary organisations were self-help groups set up by the parents of disabled children as repression of social initiatives subsided under Gorbachev. It is probable that in many areas informal groups existed for many years before 1985 and were tolerated as not being obviously dissident. Kuts (2002 p. 81) writes that the Ukrainian population continued to practice traditional philanthropy at local levels, despite the fact that they were perceived to be acting in their own interests, contradicting a régime designed to eliminate individual and community interests.

It would seem, therefore, that the closed communist system in the USSR before 1991 was probably a mass of contradictions. Propaganda promoted a clear philosophy, but in practice social problems, including the care of disabled children, were provided for in many ways, both formal and informal. Without doubt there were wide variations in provision. State control co-existed with 'a non-regulated, informal, crude and pseudo-market system' as well as a burgeoning voluntary sector (Kourktchian 1998 p. 69, White 1999). How this uncertain system changed and developed during transition in Ukraine is the focus of the next section.

DISABLED CHILDREN IN UKRAINE DURING THE PERIOD OF TRANSITION FROM COMMUNISM

The Transition

The radical change from state control of welfare to a market economy happened suddenly and in an unplanned way. Life in the cities appears prosperous. However, in the country as a whole, poverty has increased as factories and the many associated work-based facilities, including crèches and holiday camps, have closed down. The derelict holiday camps, situated by the lakes in the Ukraine countryside, are evidence of the former glories of the communist welfare provision for citizens. Those still officially employed often do not receive wages for months, but continue to go to work to protect their social security entitlements, and because they are able to obtains materials from the factories that can be sold. Professionals also report waiting for months for their wages, so that subsistence and black market economies are essential for survival.

Commentators on the transition in Eastern Europe have noted that 'the young, the dynamic, the mobile, the connected' have benefited most from democratisation and the free market, 'leaving behind the vulnerable' (Binyon 1999; Manning 1995). Increases in homelessness, delinquency, child abandonment and alcoholism underline the inadequacies of social welfare strategies (Harwin 1996 p. 172, Manning 1995). While disabled children had always been marginalised under Soviet collectivism, reduction in the value of pensions, and the acute and escalating poverty experienced by families during the transition, could only make their situation worse.

Care in the Community: NGOs and Self-Help Groups

The focus of concern for disabled children in Ukraine has centred largely on those in institutions, and on those disabled and sick as the result of the Chernobyl explosion. So far, less attention has been paid to the burgeoning voluntary sector provision, and in particular to self-help groups.

The voluntary sector defies firm definitions, remaining, in Kendall and Knapp's words (1995 p. 66) as a 'loose and baggy monster.' Voluntary organizations range in size from small self-help groups to large multi-national organizations like the Red Cross. They have in common a 'not for profit' approach, and involvement of volunteers. They usually provide for special aspects of social welfare focusing on social problems. Staffed by service users, volunteers, and professionals, they may advocate and act as pressure groups for social policy change. Thus, they combine 'the more passive role of providing a service' to individuals, families and groups with identified needs, with 'an inherently political role' of providing a 'critical voice' about public policy (Reading 1994 p. 13).

The voluntary sector in Ukraine is as diverse as in the rest of the world. Kuts (2002 p. 80) explains that 'Ukrainian philanthropy in its collective manifestation is rooted in antiquity.' Informal support from family and neighbours has always been vital, especially in rural communities. Although repressions during Soviet times and the Great Famine of 1933 damaged this traditional philanthropy, communal philanthropy recovered during the last years of socialism, and the tradition was urbanized with the rural migration into the cities in the 1960s. Kuts (2002 p. 81) reports that 'Ukrainian people still consider the community as the basic provider of social support.'

After ten years of transition, some distinct themes may be identified by Western observers about the development of informal and formal social welfare voluntary groups. The most striking features are how numerous they are, how quickly new projects spring up, and the range of problems for which they are designed. Many are set up as self-help groups, whose interests were denied under communism. Coordination between groups with the same interests in different areas seems to be lacking, and usually discouraged as there is competition for outside sponsorship.

Visitors gain an impression that a top priority for these organisations is to obtain Western sponsorship so that, instead of collaborating with each other and seeking alliances, the mood seems to be one of competition to entice visitors to their projects. While there is a real need for sponsorship, this persistent agenda stands in the way both of useful collaboration between groups with similar interests, and of the genuine exchange of ideas.

An example of this dilemma was a visit to a self-help group, with the intention of advising the leader on ways to improve the centre. She was enrolled as a part-time student on a social work course at the KMA, so the aim was to help her to apply her learning to practice. However, the opportunity for seeking sponsorship from Western visitors proved too good to miss. Thirty mothers were present at the meeting, each accompanied by their disabled child, and each child's history was told in great detail. The most heart-rending aspect to this was the knowledge that many of these children's lives could have been improved considerably with access to Western educational and medical services. The young adults would have been able to find employment in supermarkets, for example.

The priority given to fund-raising also caused some unease as the strength of corruption and duplicity is well known in Eastern Europe. Lloyd (1998) describes Russian society as 'permeated by crime from top to bottom' because in Soviet society so many normal activities were against the law. In relation to developing social welfare, Ramon (1995 p. 51) explains that 'the boundary between legitimate perks and small scale corruption is not simple to determine for Western participants, when there are cultural subtleties to which they are not party . . . and there is the argument that everyone is behaving in this way.'

Donor concerns about dishonesty were also linked to frustrations caused by the endless bureaucracy associated with any provision of aid. An example of this was the gift of a bus to provide transport for disabled children from their homes to a voluntary project. The donors discovered that, for several months, the bus could not be used because it had not been licensed, and equipment for disabled children was locked away in order to prevent it from being stolen.

There were several opportunities to examine this burgeoning voluntary sector at first hand on visits as a consultant to work-based social work students from the KMA. It became apparent that these projects were initiated by mothers in response to two main factors: Firstly they wanted to save their disabled children from institutionalisation, and secondly they wanted their children included in mainstream activities, especially education. An example of the stringency of the legal regulations, requiring the segregation of disabled children in the community, was the rule that disabled children were not allowed to swim with able children.

This caused problems for a mainstream kindergarten used outside school hours by groups of disabled children. The Department for Education was not happy with proposal for disabled children to use the pool on the premises, and was looking for Western sponsors to refurbish an unused crèche building nearby. The local school inspector explained that, apart from the regulations, she believed that the disabled children would be happier in a separate place of their own. This also seemed to be the views of parent initiators of the self-help groups.

The categories of children provided for in these specialist projects were usually identified by the disabling condition of child of the parent founder, although, in practice, many children tend to be multiply disabled. The parents had usually found accommodation in a building, previously used as a crèche in Soviet times, but shut down once the factories closed, and unemployment meant mothers could not afford day care and therefore did not need the facilities. The initiators tended to be articulate middle class women with professional training who were unwilling to accept their child's hopeless prospects in society, and set about providing alternative forms of education, treatment, and day care.

Education

Most of the projects had an education focus, being alternative schools with parents as teachers. Some of these groups had been in existence for many years, and the parents/staff were anxious about the absence of work prospects or continued training for their young disabled adults. One project was seeking funding to set up a special centre for those too old for school where they might continue to learn skills for daily living, including cooking and laundry. Underlying this proposal were the fears of parents internationally about the care of these young adults, when their parents became too old to care for them or died. Having avoided institutional care throughout childhood, there seemed no escape in the long-term.

Teaching methods in these alternative schools tended to be pedagogic as is the custom in Eastern European education. Instruction and small formal group tasks were the usual practice. For example, a teacher of art painted her version of a butterfly and pinned up her painting for a group of six children with cerebral palsy to copy. They sat round a table each with some paints and a piece of paper. The teacher then proceeded to go round to each child in turn guiding their hands so that, by the end of the lesson, each of them had reproduced a copy of the butterfly to take home.

Medical Treatment

In many centres this educational focus was combined with medical treatments. These were based on the espousal of the medical model of disability challenged fiercely by writers about the disability movement in the West, Finkelstein (1980), Oliver (1990), and Barnes (1991) for example. The underlying aim might be described as attempting to 'cure' a child, or to achieve as much 'normality' as possible, so that a child might recover sufficiently to be allowed access to mainstream services.

The treatments offered depended on the knowledge and skills of the staff. It was apparent that a range of extraordinary treatment approaches was available. Many of them appeared to have doubtful value from a Western perspective; they were difficult to understand, and seemed painful, even punitive. We were shown 'the cabinet of electric sleep' where children lay on beds in a dormitory wired up to electrodes. This treatment was supposed to produce a calming effect, as was using an electric comb. There were herbal treatments for undernourished children, and a version of speech therapy appeared to involve pulling out the child's tongue and twisting it. Entering what was called a treatment room, we discovered a group of asthmatic children sitting round covered in white sheets looking like little ghosts as they inhaled special minerals infused into the air. The worst example of both doubtful medical value, and questionable ethical practice, was the regulation that children with cerebral palsy were required, by law, to have brain surgery to insert foetal material to restore damaged brain tissue. The requirement seemed to be related to establishing eligibility for disability pensions. This raises the ethical question about the sources of this foetal material in view of the fact that abortion is the dominant form of birth control in Eastern European countries (Hyde 1999).

The continued use of outdated treatment methods in Ukraine appears to be another example of the very variable standards of treatment and care available to citizens throughout the USSR. Health, medical care and training were prioritised under the Soviet system. Semachko (1929) gave a detailed description of medical facilities including Institutes for Physiotherapy and Orthopaedics in Leningrad and Moscow, although these were intended for those wounded in industrial accidents or in wars rather than for disabled children. However, in the 1970s Moscow parents of children with cerebral palsy initiated a project to build a rehabilitation centre, which opened in 1990 (White 1999 p. 62). Currently this centre provides Western treatments including hydrotherapy and Vojta physiotherapy, treatments rarely available in rural areas of Eastern European countries. The exceptions are Western sponsored projects, including the German sponsored rehabilitation centre in Chernobyl. It seemed that, despite being charitably funded, this centre charged patients for treatment so that access was restricted to those able to pay.

All the self-help projects lacked essential disability aids like wheel-chairs and physiotherapy equipment so that conditions, with potential for improvement, were left untreated. These obvious privations were distressing to observe for those aware of possible, effective Western treatment approaches. The same could be said about educational materials including computers, paper, writing equipment, and toys. The ingenuity used by the staff to produce handicrafts out of household packaging and odds and ends was impressive. Very few children produced handicrafts for sale, although their art works and handicrafts brightened up the rather drab premises.

DAY CARE

Despite the educational and treatment aims of the staff, these centres also provided day care for the children of working parents and for those unable to cope. Some were open from 8 am until 6 pm, and cooked meals were provided. Non-participatory mothers were criticised by the staff, whose lives seemed to be devoted to their child's world and the associated problems of disability. From a more sympathetic perspective, these mothers were often single parents trying to care for their disabled child at the same time as going to work.

This raises the question of how many children cared for by their parents were actually able to attend one of these centres. In Kyiv the Education Department provided peripatetic teachers for disabled children confined to their homes. This service was not available in rural areas and appeared to be less effective than it might have been since parents reported that the teachers were unreliable. It is probable that many disabled children are confined in small city tower block apartments and in rural dwellings for a number of reasons including inadequate transport, inclement weather, attitudes of shame, and poverty.

This situation echoes that in many parts of the world, the UK being a prime example, where middle class parents fight for and provide resources for their disabled children (Bridge 1999). The increase in rural poverty with associated ignorance and superstition means that it is likely that there are still many 'hidden' disabled children. A case study presented by a student, during a consultation, involved a young adult with Down's Syndrome being kept tied up in the farmhouse while his parents worked. Initially they refused offers of institutional care by the Department of Social Protection because they had hoped he would be able to work on the farm. His violent behaviour, resulting from this captivity, meant they could no longer manage, and they agreed to accept the offer.

Therefore, despite the media attention to the plight of disabled, abandoned and orphaned children in institutions in Eastern Europe, access to Western views about the need to close them down and to develop a social model of disability towards caring for children in the community, appears to have had only minimal effect. Many authors have described projects to develop fostering and to begin the process of reducing the number of children in institutional care. However, these projects can only provide local and relatively small-scale improvements (for example, Tresiliotis 1994; Kukauskas 1999). Indeed, evidence from many sources indicates that 'numerous initiatives, buoyed by international assistance in Russia and other countries of the former Soviet Union, have not succeeded in alleviating the pressure on orphanages or in developing a coherent system of community support able to reduce the need for public care' (Harwin 1995 p. vii). It is possible that the trend reported by Bertmar (1998) for really poor families in Armenia to obtain places in institutions, by trying to have their children registered as handicapped, may also be prevalent in rural areas of Ukraine.

RELATIONSHIPS BETWEEN NGOS AND THE STATUTORY SECTOR

How projects for disabled children relate to the statutory authorities is interesting. They are working in partnership and receiving considerable assistance. The Education Department may provide premises and pays the costs of utilities. Additionally, the Department pays the teachers' salaries. It appears that voluntary organizations have to bargain with their local authority, agreeing to seek sponsorships in return for some assistance. Therefore, much depends on the interest of local authority officials, and on the bargaining power of the proposers. Concern was expressed about future mergers of local districts that might disrupt these alliances. Also, there are problems about the overlapping but extensive responsibilities of Education, Social Protection, and Health Departments.

Kuts (2002, p. 80) expresses strongly the view that the state is unable to satisfy basic social needs through 'ineffectiveness of public management.' However, it does appear that, in some areas, the statutory sector has begun to accept some responsibility for contributing to meeting needs of formerly disadvantaged groups. This could be the result of the many training opportunities offered to staff. For example DFID (Department for International Development, UK) has encouraged KMA to give priority for places on their modular courses to staff seconded from Departments of Social Protection. That local authorities are either unable or unwilling to fund projects fully has the effect of making their futures uncertain. The frustrating fundraising activity of such organizations is a constant dimension to their work. As funding is usually time-limited, these organizations will always be precarious. While the success of the organization described here is to be admired, it may be that obvious success may discourage future sponsors on the grounds that their help is no longer necessary. In this case the local authorities will either have to accept full responsibility, or witness the closure of a valued resource.

SOCIAL WORK EDUCATION

Attempting to define the role and tasks of social workers within the context of these self-help groups is not easy. Above all, it is essential to avoid taking a Western blue print for how professional social workers might be employed. In their Definition of Social Work (2001), the International Federation of Social Workers (IFSW) states that 'the holistic focus of social work is universal, but the priorities of social work practice will vary from country to country and from time to time depending on cultural, historical, and socio-economic conditions.' The challenge for those developing social work in Eastern Europe has been to stimulate social work activity appropriate to time and place in societies experiencing radical change (Bridge 1999; Slater 1995; Jack 1996; Horwath and Shardlow 2001).

From the discussion in this article, there appear to be four main areas for social work intervention. The first is on a therapeutic level with parents and with disabled children themselves. This should lead into the second, which is about promoting a social model of disability at both local and national levels. The third is about developing better understanding of multidisciplinary work, and the fourth is improving management of organizations, including fund raising. This is an ambitious list, but covers the areas discussed previously.

Experience of training social work students over this period of six years has shown that perhaps the most crucial area of learning is about management of organizations. This encompasses staff supervision and training in professional roles and their boundaries. Since the founders of these voluntary groups are usually involved as users and carers, they belicve in promoting social justice; they have knowledge of the social problem they intend to address, but they welcome training in staff management issues and in the training and management of volunteers. Staff conflicts are likely to be heightened when staff members are personally affected by the service.

Social work activity must be divided between campaigning for social and legal change, and meeting the needs of service users. Zaviršek (1999) comments about developing social work in Sovenia, that political activity is necessary to counteract seventy years of repression. For social work education to have relevance to the burgeoning voluntary sector in Ukraine, the syllabus must include both political and therapeutic dimensions.

CONCLUSION

In many ways the collapse of the Soviet Union and the end of communism has been celebrated as the end of a repressive era, and an opportunity for the people of Eastern Europe to benefit from a free market economy and access to Western ideas and achievements. In practice, those monitoring the transition over the past decade have commented unfavourably on the social inequalities that have ensued and the emergence of serious social problems, previously denied or catered for through state welfare.

Since 1991 it has become possible for Westerners to obtain a better understanding of the extent and nature of the problems concerning disabled children in Ukraine. For parents and professionals in Ukraine it has become easier to access information about alternative treatments, equipment for the disabled, and educational approaches. The leaders of the self-help groups are active searchers on the Internet as a source of both possible sponsors and of information to improve the quality of their children's lives. The courage and tenacity of the parent leaders in the voluntary sector is admirable.

However, the emotional pressures they are under have actually increased as the result of access to Western solutions. Their involvement in voluntary activity, with its associated process of seeking sponsorship through the private sector, is clearly totally inadequate to meet the needs of the large numbers of disabled children living with their parents in the community.

In addition this paper has drawn specific attention to the limited educational and rehabilitation facilities available to disabled children. In particular concern has been expressed about certain treatment methods that appeared to be 'medieval,' punitive, and of doubtful therapeutic value. It appears that the developmental, social and emotional needs of many of these children are being sacrificed in the search for improvements and cures. This is little different from the desperate searches for effective treatments by parents of disabled children throughout the world who tend to put their faith in inadequately researched treatments (see Bridge 1999 chapter 10).

Caring for disabled children in Ukraine has become a public issue as the result of increased access to Western ideas and resources. However, this process has the inevitable resulting consequences of heightening stress for both parents and their children, as they experience deep envy and frustration that resources in other parts of the world are out of their reach.

REFERENCES

Alur, M. (1989) *Practical Difficulties Encountered by Parents of C.P. Children*, Bombay: The Spastics Society of India.

Barnes, C. (1991) *Disabled People in Britain and Discrimination, A Case for Anti-discriminatory Legislation*, London: Hurst.

Bertmar, A. (1998) *Armenia. Children's Deinstitutionalisation Initiative. Beneficiary Assessment of Children in Institutions* (unpublished paper, University of Yerevan).

Binyon, M. (1999) *Maimed by embracing the market*, The Times, Monday, August 23.

Bridge, G. (1999) *Community Care for Children with Cerebral Palsy: Social Work Perspectives*, Practice, Vol. 11, No. 4, pp. 15-26.

Bridge, G. (1999) *Parents as Care Managers: The experiences of those caring for young children with cerebral palsy*, Aldershot: Ashgate.

Bridge, G. (2000) *Let's take practice teaching to Eastern Europe*, Journal of Practice Teaching in Health and Social Care, pp. 47-60.

Dalton, M. *Culture Shock: Ukraine*, London: Kuperard

Finkelstein, V. (1980) *Attitudes & Disabled People: Issues for Discussion*. New York: World Rehabilitation Fund.

FOCCUS, www.iiconnect.org.FOCCUS.html

Harwin, J. (1996) *Children of the Russian State*, Aldershot: Avebury.

Human Rights Watch (1998) *Cruelty and Neglect in Russian Orphanages*.

Hyde, L. (1999) *The Abortion Production Line. Alternative methods fail to displace state-provided abortion as dominant form of birth control*. Kyiv Post, March 18th Vol. 5, Issue 11.

Kendall, J. & Knapp, M. (1995) A Loose and Baggy Monster: Boundaries, Definitions, and Typologies, in Davis Smith, J., Rochester, C., & Hedley, R. (1995) (Eds.). An Introduction to the Voluntary Sector, Chapter 4, pp. 66-95, London: Routledge.

Kourktchian, M. (1998) Redistributing wealth and power between the state and individual entrepreneurs: Armenia, pp. 69-80 in Part ii of Ramon, S. (ed.) *The Interface between Social Work and Social Policy*, Birmingham: Venture Press.

Kukauskas, R. (1999) *Developing Fostering Services in Lithuania*, Social Work in Europe, Vol. 6, No. 2, pp. 51-56.

Kuts, S. (2002) *Ukraine. The role of the private sector of Ukraine: Social-political governance perspective*, European Journal of Social Work, Volume 5, Issue 1, pp. 79-84.

Lloyd, J. (1988) *Mafia capitalism: The warning from Russia*. Prospect, January, pp. 34-39.

Manning, N. (1995) *Social Policy and the Welfare State*, Chapter 12 in Lane, D. (ed.) *Russia in Transition*, London: Longman.

Monk, V. and Singleton, N. (1995) *Lessons from Social Work in the Czech Republic*, Social Work in Europe, Vol. 2, No. 3, pp. 42-48.

Oliver, M. (1990) *The Politics of Disability*, London: Macmillan.

Ramon, S. (2000) *Creating Social Work and Social Policy Education in Kiev, Ukraine: An Experiment in Social Innovation*, Cambridge, APU.

Ramon, S. (ed.) (1998) *The Interface between Social Work and Social Policy*, Birmingham: Venture Press.

Ramon, S. (1995) *West-East European Social Work Educational Initiatives: Continuing Dilemmas*, Social Work in Europe (p. 5). Vol. 3, No. 2.

Reading, P. (1994) *Community Care and the Voluntary Sector*. BASW, Venture Press.

Semachko, N. (1929) *Social Work in the Union of Soviet Socialist Republic*, Paris: First International Conference of Social Work, Vol. II.

Semachko, N. (1929) *La Protection de la Santé Publique dans L'Union des Républiques Socialistes Soviétiques*, Paris: First International Conference of Social Work, Vol. II.

Slater, W. (1995) *'Women of Russia' and women's representation in Russian politics*, Chapter 5 in Lane, D. (ed.) *Russia in Transition*, London: Longman.

Solomon, R. (1994) *East meets West: Developing a Community Fostering Service in Warsaw*, Social Work in Europe, Vol. 1, No. 1 pp. 11-22.

Thorburn, M. J. (1985) *The Disabled Child in the Caribbean in Childhood Disability in Developing Countries*, New York: Praeger.

Tresiliotis, J. (1994) *Setting up Foster Care Programs in Romania*, Community alternatives, 6, 1, pp. 75-92.

UNICEF (1997) *Children at Risk in Central & Eastern Europe: Perils and Promises* Economies in Transition Studies, Regional Monitoring report, No. 4.

Werner, D. (1987) Disabled *Village Children*, Palo-Alto, CA: Hesperan.

White, A. (1999) *Democratization in Russia under Gorbachev (1985-1991)* Hampshire: Macmillan.

Parents as Advocates: Stories of Surplus Suffering When a Child Is Diagnosed and Treated for Cancer

Juanne N. Clarke, PhD
Paula Fletcher, PhD

SUMMARY. Twenty-nine parents of children who had been diagnosed with cancer were interviewed through long and relatively unstructured interviews conducted via telephone by a mother whose own daughter once had cancer. Parents were asked to tell the story of their experiences during the time that they were 'going through' cancer. Parents usually began their narrative in the months, weeks, or days prior to the diagnosis. They spoke of various parts of the story. In this paper, the focus is on one topic that parents talked about a lot. We call this 'problems with the system' or 'surplus suffering.' Here parents reported on their perceptions of mistakes, and delays in diagnosis, errors, carelessness, and unkindness during treatment. They talked of how they felt they had to be on constant

Juanne N. Clarke is affiliated with the Department of Sociology and Anthropology, Wilfrid Laurier University, 75 University Avenue, Waterloo, Ontario, N2L 3C5, Canada (E-mail: jclarke@wlu.ca). Paula Fletcher is affiliated with the Department of Kinesiology and Physical Education, Wilfrid Laurier University, 75 University Avenue, Waterloo, Ontario, N2L 3C5, Canada.

[Haworth co-indexing entry note]: "Parents as Advocates: Stories of Surplus Suffering When a Child Is Diagnosed and Treated for Cancer." Clarke, Juanne N., and Paula Fletcher. Co-published simultaneously in *Social Work in Health Care* (The Haworth Social Work Practice Press, an imprint of The Haworth Press, Inc.) Vol. 39, No. 1/2, 2004, pp. 107-127; and: *Social Work Visions from Around the Globe: Citizens, Methods, and Approaches* (ed: Anna Metteri et al.) The Haworth Social Work Practice Press, an imprint of The Haworth Press, Inc., 2004, pp. 107-127. Single or multiple copies of this article are available for a fee from The Haworth Document Delivery Service [1-800-HAWORTH, 9:00 a.m. - 5:00 p.m. (EST). E-mail address: docdelivery@haworthpress.com].

Digital Object Identifier: 10.1300/J010v39n01_08

guard, and at times, to intervene in their child's care. This paper provides a picture of parental expectations and their violation during the treatment of their children for cancer. It begins to demonstrate how parents see themselves as advocates for their children in a context of fragile power relations. *[Article copies available for a fee from The Haworth Document Delivery Service: 1-800-HAWORTH. E-mail address: <docdelivery@haworthpress.com> Website: <http://www.HaworthPress.com> © 2004 by The Haworth Press, Inc. All rights reserved.]*

KEYWORDS. Narrative account, parents as advocates, children, cancer, diagnosis and treatment, suffering, mistreatment by medical system

THE ACADEMIC AND PROFESSIONAL LITERATURE

Whatever the specific diagnosis, it must be understood and accepted that the child who was previously thought to be well and happy must now face a lifetime of uncertainty and considerable physical pain. (Eiser, 1996:146)

The future is severely compromised, as are parental expectations. (Eiser, 1996,146)

Learning that one/one's child has a life-threatening disease is now included as a qualifying event for post-traumatic stress disorder (PTSD) with Diagnostic and Statistical Manual of Mental Disorders. (4th Edition; DSM-IV; American Psychiatric Association)

WORDS OF THE PARENTS

You are fighting for the survival of your own child. (a parent)

I learned early on that I had to be an advocate for her. (a parent)

It is instinct too; you will do anything for these children. (a parent)

INTRODUCTION

The origin of this research is an involuntary ethnography, which resulted from a sudden immersion into the world of childhood cancer when my daughter, at seventeen, was diagnosed with Acute Lymphoblastic Leukemia (ALL). This experience led to the book *Finding Strength: A Mother and Daughter's Story of Childhood Cancer* (Clarke and Clarke, 1999). Writing the book led me to ask a number of questions of the sociological and psychological research literature about why our family experienced what it did. I was startled by how alien the focus of the research literature was to our experience, questions, and ideas. But I recognized that my story was just that. It was in many ways unique; thus, this paper is based on an extension of my involuntary ethnography to a more systematic study of other parents whose children had been diagnosed with cancer within the previous five years in Ontario, Canada.

The research discussed in this paper is based on an inductive model of the process of theory building. In this model, the theory and the accompanying review of relevant literature occur after the detailed collection of data regarding an aspect of the social world under investigation. In keeping with this, the logic of the paper follows the logic of inductive theorizing. First, the sample and the method used to collect the information, then the data analysis strategies, will be described. Finally the paper will analyse the data in the context of available literature and offer theoretical interpretations.

METHODOLOGY

Sample

The sample is a non-representative volunteer and quota sample. The initial population pool was a list of individuals whose names were given as contacts for regional parent support groups in Ontario through the organization of OPACC (Ontario Parents Advocating for Children with Cancer). Every person listed was contacted by telephone including the representatives of larger organizations such as Childcan and Families for Children with Cancer. All of those contacted were asked to take letters of explanation, introduction, and solicitation to parent support groups at their next regular meeting and to ask for volunteers for parents who had had children treated for cancer within the previous five years in Ontario. Those who were willing to be interviewed indicated to the group leader who informed the research assistant of their names and telephone numbers. This resulted in 27 names of parent volunteers across the province but excluded people from Northern Ontario where the population is much less dense. Several phone calls to the North resulted in no volunteers. Thus the researcher contacted the North Eastern Ontario Regional Cancer Centre directly and after receiving ethics clearance, three parents from the treatment center volunteered to be interviewed. This resulted in three more names. A total of 34 parents initially responded and indicated that they were willing to be interviewed, but five were not interviewed. Two parents declined when they were re-contacted (one offered no explanation, and the other said that she did not wish to relive her experience at this time). One parent could not be contacted, and the final two had children whose health had suddenly deteriorated and were not available to be interviewed.

Sample Description

There were twenty-nine respondents altogether, four fathers and twenty-five mothers, of children who had been diagnosed with cancer. The average (median) age of the respondents was 39.7 years. The average age of their children at the time of diagnosis was 5.4 years old. Seven of the children who once had cancer were female and twenty-two were male. The family sizes varied: Two families had no other children, thirteen families had one other child, twelve had two other children, and two families had three other children. Each of the families spoke English. Additionally, six families were bilingually French, one family was also Philippino, and another family was Polish. The occupations of both mothers and fathers were varied. Most of the fathers were blue-collar workers who engaged in employment such as pipefitting and contracting. In comparison, a few were white collar workers including a teacher, real estate agent, and mechanical engineer. The occupations of the mothers ranged from stay-at-home moms (seven) to nursing, teaching, secretarial work, and hairdressing. Thirteen of the families within this sample indicated that they had lost income as a result of their child's illness; however, all were able to access extended health care support to pay for the drugs that their children were prescribed. In some cases this coverage was only 80% of the total cost. Nine of the fathers had post-secondary education including community or technical college and university. Other fathers had completed high school while a few had apprenticeships. The mothers were more likely to have completed community college (eight) or university (nine).

Data Collection

The data were collected by telephone by a mother whose child had had cancer and was finished with treatment. All of the participants were informed that the study was being conducted by a mother who had had a child diagnosed with cancer and that the interviewer, too, was a mother whose child had once suffered through cancer. The interviews varied in length from one to four hours. The time chosen for the interview was at the convenience of the interviewed parents who were all interviewed by telephone while they were in their own homes. The interviews were open-ended and the topics were, as much as possible, determined by the interviewees. The general topic was parent's views of the experience of having had a child treated for cancer. Parents were asked to tell their stories beginning with their remembrance of the things that had led up to the diagnosis (e.g., symptoms), and then following through with the issues that they considered relevant during the whole process of treatment. The interviewer had been trained by the principal investigator to complete open-ended interviews and at the same time been given a list of possible questions/topics for discussion should she need these questions. The interviewer was directed to ask as few questions as possible and instead was directed to ask respondents to "expand" and "clarify" by saying, for example, "please tell me more about that." In reality the mother/interviewer became involved in the process and actually discussed and shared her own experiences when she thought they were relevant. The interviewer became passionate about listening to and enabling the telling of the stories of parents whose children had had cancer. All interviews were taped and later transcribed by a typist who was briefed in issues of confidentiality and privacy.

This qualitative method is consistent with a growing body of literature in the social and behavioral sciences. It values and emphasizes the narrative account of the research participants who are asked to describe an event or an aspect of their life in rich detail and with the level of intimacy that they find comfortable. Evidence suggests that significant experiences in life (such as having a child diagnosed with cancer) can be transformative; they change the ongoing life story that human beings create as they live and make meaning of their lives. Such experiences are best "captured" by qualitative and narrative methods that give to the research participant the power of self-definition and storytelling. Not only is this a method that tends to elicit stories which emphasize the issues most salient to the individual, it is also a method that offers something immediately back to the participant. All of the participants in this research (and in my experience most in all research of this type) thanked the interviewer for listening. Many also commented that it was very helpful to have the opportunity to share their experiences with another. Although this had not been systematically investigated, I suggest that there may indeed be human benefits to such research.

In addition, all parents who contributed to the research via interviews answered a questionnaire. This questionnaire asked about topics such as the socio-economics, ethnicity, and educational status of the parents as well as the financial costs of treatment and the use (or not) of complementary and alternative medicines. Highlights of the questionnaire responses are reported in the 'description of the sample' portion of the paper.

DATA ANALYSIS

The interviews were taped verbatim although punctuation was added by the transcriber who herself made 'common sense' of what was being said and thus constructed sentence and paragraph formats. The transcribed interviews were read by two researchers and a research assistant who assessed the work for common themes. After a preliminary meeting confirming common themes, the team coded a selection of interviews, then met again to confirm parallel coding decisions and to explicate any differences in coding decisions through discussion. Once the general themes (and their indicators) were agreed upon, the research assistant completed the coding. Excerpts from the transcripts reflecting specific themes were then cut and pasted into files. Some of the resulting themes were "communication," "end of treatment," and "support." The researcher/writer then read through these theme files and developed sub-themes and coded, numbered, and listed these as an index to the themed excerpts. Additionally, the researcher re-read all of the transcripts, after a period of time, to confirm and elaborate on the original interpretations and coding decisions.

One of the themes that seemed to have the most salience, in the sense that many people spent a great deal of time talking about it and returned to it a few times during the interview, was what we call "problems with the system" or "surplus suffering." This topic included a variety of issues, but the major ones were the perception of mistakes and delay in diagnosis, carelessness and unkindness during treatment, and the corresponding view that parents needed to be on guard and to intervene in order to protect their children during their care.

The next section of the paper presents examples of the stories told by parents in order to illustrate this theme of "problems with the system" or "surplus suffering." This is followed by a theoretical interpretation and analysis.

PROBLEMS AT DIAGNOSIS

Sometimes the sick children were diagnosed very quickly after doctors felt for and found 'typical' signs of childhood cancer such as lumps, swollen liver or spleen, tiredness and bruising, or pallour and then ordered blood and other diagnostic tests. Other times, the transition to a diagnosis was an arduous one in which parents felt they had to fight to have their perception that their child was really sick taken seriously and then finally acted upon. The diagnostic process, as described by these parents, took up to months of repeated visits to the doctor (or doctors) and misdiagnosis after misdiagnosis. Following is one mother's story of a slightly delayed diagnosis and her feeling that this was because of the physician's biases about daycare.

> Annie was diagnosed in January of 1996. I first noticed something amiss in November of 1995. She was getting sick all of the time but she looked OK. She had ear infections. I took her to the pediatrician who was kind of against daycare. I had my daughter in daycare and she was of the mind that you stay at home and have one caregiver until the child is three. She kept saying 'you know you have her in day care this is what you get. You get sick children.' I thought OK I guess this is typical that they are more sick than they are healthy. I thought that was typical and she was my oldest daughter so I really didn't have a benchmark and then it accelerated.

> Around the third week in December I noticed she was really ill. I was bathing her one time and I noticed her lymph nodes were big just behind her ears. At the time, the pediatrician's office was closed as it was officially the Christmas holidays. I took her to a walk-in clinic right after her bath. It was still open. It was, 'well she has a virus, here are some antibiotics.' They never told me the source of the virus or anything but said the swollen lymph nodes were indicative of an infection. So antibiotics it was. She had been

on so many antibiotics since November it wasn't even funny. Again, I didn't have a benchmark so I said fine.

I remember taking her to a party on Christmas Eve and actually put blush on her. She was beyond pale. She was gray and she had no color in her lips. After Christmas her face got really puffy and she was crying all of the time. I thought 'I am not taking her back to the clinic, and the doctor's office is closed right through New Year's.' I thought 'at least I am here.' She was still on the antibiotics and this was the third week in December. I thought that would be sufficient until I got her to the pediatrician but by the time I got her to the pediatrician, it was like the world opened on the third of January. Her appointment was on the fifth. By then I thought 'all right, you know I am a layman but she needs blood work, she is so white.' I walked her into the pediatrician and said 'she is white, she is not herself, she is crying all of the time.' 'I know she is in daycare,' and I was prepared for a fight actually, saying 'she needs to have blood drawn' and the pediatrician said 'yes she does.' She wrote the requisition form that said STAT and I knew what STAT meant.

Another mother, this time the mother of a teenage girl, described how she finally asked for a blood test for mono after months of treatment with antibiotics. The blood test led to the diagnosis of cancer.

Susan was diagnosed in October 1996. I think the cysts started to appear in the summer previous to that. I noticed that she was more lethargic than usual. She had been a competitive swimmer. In the summer, she would always be swimming and very active. She was lying around a lot and seemed uninterested in activities at our cottage. I blamed it at that point on the fact that she was fourteen and was at the age where they can be difficult. She then developed something on her foot and that summer, we thought she may have stepped on something in the water. It was like a cut or something. We went to the emergency about it because she was in a basketball camp and it was hurting her to run on that foot. I think they tried to drain it and nothing would drain and they seemed a little perplexed as to what it was. I think that it was probably a cyst that had something to do with the leukemia.

That fall, she went into high school and tried out for the basketball team. Again she was feeling tired quite often and would come home from school and sleep, which was totally unlike her. Then she developed what looked like a cyst on her knee. It became irritated, red, and it bothered her. I phoned the family doctor and couldn't get her in that day or the next. I then took her to the hospital and they looked at it in emergency and they knew about the foot. I think they opened it up which was the worst thing that could have been done. Again nothing really drained and they weren't sure if there was something under the skin and they sent her home. They put her on antibiotics for it.

When she was on the antibiotics, she seemed to improve. The other thing she started getting was headaches and sometimes a bit of a fever that would come and go. It was like flu symptoms . . . When the antibiotics stopped, everything came back again and she was looking very pale at this point and she was tired. Sometimes she would call home from school to be picked up so I took her to the family doctor again. He was ready to send us home because he felt it was just a bug and I said 'could it be something more like mono.' He didn't think so but just in case he wanted a blood test. He took blood and then the following morning he called. I was alone. As soon as he phoned I sat down because the doctor doesn't phone you unless something is wrong.

I remember him clearly asking me if I was sitting down. I said "yes I am." He said 'well, we have the results back from the blood work and it looks like leukemia.' He said 'I want her to be treated immediately.'

One mother 'knew' her child had relapsed before the tests had been done.

The relapse, well I knew he was sick. I have always known. He had a severe pain in his shoulder blade. I said, 'I am not leaving here. I'm dropping my son off [at the hospital] unless you do something.'

Another parent had been carrying her two and a half year old son around. He had had intermittent high fevers and was pale. The fevers came and went and it wasn't until his temperature reached 105° F that the parents took their child to the emergency department where the doctors said it was a virus and sent him home. It was only after a few more weeks of intermittent fevers, being carried, complaining of sore legs and eventually the appearance of tiny bruises, when she and her son were watching Charlie Brown, that a different diagnosis became a possibility. She describes this 'discovery' as follows:

> This was a Charlie Brown I have never seen in my life. What is this? I am watching Charlie Brown and it is about a little girl who has leukemia. A voice in my head, my voice or God, I don't know, said 'Alex has leukemia.'

The next day, she insisted on blood tests which indicated the probability of leukemia.

MISTAKES, CARELESSNESS, AND UNKINDNESS DURING TREATMENT

The next section illustrates a few of the problems that parents reported they experienced during their child's treatments for cancer. Some of the problems the parents considered mistakes, some carelessness, and others' unkindness. One of the concerns that several parents raised was that they felt very frustrated and uncertain because many of the doctors and nurses seemed to have policies which they had at one time or another explicitly stated but which they later ignored. They were troubled by their experience that although there were known rules, they were not necessarily followed. In this situation parents felt unsure about whether to trust that other parts of their children's treatment was actually proceeding along the lines that they had been told they would.

> Another thing that was a problem was they don't respect their own policies. They say visiting hours are over at eight, one person maximum to a room, I had my co-owners of my room set up a bed to go to sleep at midnight and have five people in the room until then. The next day I was so mad I was slamming all the doors and being so noisy. They say from 12:30-1:30 is nap time and their kid fell asleep at 3:30. I did something I have never done before, I turned on the TV really loud and the Nintendo machine really loud and we were talking and laughing and making noise. I heard grandpa say don't they realize that C. is trying to sleep. I think they got the message but I don't think it was my business to give it. The nurses should say it's 8:30 and you should go.

Another thing my wife carried Katey down to the room for an LP and the one nurse dropped one of the instruments on the floor and she picked it up and she was going to use it again and my wife said that has been on the floor. The two nurses and doctor were contemplating whether it was sterile or not. My wife said if you are going to argue about it, I am going back. She put her arms around Katey and started heading back and then they decided it was non-sterile. That was one big incident.

One mother tells how her son almost died as the result of his misdiagnosis or mistreatment of chicken pox while he was known to have and to be under care for leukemia. She also notes how, had she not become assertive about her son's treatment, he might have died. Interesting, too, is the fact that this is one of two situations in which a parent actually made a complaint to a higher authority about an aspect of care.

When we were at home on a weekend, Bobby was having abdominal pains, severely. We called and it was the other oncologist and it wasn't ours. She said he was constipated and to keep him at home. I ended up with a counter full of medication and Tom rushed him into Emergency in the middle of the night. The child was like a woman in labor without an epidural. His eyes were dilated and you could see the contraction coming. Tom brought him in and we found chicken pox on his abdomen. Tom brought him in at 4:00 in the morning and Emergency sent him home with a prescription, which you administer, intravenously for a child with a suppressed immune system for chicken pox. We were sent home and for all the time I had spent with the hospital, there are posters everywhere, saying what a serious virus chicken pox is, and they send him home. He had chicken pox. I called the oncologist again and she said did they do his blood work and I said yes. He has chicken pox and he is having contractions every two minutes. Finally on the second time I called the hospital and I said my name is J., I am bringing my son in now and you can look up your records from last night in Emergency. He has leukemia, he has the chicken pox and he is experiencing severe abdominal pains. My husband is in the car now, he is seventeen minutes away from you now, and I am following him in half an hour. This is his OHIP number but you may not even be worried about that.

He was admitted right away, he was hooked up, his bowels had shut down, his liver and kidneys were becoming infected, and we nearly lost him, it was very close. He still has, it looks like beauty marks, and his back and front are covered with them from severe chicken pox marks. It took the oncologist a day to come near us and Tom said to her, she had six people following her; we don't want anybody in here. Bobby had tubes in and out of him and he was fighting for his life. Our family was coming from Toronto and Ottawa. Tom raised his voice and she said if you are going to talk to me like that then I am going to leave and he said you know what, you better leave. Tom addressed the administrator of the hospital totally. He said you guys are damn lucky that this isn't going any further. We had the best care for the next ten days that you could possibly imagine.

In the following excerpt, a father describes, a not uncommon situation, in which, were it not for the presence of his wife, he believes that his child would have been given the wrong drug.

They were going to give Cathy some different medication that she had not too long ago. The other patient's name was Cathy and they may have given it to the wrong person if it wasn't for my wife being there. We figured they would have. They weren't checking.

The following is another story of a drug-related mistake.

Darcy was also given a fairly serious overdose of antibiotics and it could have caused him permanent damage. I felt to a large degree it was because of poor communication amongst staff members and things. I can't prove that but that was my feeling. After that I refused to go back there. They reversed the gentamicin and the tetrocillin dosages and they are hugely different. Gentamicin is extremely toxic. I wasn't real happy with the care there.

PARENTS AS GUARDS AND ADVOCATES

Parents often felt powerless. This was sometimes frustrating because they felt that they cared more for their child and their child's well-being than the health care team and therefore had sometimes to be assertive to ensure that their child received what they considered to be appropriate treatment. The following four excerpts describe how parents spoke of how they felt the need to intervene, be persistent and sometimes aggressive.

> I know some of the moms once we got into the Cancer Center and you know yourself some of the stories are just unbelievable. I remember moms telling me they would take their kids in and say they are tired and they would say oh they are just growing or they are just too active. They had nothing to show to say look they were just going on their mother's instincts like that isn't good enough for them. Or they say she is just an overprotective mother or the mother that complains about her kids that have had headaches. Basically they give the CAT scan to the kid to shut the mother up. I think it boils down to how persistent you are if you know something isn't right. I am fairly aggressive.

After being sent home from the doctor's office a number of times, with a very sick child, the following mother provided this account.

> When I went into the Children's Outpatient Center you have all these residents and clerks and I said you can all get the hell away from me because I am only doing this once and I am speaking to someone who does this. I didn't make a very good impression coming in because I was coming in as a big bull moose. Something is wrong with her guys so tell me what. The pediatric oncologist said I am going to send you for a CAT scan, which in my eyes was like hello. I am going to book you for a CAT scan but in the meantime the CAT scanner was broken. This is the only part I do know, I said well you are going to admit him to the hospital because the chances of getting a CAT scan are better when you are an inpatient than an outpatient. She admitted us to the hospital.

Another mother felt she needed much more medical support than she seemed to be receiving.

> They tried to cut back on the nurse coming [to the home], which was already very little. It was just a nurse coming and hooking up bags and they would want me to do everything so they wouldn't have to come. I was not ready to leave (the university hospital).

Just before Christmas they wanted Sara to leave the university hospital and to come to "the community hospital" because they try to reduce the number of patient beds before the holidays. At that point she was doing fairly well. I said no I don't want to go back because the pediatric hematologist was going to be away for three or four weeks over Christmas. I am not going to be there and have to deal with residents. I am not a very assertive person but I really put my foot down on that issue. I remember Dr. C. being very angry about it and he said there was no reason for her to be here and she would be looked after and I said no I refuse to go. Finally they gave in and said she could stay and he said to me after that ICU incident it is a good thing she stayed here. I learned early on that I had to be an advocate for her.

In the following incident, a mother watched while her daughter's wishes were being disregarded until she finally gave in and stood up for her.

When Melody had her port accessed she would always sit up to do it. The nurses said if that is how she wants to do it then that is fine. We had one nurse in and she wouldn't let Melody do that and she said lie down. I said look she doesn't want to do it like that and she screamed as soon as they came at her with the needle. She would not let her sit up. She tried to access her port three times. I said if you don't get someone in here to do it the way she wants it done then you are not going to be able to do it.

Aside from mistakes, carelessness, and unkindness, there were other times that parents expressed frustration and in the following excerpt, a parent witnesses an argument between two doctors, one of whom is saying he does not have time to do the procedure with her child that was already underway.

The anesthesiologist was arguing when Cory was on the bed for her LP that he had no time and he had to be somewhere else for two o'clock.

Another mother felt hurt by a comment made by a doctor about her mothering.

The doctor made a really nasty comment to me something to the effect of you should put this all into perspective and think about your son; he does have leukemia as if I was not thinking about him. I just lost it with him. He apologized later and said he should not have made that comment.

Repeatedly, parents emphasized that they felt they were responsible for their children and yet they lacked control or knowledge about what was happening or what was planned. They knew the lives of their children were in danger, and they wanted to do what they could but were not always informed clearly, carefully, and without mistake. A typical comment follows.

I had to advocate for him because you have to fight for them. I remember having to fight one day because there were no beds for chemo. They had to delay chemo for one week and I went ballistic. What is going on here? This is ridiculous. This is my child here and you can't delay chemo for a week, this thing can grow.

DISCUSSION AND CONCLUSION

Most of the available literature on parents focuses on psychopathology. This has certain advantages. It is aimed at providing understanding of the psychosocial suffering that parents undergo when their children have cancer. It provides information for people in the helping professions that may enhance their ability to understand the experiences of parents with whom they work and to design helpful interventions such as parents' groups and individual counseling. The designating of parental experience as a psychiatric disorder allows treatments to be managed by psychiatrists and covered by medical and various health policies. However, there is a way in which focusing on the psychosocial characteristics of the parents neglects what might be a more useful strategy eventually, the understanding of the most important issues facing parents from their own perspective and contextualized within their relevancies.

Iatrogenesis refers to the suffering caused by treatment. I prefer the phrase *surplus suffering* because it emphasizes the idea that there is physical suffering that results from the disease and its medical treatment, and there is mental/emotional suffering that attends watching a child suffer; however, there is additional unnecessary surplus suffering that results from the health care and other institutions and systems themselves. This paper has focused on parents and some difficulties resulting from medical treatment itself. Some aspects of this suffering come from the difficulties that result from the failure of staff to follow hospital policies, mistakes made by medical professionals, occasions when medical professionals act in an "unprofessional" manner, when medical staff do not appear to be qualified/experienced with the particular procedures they undertake, and what appears to parents to be a lack of responsible caring by the professionals.

It is not that parents are not grateful for excellent medical care when they feel that they receive it but that they feel that they are ultimately responsible for their children. Usually they noticed the early symptoms that led them to take their child(ren) to the doctor. Sometimes doctors ignored these early signs, and parents had to be positive and demanding about their perspective and their view that all was not well with their child(ren). From this early pre-diagnosis to diagnosis, to in-hospital, outpatient, and in-home care parents described how they fulfilled their responsibilities. Sometimes this was through a process of straightforward collaboration, but often it involved them in continuous interventions and assertions against what they saw as medical mistakes, wrong-doings, and failures or their potential. They saw themselves as advocates for their children against the surplus suffering caused not by the disease and the physical treatment per se but from the contradictions and confusion within the medical system. These parents' stories did not emphasize their own emotional devastation or pain. It is not that they did not mention their sorrows, angers, fears or frustrations, but rather that they focused on how they worked to ensure what they believed to the best for their child(ren).

These findings, which portray parents as advocates and even heroes in their own stories, are particularly interesting for a number of reasons. Some of these reasons pertain to the substantive literature in psycho-social oncology regarding parental experiences when a child has cancer. Others pertain to related theoretical and methodological issues.

First with regard to the substantive literature, there is a significant disjuncture between the preponderance of research and parental perceptions. Rather than their own psychological difficulties, parents focus on their commitment to their children and their ability, willingness, and necessity to be 'good' parents and to care for their children even in the most dramatic of situations and even against, sometimes, very heavy odds. Parents did not spend time talking about their depression, anxiety, stress or other psycho-pathologies, instead they spent time talking about what they had to do and what they did do for their children. In fact, they felt that they demonstrated strength, courage, and intelligence when they guarded and protected their children from perceived mistakes, carelessness and unkindness that their children would otherwise have experienced at the hands of the medical system. Parents saw themselves as necessary advocates in the face of surplus suffering.

The dominant themes in the psycho-social research literature reflect the assumption that having a child with cancer is usually regarded as "one of the most stressful experiences that a family can have" (Kazak and Nachman, 1991:462). In fact, with childhood cancer "the child who was previously thought to be well and happy must now face a lifetime of uncertainty and considerable pain, as must the parent" (Eiser, 1996:146). Much of the research on parents has focused on their adjustment, coping, depression, anxiety, and psychopathology (see Grootenhuis and Last, 1995, for a review of studies of coping and adjustment among parents whose children have been diagnosed since 1980). Some studies have documented variations in adjustment and coping, in anxiety and depression as much as 10 years after diagnosis and the end of treatment. These studies demonstrate that researchers have focused on the psychological impact of childhood cancer in parents. However, psychological scores among these parents such as depression, anxiety, stress and so on are not much different than those of other adults in "normal circumstances." Moreover, these parents' scores may move up and down over time. For instance, diagnosis is often a period of exacerbated stress/depression/anxiety, as are relapse and acknowledging a terminal phase of illness.

These published studies are not entirely comparable nor conclusive because they are based on various samples, ages of children, diagnoses, ethnicities of parents, differing medical and national contexts, differing measures and so on. They do, however, point out what has been absent in such research. They tend to treat the parental/family system in a vacuum characterized, solely or chiefly, by the common (assumed independent) variable, the presence of childhood cancer in the family. The fact that the diagnosis itself is the cause of the stress is so widely assumed that it has become a psychiatric diagnosis. Learning that one/one's child has a life-threatening disease is now included as a qualifying event for post-traumatic stress disorder (PTSD) in the *Diagnostic and Statistical Manual of Mental Disorders* (4th Edition; DSMIV: American Psychiatric Association, 1994:424). There is very little discussion in the literature of the significance of the process of diagnosis, the degree of impairment, communication, the prognosis, the interaction with the medical care system, or socio-economic variations such as income, education, marital/family structure, age of parent/age of child, culture/ethnicity. In short, the social structural, cultural, and medical context of the diagnosis is, relatively speaking, ignored.

One study, an exception to the argument, by Lozowski et al. (1993) described parental involvement in medical care. They found that parents play an active and assertive role in their child's treatment. Fifty-six percent of the parents studied reported intervening at some point in the treatment process to prevent or correct a medical mistake. Among the reasons for the intervention were the following: (A) erroneous administration of drugs; (B) reminders to staff of correct/incorrect procedures; and (C) alteration of intravenous procedures being used by staff interaction. As the authors note, "many parents become, and are compelled by circumstanced to act as lay experts in the treatment of pediatric cancer" (Lozowski et al., 1993:82). The authors also suggest a cause for conflict resulting from the fact that medical staff are used to "asymmetrical" relationships.

The notion of asymmetrical relationships is one that, in light of the data from the present study, deserves further exploration and takes us to the methodological and theoretical issues the parents comments raise. Power is a central issue in all human relationships (Turner, 1978). Sometimes it is manifest and then it is demonstrated through a show of force or its potential. Other times it is latent and shown, for instance, through subtle conversational techniques such as interruption, a refusal to take a conversational turn, or perhaps the censoring of topics (Fox, 1994). Some social theorists have examined this aspect of human relationships to suggest that all relationships are precarious because of the dynamics of power and exchange and moreover, that these "differences in power inevitably create the potential for conflict" (Turner, 1978:254).

When the more powerful in a relationship conform to the norms and expectations of the situation, their power will be seen as legitimate and conflict will tend to be avoided (Blau, 1955:255). However, when the more powerful in a relationship violate or are perceived to violate expected norms, their power will be seen as illegitimate and conflict (Blau, 1955:255), disappointment, or suffering are possibilities. These transcripts suggest instances of perceived illegitimate use of power, norm violation, conflict, and potential for conflict.

In one sense, parents and the medical care team have the same goal, the return to health and the minimizing of suffering of a child with cancer. The means to attain this goal, however, is understood differently by parents than by the medical professionals. In the real world, moreover, people make mistakes and fail to meet normative expectations. Norms are routinely broken. In fact, there are times when their presence is only known because they have been broken. In this situation, characterized by the unequal position of parents and health care professionals, norm violation can lead to conflict and the delegitimization of the authority of the more powerful party. Power is not stable or static. Thus violation of its norms can lead to power's demise. Power must be continuously legitimated by parties to it (Blau, 1955:255).

Finally, with respect to methodology, previous research has tended to be done by professional psychologists, social workers, and nurses who have the vantage point of care providers. From this perspective, they have tended to study parental adjustment, stress, anxiety, depression, and to have compared the scores of parents of children with cancer with adults in 'normal' situations. In keeping with the positivist model of science, this research is considered to be cumulative and standardized measures, which allow for generalizable and comparative findings, tend to be used. By contrast, this study was designed by a parent who had a child diagnosed with cancer (and who was also, by chance, a medical sociologist) and the data were collected by open-ended and focused telephone interviews by another parent whose child had had cancer. The focus was not building or extending the professional literature but rather on the narratives of parents and what they emphasized as the salient aspects of their experience. That the findings here emphasize the advocacy and protection work of parents, their strengths and even heroism rather than their anxieties, fears and depression may relate to the particular vantage point of the researcher and interviewer. That the parents did not talk of their suffering, does not mean that it is irrelevant or it did not occur. It does not mean that this other literature should be ignored. Rather, there is validity in both types of findings and both research paradigms and the findings of both provide a fuller picture than does either alone.

CONCLUSION

It is important to note that this study has many limitations. It was based on a small sample of 29 mothers and fathers of children who had been diagnosed with all sorts of cancer within the five years previous to the research. The qualitative open-ended interviews were conducted by one parent who had had a child diagnosed and successfully treated for cancer in the previous five years and would, subtley yet inevitably, through her interaction and reflections have affected the results. Reliability is somewhat compromised because a different interviewer or an interview conducted at a different time and place might very well have led to a somewhat different emphasis. It is important to note in this context, however, that all interviewed parents expressed satisfaction with the interview process and indeed thanked the interviewer for listening. Some said they were particularly grateful because this had been the first time they had had an opportunity to tell their whole story, in an uninterrupted fashion to another person.

In addition, the interviews were based on retrospection. Parents were asked to reconstruct the stories of their experiences with their child's diagnosis, illness, and treatment. Some of the events described took place several years prior to the interviews. Thus, it is likely that they were edited and recontextualized by the time of the actual interview. Second, these data are verbal. Observation of the described situation would undoubtedly tell a somewhat different story than that of the perspective of the interviewed parent. Indeed, the perceptions of the nurses, doctors and the children, among others, are not included in these data. Further, studies using narrative approaches and based on the perspective of the other important actors in these stories are necessary and important in order to include a full account of the situation at hand. The social desirability effect is always a potential problem when participants are asked to recreate and relay their stories. Another limitation of this research is its lack of generalizability across time, place or parents. The stories relayed here are not claimed to be any more than the stories of these particular parents captured at one time and place. The majority of the parents who volunteered were women and from certain ethnic, educational, and socio-economic status groups.

Despite the limitations, this study does suggest that the experiences of parents whose children have cancer are related not only to the reality of the diagnosis of cancer in their children and its treatment. Instead, their experiences are linked, as well, to their experiences of surplus suffering, because of what they see as various problems with the medical system. It points too, to the fragility of the relationships between parents and health care providers in a situation in which there is a lack of shared meanings regarding health and its achievement and power differences in a situation lacking clear specifications of mutual roles and responsibilities. The paper reveals the particular notion that power/knowledge conflicts are central to the suffering of parents when their children have cancer. Parents feel relatively powerless when they are in the midst of the medical system, yet they feel they have to take power, be advocates, and guard their children against mistakes, carelessness, and unkindness.

REFERENCES

Blau, P. (1964). *Exchange and Power in Social Life.* New York: John Wiley & Sons.

Clarke, J.N. & Clarke, L.N. (1999). *Finding Strength: A Mother and Daughter's Story of Childhood Cancer.* Toronto: Oxford University Press.

Eiser, C. (1996). Comprehensive care of the child with cancer: Obstacles to the provision of psychological support in paediatric oncology: A comment. *Psychology, Health & Medicine, 1*(2), 145 157.

Fox, N. J.(1994). *Postmodernism, Sociology and Health.* Toronto: University of Toronto Press.

Grootenhuis, M.A., & Last, B.F. (1995). Adjustment and coping by parents of children with cancer: a review of the literature. *Supportive Care in Cancer, 5,* 466-484.

Kazak, A.E. & Nachman, G.S. (1991). Family research on childhood chronic illness: Pediatric oncology as an example. *Journal of Family Psychology, 4*(4), 462-483.

Lozowski, S., Chesles, M.A., & Chesney, B.K. (1993). Parental intervention in the medical care of children with cancer. *Journal of Psychosocial Oncology, 11*(3), 63-88.

Turner, J.H. (1978). *The Structure of Social Theory.* Homewood, Illinois: The Dorsey Press.

The Long-Term Psychosocial Effects of Cancer Diagnosis and Treatment on Children and Their Families

Suzanne Quin, BSS, CQSW, MA (Social Work), PhD

SUMMARY. Using both qualitative and quantitative methods, a study of 77 families was undertaken to examine the long-term psychosocial effects of cancer on children and their families. This paper focuses specifically on the findings in relation to the parents' subgroup of the overall study. Key findings were that the majority of parents and their children readjust to ordinary family life following completion of treatment. Gender differences in parents' coping mechanisms emerged. The period immediately following the cessation of treatment can create feelings of isolation and vulnerability, and many parents have ongoing worries about their child's continued well-being. *[Article copies available for a fee from The Haworth Document Delivery Service: 1-800-HAWORTH. E-mail address: <docdelivery@haworthpress.com> Website: <http://www.HaworthPress.com> © 2004 by The Haworth Press, Inc. All rights reserved.]*

Suzanne Quin is affiliated with the Department of Social Policy and Social Work, University College Dublin, Belfield, Dublin 4, Ireland (E-mail: suzanne.quin@ucd.ie).

This study was a joint research project carried out by the Oncology Unit, Our Lady's Hospital for Sick Children, Crumlin, Dublin and the Department of Social Policy and Social Work, University College Dublin. It was funded by the Children's Research Centre, Our Lady's Hospital for Sick Children, Crumlin, Dublin, Ireland.

[Haworth co-indexing entry note]: "The Long-Term Psychosocial Effects of Cancer Diagnosis and Treatment on Children and Their Families." Quin, Suzanne. Co-published simultaneously in *Social Work in Health Care* (The Haworth Social Work Practice Press, an imprint of The Haworth Press, Inc.) Vol. 39, No. 1/2, 2004, pp. 129-149; and: *Social Work Visions from Around the Globe: Citizens, Methods, and Approaches* (ed: Anna Metteri et al.) The Haworth Social Work Practice Press, an imprint of The Haworth Press, Inc., 2004, pp. 129-149. Single or multiple copies of this article are available for a fee from The Haworth Document Delivery Service [1-800-HAWORTH, 9:00 a.m. - 5:00 p.m. (EST). E-mail address: docdelivery@ haworthpress.com].

Digital Object Identifier: 10.1300/J010v39n01_09

KEYWORDS. Parents, children, cancer, survival, siblings, family, effects

INTRODUCTION

The study discussed in this article was concerned with the long-term psychosocial effects of cancer diagnosis and treatment on children and on their families. With over two-thirds of children who develop cancer now achieving disease free survival, the emphasis is shifting from preoccupation with treatment and palliative care to survival and coping with the aftermath of the disease and its treatment. The focus of the study was the psychosocial effects of the disease and its treatment on the children, on other family members, and on the family as a whole. Impetus for the study came from the social workers in oncology based in one of the major children's hospitals in the Dublin area who approached the Department of Social Policy and Social Work in University College Dublin, Ireland, to set up a research project. Hence, a research plan was jointly designed to answer the questions raised by practice and, in turn, to inform future practice.

In itself, survival following diagnosis and treatment of cancer for children or adults does not ensure quality of life. Along with increased survival rates, therefore, has been "growing concern about the biological and psychological late effects of childhood cancer and its treatment" (Friedman and Mulhern, 1991). Cincotta (1993) describes a child's cancer as being a family disease since it affects everyone within the family system. Indeed, the child's adaptation to illness is inevitably complicated by the coping responses of the adults and children who are part of the child's world. Ultimately, then, the challenge of caring for children with cancer extends beyond those children in active treatment and must take account of all the psychosocial aftermath for parents and children.

This finding echoes a study of twenty-one adolescent survivors by Schroff-Pendley et al. (1997) indicating that children diagnosed during middle childhood or adolescence are more at risk of psychological difficulties than those diagnosed in their infancy. Roberts et al. (1998:16) argue that adolescent cancer patients are "uniquely challenged by cancer treatments as they must confront their own mortality and worry about their health while their peers are typically ignoring or denying these realities."

The importance of the family in the coping process of childhood survivors of cancer cannot be underestimated. A study by Kupst et al. (1995)

found that the most significant predictor of the child's coping and adjustment was the coping ability of its mother. Knowledge about the father's role in coping is less documented on account of their lower participation rates in studies relative to mothers (Janus & Goldberg, 1997). Pelcovitz et al. (1996) suggest that the tendency of fathers to use avoidance as a coping strategy to deal with chronic illness in their child may put them at significant risk of developing Post Traumatic Stress Disorder. Findings by Dalquist et al. (1996) indicate that fathers tend to rely on their spouses as their sole means of support, whereas mothers have broader social support networks to turn to when their child develops a serious illness. This concurs with findings in an earlier study by Leventhal-Belfer et al. (1993) that mothers often share such concerns more with friends than with their spouses while fathers did the opposite. Dalquist et al. (1996) suggest that psychosocial interventions focusing only on the mother can run the risk of ignoring the psychological impact of illness on the father. In addition, his potential contribution as a source of support and affirmation for his partner may be lost which can be an important contributor in parental adjustment during a child's illness. Elliott Brown and Barbarin (1996), in their study of gender differences in parental coping with childhood cancer, suggest that fathers may need 'permission' to articulate their emotional responses to their child's illness. At the same time, social workers need to take account of the importance for fathers of having a sense of control in such a situation of intense stress.

Cincotta (1993) viewed cessation of treatment as a time of transition. Hence, the time when treatment ends may rekindle feelings that have been suppressed since the time of initial diagnosis and bring with it fears about the possibility that the cancer could reoccur. Findings by Van Dongen-Meldman et al. (1995) support the significance of this stage for parents. Their study indicated the presence of late psychosocial effects on parents after treatment ends. On the basis of their results, Van Dongen-Meldman et al. (1995) recommended routine psychosocial follow-up consultations for parents in medical follow-up programmes. Mothers, in particular, may find the post treatment phase particularly stressful. A study by Leventhal-Belfer et al. (1993) found that mothers exhibit a much stronger desire to maintain contact with the health care professionals after their child's treatment is completed than do fathers. The researchers suggest that this is as a result of mothers more usually acting as intermediaries between health care professionals and the family throughout the period of the child's diagnosis and treatment.

Heffernan and Zanelli (1997) highlight the tendency to limit research on coping strategies to parents (particularly the mother) and the child with cancer while all but ignoring the siblings in the family. It is only recently, they point out, that research has begun to incorporate siblings in studies of children who survive cancer. Their study found siblings as experiencing major stressors where cancer occurs, resulting in feelings of anger, guilt, fear, anxiety, embarrassment, and frustration. This supports an earlier view put forward by Rollins (1990) who referred to siblings as "the forgotten ones." Cincotta (1993) suggests that siblings may be at greater risk of psychosocial difficulties than their ill brothers or sisters, a view supported by other studies such as Adams and Deveau (1998), Martinson et al. (1990), Eiser and Havermans (1992), and Chesler (1992).

Hamama et al.'s recent study (2000) indicates that siblings who are young at the time of diagnosis and treatment may be at greater risk of ongoing stress than older children. The latter, they suggest, may have the relative advantage of being able to understand better what is happening during the illness and have more developed emotional and social skills as well as peer support to help them cope. A study by Shields et al. (1995) of family needs when a child has cancer indicates that parents are likely to need assistance in helping them to discuss the situation with other children in the family.

A life once challenged by a potentially fatal illness may never be quite the same again for the individual concerned and, particularly in the case of a child, for other family members and for the family as a whole. Childhood cancer is indeed a family disease that has far reaching psychosocial consequences for all family members. As more children survive it becomes all the more important to understand the psychosocial effects of cancer diagnosis and treatment. Initially, research tended to focus on the children themselves and their mothers, the latter tending to be the 'significant other' in the treatment process. Increasingly, attention is being directed at siblings of the child with cancer and on the roles and responses of fathers. However, the latter is still poorly represented in studies of parents in this context. Even less is known about the role of extended family members in helping parents and children cope with the experience of cancer and its aftermath.

RESEARCH DESIGN

In Ireland, figures from the National Cancer Registry show an average of 130 cancer cases per annum for children less than fifteen years of age. This shows the small population to be researched. Our Lady's Hospital for Sick Children in Dublin, Ireland, is a national centre for paediatric oncology. It provides inpatient and outpatient treatment for children throughout the twenty-six counties of the Republic of Ireland. Using a stratified random sampling technique, a nation wide sample of 100 families was selected from a total population of 249 children from the medical records in the paediatric oncology unit in Our Lady's Hospital. The sample was stratified on the basis of geographical location and to ensure that children with different types of cancer were represented. All children with cancer are treated in the public hospital system that is free, as are the drugs and clinic visits required. The sample selected had the following three criteria: they were children who had survived cancer, they had attended the Oncology Unit since 1992, and they were at least two years post treatment. A letter from the paediatric consultants introducing the research was sent out to each family. This was followed up by a phone call from the researcher to establish whether or not the family was willing to participate and, if they were, to arrange date, time, and venue for the interviews. Home interviews were the preferred option for over 95% of the research sample. Out of the sample of 100, a total of 77 families took part in the research. Of the remaining 23 families, 19 were not contactable, being away at the time of the study or having moved with no forwarding address, and four families refused to participate. The ages of the children ranged from 3 years to 21 years at the time of the study (mean age 12 years). The children's parents, their siblings living at home, and extended family members (grandparents, aunts/uncles) who had close ongoing contact with the family during the illness were invited to participate in the research.

The methodology included both qualitative and quantitative elements. The quantitative research instruments were chosen to incorporate a broad spectrum of data on the psychosocial effects of cancer diagnosis and treatment on children and their families. The results discussed below focus on the parents' subgroup with particular emphasis on their experiences, ways of coping and views about the effects of cancer diagnosis and treatment on themselves and their children.

The study used a range of standardised tests with the children who had cancer, the parents' assessment of their children, and the parents' own coping strategies. The COPE (Carver et al., 1989) and General Health Questionnaire (Goldberg, 1981) was used for the parents in order to identify their coping strategies and their self-perceived health status. For the parents' assessment of the children, the Social Skills Questionnaire-Elementary and Second Level (Gresham & Elliott,

1990) was utilised. The tests selected for the children were: Culture Free Self Esteem Inventory (Battle, 1982); Children's Loneliness Questionnaire (Asher, 1985) for the younger children, and the Offer Self Image Questionnaire Revised (Offer, 1992) for the adolescents.

As well as standardised measures, in-depth interviews were carried out with the research participants. Interviews took place in the family home or in an alternative setting such as the hospital, depending on what suited the family. Fathers and mothers were invited to participate in the interviews as well as completing the standardised instruments outlined above. The children and their siblings who had sufficient language skills also participated in the in-depth interviews. For younger children and their siblings, simple drawings of hospital scenes were used to stimulate discussion. In addition, the children and their siblings were asked what would be their three wishes. The purpose of this was to gain some measure of the immediacy of health in relation to other aspects of their lives at the time of the study.

RESULTS

Altogether, a total of 74 mothers and 46 fathers took part in the research as well as 38 siblings and 13 other relatives. Forty-two of the children who survived cancer were interviewed. Thirty-one percent of families lived in the greater Dublin area reflecting the population distribution whereby almost one-third of the total population reside in the area. The remainder resided throughout the rest of the country. Only a very small proportion (3%) of the children were only children; the majority (80%) had 1-3 siblings, while 17% had 4 or more siblings. As paediatric oncology is provided only through the public health sector, all socio-economic groups were represented in the sample. The breakdown for this was as follows: 4% professional workers; 12% managerial and technical; 19% clerical; 23% skilled manual; 14% semi-skilled; 5% unskilled; 9% farmers, 9% unemployed; 2% pensioners, 2% students, and 1% attending a training scheme. Over 90% of the parents were married and both were the child's natural parent. Ireland has until very recently been a mono-cultural society. This was reflected in the survey population whereby all of the sample were Irish born and of Irish descent. It is likely that if such a study were to be repeated a decade on, the changes in emigration with increasing numbers of refugees/asylum seekers would be apparent. In relation to diagnosis, a wide spectrum of cancers was represented with a total of 18 different diagnostic categories. The most prevalent cancers were Acute Lymphoblastic Leukaemia (19%), followed by Hodgkins Disease (9%), Wilms Tumour and Neuroblastoma (8% each), and Rhabdomyosarcoma (6%).

QUANTITIVE FINDINGS–PARENTS

COPE Scale

COPE is a measure used to assess both levels of coping and methods of coping of adults. In this study the COPE Scale was used to assess how well the parents coped in relation to the population in general. The Scale, which is self-administered, addresses both the thought process and the actions in relation to coping. Parents were asked to relate each item to their own experiences and score each on a level of 1-4 with each score having a related value from 1 *'I usually don't do this at all'* to 4 *'I usually do this a lot.'* Scores were divided into 15 component scales and then compared with norm mean scores from the COPE manual.

As can be seen in Table 1, overall, the results showed that parents in the study have average levels of coping in relation to the norm levels. A clear exception was the positive relationship between having a child with cancer and seeking comfort through increased involvement in religious activities, the norm for this item being 8.82 with 11.55 the score for the parental sample. The sub-sample of mothers with a mean of 12.58 had highly significant results in this respect.

More detailed examination of the sub-scales identified some interesting findings, particularly in relation to gender differences. While the parents overall sought external support less than the norm, mothers in the study made greater use of many coping strategies, internal and external, than did fathers. In relation to seeking instrumental social support, the parents as a whole scored .77 below the norm of 11.5 while fathers in the sample were 1.7 below it. As regards seeking emotional social support, there were even greater differences (with the norm of 11.01, parents as a whole scored 1.6 below the norm with the sub-sample of fathers scoring 3.23 below it). Indeed, the most striking differences was the mothers' higher use of many coping strategies both internal and external and the fathers' tendency to rely on mental disengagement (norm 9.66, sample as a whole 7.97, sub-set of fathers 7.49), denial (norm 6.07, sample as a whole 6.74, sub-sample of fathers 6.86), and the use of alcohol/drugs as coping mechanisms (norm 1.38, sample as a whole 2.68, sub-sample of fathers 2.91). On the other hand, mothers

TABLE 1. Mean Scores for COPE by Gender of Sample

Scale	Norm for Scale	Entire Sample	Mothers	Fathers
Active Coping	11.89	11.51	11.68	11.29
Planning	12.58	11.42	11.78	10.96
Seeking Instrumental Social Support	11.50	10.73	11.46	9.80
Seeking Emotional Social Support	11.01	9.41	10.64	7.78
Suppression of Competing Activities	9.92	10.72	11.60	10.29
Turning to Religion	8.82	11.55	12.58	10.57
Positive Reinterpretation and Growth	12.40	11.79	11.98	11.55
Restraint Coping	10.28	10.35	10.52	10.13
Acceptance	11.84	12.50	12.76	12.17
Focus on and Venting of Emotions	10.17	8.97	10.08	7.57
Denial	6.07	6.74	6.65	6.86
Mental Disengagement	9.66	7.97	8.34	7.49
Behavioural Disengagement	6.11	6.89	7.34	6.31
Alcohol/Drug Use	1.38	2.68	2.49	2.91
Humour	N/A	6.19	6.06	6.35

had higher levels of suppression of competing activities than did fathers (norm of 9.92, sample as a whole 10.72, sub-sample of mothers scoring 11.06 in comparison to the fathers' score of 10.29). A likely explanation for this is that the mother's focus has continued to be on the child's on-going emotional and physical needs. Comparison of the data in relation to socio-economic status and marital status of the participants did not yield any statistically significant differences. Overall, the results indicated that mothers have an increased tendency to cope better and more effectively than fathers in circumstances of their child developing and surviving cancer.

General Health Questionnaire

The General Health Questionnaire is a 28 item self-administered questionnaire divided into four scales that assess four different elements of general health: (A) general level of health, (B) sleep problems, (C) sense of control, and (D) feelings of self worth. It measures respondents' perceptions of their current physical, mental, and emotional well-being, through the use of negative and positive questions which are scored on a Likert score scale from 0 to 3 for four possible response items.

As can be seen from Table 2, the total sample scored a mean of 18.4 with an individual item mean of 0.66. Hence, the mean Likert score per item for this population was 1 that denotes the 'same as usual' health levels or 'no more than usual' negative health levels. Within this total, fathers scored a total mean of 16.8 while mothers scored 19.5. This difference of 2.7 in the total mean between them indicates a significant relationship between gender and health perceptions in the study population. Comparison of the respondents in relation to socio-economic status and marital status found no significant differences within the study population.

The results showed the parents did not regard their current state of health as any different than it had been in the past. It should be noted that the questionnaire relates only to current perceptions of health levels and is neither retrospective nor prospective. The parents' perceptions of their own health status at the time of the child's illness is, therefore, unknown. However, the results indicate that the health levels of the parents of a child with cancer undergoes no lasting change and that health status returns to the normal for most parents. When gender differences were taken into account, it was found that mothers reported sleep difficulties more frequently than did fathers. In addition, the fathers were more likely to consider their general health as normal in comparison to the mothers who perceived themselves as having relatively more negative health status. An examination of those who scored badly on both the COPE and the GHQ (i.e., poor health and poor coping) showed no consistent minority group emerging other than the fact that all were female.

QUALITATIVE RESULTS–PARENTS

A total of seventy-four mothers and forty-six fathers took part in the qualitative interviews. The participation rate for fathers was a particu-

TABLE 2. Mean Likert Scores for GHQ Scales A-D by Gender

Scale	Total Sample	Mothers	Fathers
A	4.6	5.0	4.3
B	5.5	6.1	4.4
C	6.5	6.4	6.6
D	1.8	2	1.5
Total	18.4	19.5	16.8

larly positive feature of the research overall as studies of parents tend to either not include fathers or report a very low participation rate for fathers. Although some parents did find it upsetting to talk about their child's illness, particularly the diagnosis and critical stages in the illness trajectory, all wished to continue with the interview. In fact, many families openly welcomed the opportunity to sit down as a family and speak openly about their experiences. An Interview Guide was developed based on the literature review and discussions with professional staff and a small group of parents who were not selected for the research sample. The guide was divided into the following themes: experiences of diagnosis and treatment including information and support available to the family; perceived changes in the child as a result of cancer treatment; effects on the family as a whole, on the marital relationship, on the child and on their siblings where relevant; current perceptions about the ongoing effects on the child, and anticipations for their future.

Memories of Diagnosis

All parents had vivid memories of the time of diagnosis. Over three-fifths commented specifically on their immediate reactions. Feelings of shock, despair and fear predominated: '*I suppose my initial reaction was shock, disbelief and after that it turned to a certain amount of anger as well.*' A common experience was feeling 'blank' and difficulty remembering exactly what was said or what they had been told when their child was first diagnosed. '*I think we heard the word cancer and we could hear nothing else.*' Parents equated the experience with a nightmare and fear of the unknown. A small number of parents reported that they had wanted to be left alone and not to have to talk to anyone on hearing the news because they felt physically and mentally unable to communicate. Medical jargon had to be deciphered also: '*I got on the phone (to my husband) and told him to come quickly. I said I'm in an on-*

cology unit and I haven't a clue what that means at this moment but I think it's something bad.'

While negative emotions not surprisingly predominated, just under a quarter of parents reported feeling very upset but, at the same time, not surprised or even somewhat relieved on hearing the diagnosis. *'Something kept telling me that something bad was wrong with him. I wasn't one bit shocked.' 'Shocked but relieved as well because I knew that whatever they could do they were going to do.'* Almost all had considered the possibility that their child might die, the word 'cancer' being equated to a death sentence for many of the parents. *'I thought she was dying, no I thought she was dead actually . . . Once she (the doctor) said 'cancer' that was it. As far as I was concerned she was finished, gone.'*

Adequacy of Information Received

Just under one-half of the parents felt they had been given adequate information during their child's illness. *'He (the doctor) was open and honest with me. He gave me all the information I needed. He held nothing back and I think that is what gave me the strength to cope.'* The rest of the parents, who were in the majority, were dissatisfied in this respect, largely in relation to the quantity of information received as well as the lack of opportunity to ask questions and get answers that were intelligible to them. *'I think they should have been able to tell us better or in a different kind of way. Maybe gear it up better for us. It was very blunt and short.'* A small minority of parents considered that they had been given more information than they would have wished to receive. *'I wouldn't want to know all these details . . . I remember they gave me booklets to read and I remember opening them and it was horrendous.'*

Experiences of Treatment

Not surprisingly, all of the parents had graphic memories of the treatment phase and its effects on the child. Seeing their child experiencing the physical effects of treatment such as weight and hair loss, the emotional effects of paranoia, aversion to medication, depression and unease as well as watching them endure treatments that were painful and distressing was very traumatic for parents. They also recalled their own feelings of worry, depression and a sense of being in a constant state of disarray. *'You felt it, you slept it, you'd eat it.'* Seeing other children on the ward who were very ill added to the overall state of distress *'You'd get attached to some of the little kids and they pass away and you feel lousy that they're gone.'* For parents living a distance from the hospital, travelling added further to stresses *'It's a long journey and with a sick child, it's longer again.'*

Two-thirds of parents had more positive than negative views about hospital personnel during the treatment process. What they valued most was being included in the process, encouraged to ask questions, and having their opinion valued and the caring approach of staff. *'They were always ready to talk to you which meant an awful lot. There was always somebody's shoulder there for you and it didn't matter whether it was during the day or three o'clock in the morning, which was great.'* One-third of parents had more negative views, the most common complaint related to the staff being too busy to talk to them. Another common grievance was the quality of the facilities in terms of environment, accommodation and food.

Looking back at the treatment stage, several parents remarked on how quickly the time had gone by: *'They were the quickest six months I've ever known but each day was the longest day of my life.'* The love-hate relationship felt by the majority of parents about the oncology unit was encapsulated by one parent's comment that *'we love the place but we never want to see it again.'*

Sources of Support

In terms of support to help them get through the time of diagnosis and treatment, members of the extended family were seen as the major source of support. *'I would never forget my family. I couldn't have got through it without them.'* Another parent commented *'I have one sister . . . she was great. She took the kids and everything and gave us a break.'* Next in ranking order came other parents who were also going through the experience of their child being treated for cancer. The sense of bonding and the sharing of knowledge were key elements in this. *'You were in the same situation and they (other parents) were the only ones who understood.'* Neighbours and friends came next, followed by professional staff within and outside the hospital context including such diverse personnel as the family dentist, pharmacist, lab technicians as well as doctors, nurses, and social workers. Specific reference was made to the key role that religious beliefs played for over one-half of the parents, particularly mothers, which is consistent with the results of COPE described above.

Support of professional staff was something that was greatly missed when the child was discharged from treatment. In fact, once the euphoria of discharge had passed, parents found the sense of isolation and aloneness post treatment to be very difficult. *'You come home on cloud nine but just after finishing chemo(therapy) is the worst part–for the parents anyway.'* *'When you bring your child home, that's when you're totally alone.'* It was strongly felt that a support service would have been of enormous help at this crucial time. *'I had all this information in my head. It would have been nice if there was someone there that would be able to talk to me in that language.'* What, to outsiders, was regarded as a success story was not necessarily so from the parent's viewpoint, and this could increase their sense of isolation and need: *'It's harder for the one (parent of a child) that lives. It's like a life sentence. I think they need help as much as if a child dies.'* It is of particular note that the negative psychological effects of the experience on the parents themselves were seen to emerge most often when treatment was completed.

Impact on Family Relationships

In hindsight, one-third of the parents regarded the experience as having had an overall positive effect on family relationships in the sense of becoming closer, living in the present, and being less preoccupied with material things. *'We go out and about and do things, not put them off.'* On the other hand, just over one-quarter saw the experience as having had an overall negative effect. The parents had focused on the sick child to the detriment of their other children, and there remained a general feeling of insecurity, worry, and fear. *'I don't know if we will ever be the same again.'* *'You're not as secure in your life. You realise that things can go very wrong.'* The remainder considered that the illness, while very traumatic at the time, had had no long-term effects on the family. *'Our everyday life is the same as any other normal family–if there is a normal family, if there is such a thing.'*

Impact on the Parents and the Marital Relationship

The majority of parents interviewed (almost three-quarters) saw their own relationship as having strengthened as a result of their child's illness. As one parent described it, *'I'd say it definitely grew us closer in our marriage. We just realised that we needed each other to get through it.'* Less than one-quarter of the parents considered that the experience of having a child with cancer had had some negative impact on their couple relationship, while a small minority found the strain on their marriage as intense, leading to breakdown and near breakdown in a few instances '. . . *(my husband) . . . was an alcoholic from the time we got married and we always had problems and I think (child's) illness blew it all up. That was the end of it, I had enough.'* Only a very small proportion regarded it as having neither positive nor negative effects.

The fathers interviewed had less to say than did the mothers about how the child's illness had affected them individually and as a couple. Just over one-fifth of fathers reported it had had no effects; the remainder considered the experience had affected them in a number of ways. The most common reaction was a change of perspective and priorities: *'It would teach you a lesson and give you a different outlook on life. You soon learn, I don't worry about work any more.'* The experience had, they thought, made them more patient, more over-protective of their children and more attentive towards them: *'It makes you softer.'* A minority considered that it had affected them in a negative way only, leaving them with feelings of anger, bitterness, depression, short-temper and fear of the future.

Only a tiny minority of mothers felt that they were personally unaffected in the long term. While mothers had more to say than fathers about the effect of the child's illness on themselves, the responses of both were similar in many respects. The most common effect was a change in life-perspective: *'It changed my whole attitude to life, to be honest. You realise how precious life is.'* Being over-protective of the child and more likely to 'spoil' them was another shared reaction. Some differences between fathers and mothers were that the latter specifically mentioned both the positives of becoming more self-confident, independent, and self-motivated and its negative effects on their physical and mental health. Negative physical effects identified by mothers were weight loss, sleeplessness, nausea, and premature ageing.

Perceived Changes in the Child

Virtually without exception, the parents believed that their child had changed in some way as a result of the illness. The perceived changes varied widely and ranged fairly evenly from very positive to very negative. *'Withdrawn,' 'introverted,' 'difficult,' 'disinterested'* were some of the terms used to describe the negative effects while others were viewed as having become more *'outgoing,' 'caring,' 'mature,'* and *'confident.'* The experience of illness had left its effects in terms of aversion to medication of any sort, fear of becoming ill again, fear of medical personnel and medical environments, and generalised anxiety *'She's a terrible worrier, she's afraid something might happen to her and we won't be there to mind her.'* The very few parents who saw no changes attributed this to the very young age at which the child's cancer was diagnosed and treated. *'He had one of the best defences of the lot, lack of knowing.'*

Regarding the children's current health status, three-quarters reported their child as having physically recovered fully from the cancer and its treatment. *'I look on her now as being cured and safe because she's growing and all the normal things seem to have happened.'* The remainder cited ongoing physical effects such as low energy levels, eyesight or hearing problems, bowel problems, and the issue of future sterility. *'When he grows up and realises he's sterile and he might never have a sex life . . . we'll have to deal with it in the future.'*

Effects of the Illness on Siblings

All of the parents were conscious of the effects of the illness on their other children. Again, there was a mixed response in terms of positive and negative effects although, in this respect, the negatives outweighed the positives. Indeed many of the parental responses were permeated with a sense of guilt about the other children in the family. Parents spoke about being focused on the child with cancer at a cost (to their other children) of time spent with them and attention paid to their needs. *'She really lost two years with us . . . She really lost out on a lot.'* Changes reported in siblings included fear, resentment, attention-seeking, guilt, worry, independence, and ongoing protectiveness in relation to the ill sibling. Problems at school, bed-wetting, and increased physical ailments were reported also.

In some respects, the parents felt that the siblings had suffered more than had the child with cancer. *'She (sister) was actually worse and I think she suffered worse. She's more insecure . . . probably she had to learn a hard lesson.'* This quote reflected the fact that the impact of the experience was often seen as ongoing. For example, another parent found herself shocked by a question posed by the brother of the child who had cancer years previously. *'It was only last year that he said he was worrying and asked 'Was it me that caused the cancer?' I knocked him.'* Relationship issues were linked to the siblings' experiences during the illness. One parent commented *'She kind of got very independent and even to this day, she sort of doesn't need anybody. She's very hard, actually. She doesn't like cuddles . . .'* In another family, the sibling was seen to take on *'a very responsible role. She maybe hid a lot of what she was feeling from us.'* In the parents' view, siblings coped best if they got as much attention as possible, were kept informed and involved in the illness process, and had other family members to give them the extra attention needed at the time *'She got so much attention, she coped very well. She had her Granny.'*

Parents were very aware of whether or not they treated the child with cancer differently from their other children. There was an equal division between those parents who had made a conscious effort not to give any sort of preferential treatment and those who felt that a child who had had cancer needed extra attention and care. Having a very ill child was seen to strengthen the parent-child bond, increase awareness of the uniqueness of the child within the family, and making the parent more 'tuned in' to the child's needs: *'It couldn't be just a normal relationship. We spent an awful lot of time together.'*

Anticipations for the Future

In relation to their own feelings about the child's future health, over two-thirds of the parents felt positive while the remainder expressed worries about some or all aspects of their child's health. Concern for the child's future focused on fears about survival as well as on the development of personal relationships, education, and employment. *'You see–it's over but it's not over. That's the worst of it now. I think that's the hardest. I know cancer can reoccur.'* In this context, searching for a cause, self-blame, anger, and guilt were ongoing preoccupations for this group of parents for whom the experience was still a dominant factor in their lives. *'You often say to yourself 'Why did it happen?' 'What did I do?' You'd be blaming a lot of things for it.'*

Interestingly, half of the parents stated that the child's illness and treatment was never discussed within the family. Most of these ascribed this to the children themselves not wanting to talk about it *'. . . he never mentions it. He seems to have put it completely to the back of his head, he doesn't want to know about it.'* Another commented *'. . . she doesn't want any of her friends to know that she was sick.'* In some cases, the parents stated that they avoided mention of the illness on account of feelings of guilt and/or denial.

Three Wishes

In the interviews with the children with cancer and with their siblings, they were asked if they could have a magical three wishes, for what would they wish. The purpose of this was to find out the extent to which illness was reflected in their wish list. This question produced interesting results. While a wide range of wishes were expressed by the children with cancer, they could be broken down into categories relating to: material changes (*'be rich,' 'live in a mansion'*); having new things (*'a TV in my room,' 'a computer game,' 'a horse'*); meeting famous people (*'Michael Schumacher,' 'Boyzone'*); going on special holidays (*'go to Eurodisney,' 'visit cousins in Canada'*); ambitions (*'be a singer,' 'play for Manchester United'*); changes in the self (*'be thinner,' 'have longer hair'*); and those specifically relating to illness (*'that never got a tumour,' 'get better,' 'illness never to happen again'*).

The wish list of siblings was equally wide ranging and reflected the same broad areas. The siblings' wishes in relation to illness reflected their experience of illness within the family (*'that he was never sick,' 'for it (cancer) never to happen to kids,' 'to have nobody sick,' 'that she gets well properly, no hospital, no moods'*). Table 3 shows the percentage of wishes relating to illness for the children with cancer and their siblings. Given the context in which the wish question was asked, it could be expected that wishes in relation to illness would be expressed. It is interesting to note the overall percentage of children who expressed wishes relating to illness and that it was the siblings, rather than the children with cancer, who expressed such wishes more often.

DISCUSSION

The realisation that your child has cancer is likely to be one of the most stressful life events a parent will experience. An overwhelming sense of despair can disrupt the lives of each member of a family at an emotional, physical, and practical level. Professionals in the field of paediatric oncology are witness to such effects on families. Social workers, in particular, on account of their family oriented involvement, are aware of the degree of upset and disruption a diagnosis of cancer can have on the family unit. Fortunately, the success rate in treating children with cancer is improving. More will now survive the disease than will die. Of increasing concern, therefore, is whether or not diagnosis and treatment of cancer will have long-term psychosocial effects on the child, the parents, siblings, and on the family as a whole. One means of assessing this is through the use of standardised instruments in relation to pertinent areas such as coping and perceived health status. Increasingly, however, the importance of incorporating the respondents' subjective experiences and views is recognised.

TABLE 3. Percentage of Wishes Relating to Illness for Children with Cancer and Their Siblings

	Children with cancer	Siblings
1st wish	15%	13%
2nd wish	7%	32%
3rd wish	13%	13%
Total	12.5%	19%

The use of qualitative and quantitative methods in this study provided a rounded picture of the children and their families after a substantial time lapse since completing treatment. The fundamental question was whether the diagnosis and treatment of cancer had had serious long-term effects on the children's psychosocial development. Overall, a positive picture emerged from this study of the majority of children and families able to move on with their lives in the aftermath of cancer. However, within these very positive findings, there is evidence of a small number of children and their families who have ongoing difficulties. Analysis of the data by diagnostic group, socio-economic circumstances, family composition and gender did not show any significant differences. The only factor in the children's adjustment seemed to be one of age indicating that those approaching or having reached adolescence may benefit from psychosocial follow-up.

A particular feature of this study was the relatively high participation rate of fathers. Our findings on the coping strategies of mothers and fathers were similar to the studies cited above. The results of the COPE Scale and the qualitative interviews showed that fathers typically used the coping strategies of avoidance and dependence on their spouses as their sole means of emotional support. Knowledge of such differences is important for understanding how each cope with stressful situations and indicates how professionals can use this knowledge to involve both parents meaningfully in the treatment process. It is also noteworthy that the parents in this study identified the period immediately following the cessation of treatment to be particularly stressful.

Only a small number of grandparents took part in the study. Those who did participate saw their role as being supportive to their own child, the parent of the child in treatment. However, the grandparents indicated a very negative view of cancer, regarding it as a death sentence. If they can be helped in their role as providing appropriate emotional and practical support, it would be important that they be provided with up to date information on improved treatment outcomes.

In hindsight, one of the parents' major concerns was the impact of the illness on the siblings. At the time of diagnosis and treatment, parents were aware of the problems for siblings but were often unable to deal with their needs effectively on account of the physical and emotional demands of having a child with cancer. From the interviews it was evident that feelings of neglect and of being of lesser importance on the part of siblings do not necessarily diminish when the treatment has ended successfully. Such findings indicate the need for them to be included as much as possible at the treatment stage and that parents are helped, in terms of information, support, and practical help, to respond to the needs of siblings in these circumstances. Support services for siblings, both at the time of treatment and subsequently, could offer help to this subset of the family who would seem to be particularly vulnerable.

Carrying out the research in the families' homes inevitably led to the dangers of distraction and interruption of the research process. However, this was well compensated by the fact that it was carried out in the respondents' own familiar setting. While the response rate was very high, there was a sizeable percentage of the original sample (19%) that was non-contactable and a further 4% who refused the invitation to participate. The question arises as to whether or not this subset would have been different those who participated in the study. The importance of social support for families where a child is seriously ill is evident in the results. The particular role played by close family members in providing support is clearly important. The grandparents who participated in the study provided interesting insights into their role and perspectives. However, the overall numbers of grandparents who participated was relatively small.

The results of this study overall indicated that most of the children were well adapted and coping effectively with all aspects of their lives. Further, in recollecting the period of diagnosis and treatment, the children's memories were by no means only negative. Parents for the most part were able to put the experience in the past in spite of some ongoing concerns about future implications for the child of having had cancer. Many of the parents were also able to identify some positive effects on themselves and on their family as a whole in the sense of changing priorities and bringing the family closer together. These findings are most encouraging for children currently undergoing treatment or recently post-treatment.

REFERENCES

Adams, D.W. & Deveau,E.J., 1988, *Coping with Childhood Cancer: Where Do We Go From Here?* Canada: Kinbridge Publications.

Asher, S.R. & Wheeler,V.A., 1985, Children's Loneliness: A Comparison of Rejected and Neglected Peer Status, *Journal of Consulting and Clinical Psychology*, Vol. 53, pp. 500-505.

Battle, J., 1992, *Culture-Free Self-Esteem Inventories*, Austin: Pro-Ed.

Carver, C.S., Scheier, M.F. & Weintraub, J.K., 1989, Assessing Coping Strategies: A Theoretically-based Approach, *Journal of Personality and Social Psychology*, Vol. 56, No. 2, pp. 267-283.

Chesler, M., 1992, Introduction to Psychological Issues, *Cancer Supplement*, Vol. 17, No. 10, pp. 3245-3268.

Cincotta, N., 1993, Psychosocial Issues in the World of Children with Cancer, *Cancer Supplement*, Vol. 17, No. 10, pp. 3251-3260.

Dalquist, L., Czyzewski, S. & Jones, C., 1996, Parents of Children: A Longitudinal Study of Emotional Distress, Coping Style and Marital Adjustment Two and Twenty Months after Diagnosis, *Journal of Pediatric Psychology*, Vol. 21, No. 4, pp. 541-544.

Eiser, C. & Havermans, T., 1992, Children's Understanding of Cancer, *Psycho-Oncology*, Vol. 1, pp. 169-181.

Elliott Brown, K.A. & Barbarin, O.A., 1996, Gender Differences in Parenting a Child with Cancer, *Social Work in Health Care*, Vol. 22, No. 4, pp. 53-71.

Friedman, A. & Mulhern, R., 1991, Psychological Adjustment among Children who are Long-term Survivors of Cancer in Johnson, J.A. & Johnson, S.B. (Eds), *Advances in Child Health Psychology*, University of Florida Press.

Goldberg, D., 1981, *General Health Questionnaire*, NFER-Nelson.

Gresham, F.M. & Elliott, S.N., 1990, *Social Skills Rating System*, Circle Pines: American Guidance Service.

Hamama, R., Ronen, T. & Feigin, R., 2000, Self-Control, Anxiety, and Loneliness in Siblings of Children with Cancer, *Social Work in Health Care*, Vol. 31, No. 1, pp. 63-83.

Heffernan, S. & Zanelli, A., 1997, Behavioural Changes Exhibited by Siblings of Pediatric Oncology Patients: A Comparison Between Maternal and Sibling Descriptions, *Journal of Pediatric Oncology Nursing*, Vol. 14, No. 1., pp. 3-14.

Janus, M. & Goldberg, S., 1997, Factors Influencing Family Participation in a Longitudinal Study: Comparison of Pediatric and Healthy Samples, *Journal of Pediatric Psychology*, Vol. 22, No. 2, pp. 245-262.

Kupst, M., Natta, M., Richardson, C., Schulman, J., Lavigne, J. & Lakshmi, D., 1995, Family Coping with Pediatric Leukaemia: Ten Years After Treatment, *Journal of Pediatric Psychology*, Vol. 20, No. 10, pp. 19-41.

Leventhal-Belfer, L., Bakker, A. & Russo, C., 1993, Parents of Childhood Cancer Survivors: A Descriptive Look at Their Concerns and Needs, *Journal of Psychosocial Oncology*, Vol. 11, No. 2, pp. 14-41.

Martinson, I., Gilliss, C., Colaizzo, D., Freeman, M. & Bossert, E., 1990, Impact of Childhood Cancer on Healthy School-Age Siblings, *Cancer Nursing*, Vol. 13, No. 3, pp. 183-190.

Offer, D., Ostrov, E., Howard, K.I. & Dolan, S., 1992, Offer Self-Image Questionnaire Revised, California: Western Psychological Services.

Pelcovitz, D., Goldenberg, B., Kaplan, S., Weinblatt, M., Mandel, F., Meyers, B. & Vinciguerra,V., 1996, Post-traumatic Stress Disorder in Mothers of Pediatric Cancer Survivors, *Psychosomatics*, Vol. 37, No. 2., pp. 116-127.

Roberts, C.S., Turney, M.E. & Knowles, A.M., 1998, Psychosocial Issues of Adolescents with Cancer, *Social Work in Health Care*, Vol. 27, No. 4, pp. 3-18.

Rollins, J., 1993, Childhood Cancer: Siblings Draw and Tell, *Pediatric Nursing*, Vol. 16, No.1, pp. 21-27.

Schroff-Pendley, J., Dalquist, L. & Dreyer, Z., 1997, Body Image and Psychosocial Adjustment in Adolescent Cancer Survivors, *Journal of Pediatric Psychology*, Vol. 22, No. 1, pp. 29-43.

Shields, G., Schondel, C., Barnhart, L., Fitzpatrick,V., Sidell, N., Adams, P., Fertig, B., & Gomez, S., 1995, Social Work in Pediatric Oncology: A Family Needs Assessment, *Social Work in Health Care*, Vol. 21, No. 1, pp. 39-54.

Van Dongen-Meldman, J., Pruyn, J., DeGroot, A., Koot, M., Hahlen, K. & Verhulst, F. (1995), Late Psychosocial Consequences for Parents of Children Who Survive Cancer, *Journal of Pediatric Psychology*, Vol. 20, No. 5, pp. 567-586.

Coping and Resilience of Children of a Mentally Ill Parent

Pirjo Pölkki, PhD
Sari-Anne Ervast, MSSc
Marika Huupponen, MSSc

SUMMARY. This paper examines the needs and stress reactions of children of mentally ill parents, as well as coping and resilience. The study is based on the interviews of six 9-11 years old children and narratives of seventeen female grown up children of mentally ill parents. The younger and older children of the mentally ill parents had not been informed about their parent's illness. The illness of the parent aroused a variety of emotions in them. The children used both practical problem solving and emotional coping mechanisms. Informal social support was available to them but seldom from the public services. It is recommended that professionals in mental health and child welfare services

Pirjo Pölkki is Professor, University of Kuopio, Department of Social Work and Social Pedagogy, Kuopio, Finland. Sari-Anne Ervast is Social Worker, Helsinki City, Finland. Marika Huupponen is Social Worker, Rantasalmi Municipality, Finland.

Address correspondence to: Pirjo Pölkki, PhD, University of Kuopio, Department of Social Work and Social Pedagogy, P.O. Box 1627, 70211 Kuopio, Finland (E-mail: Pirjo.Polkki@uku.fi).

The authors are indebted to the Central League of Mental Health in Finland for allowing the use of their material for the study. The authors offer thanks to both the younger and older children for their kind assistance.

[Haworth co-indexing entry note]: "Coping and Resilience of Children of a Mentally Ill Parent." Pölkki, Pirjo, Sari-Anne Ervast, and Marika Huupponen. Co-published simultaneously in *Social Work in Health Care* (The Haworth Social Work Practice Press, an imprint of The Haworth Press, Inc.) Vol. 39, No. 1/2, 2004, pp. 151-163; and: *Social Work Visions from Around the Globe: Citizens, Methods, and Approaches* (ed: Anna Metteri et al.) The Haworth Social Work Practice Press, an imprint of The Haworth Press, Inc., 2004, pp. 151-163. Single or multiple copies of this article are available for a fee from The Haworth Document Delivery Service [1-800-HAWORTH, 9:00 a.m. - 5:00 p.m. (EST). E-mail address: docdelivery@haworthpress.com].

clarify their roles when working with mentally ill parents. The best interest of the child and the parenting they need should be carefully assessed. Open care measures should be offered to families early enough to prevent serious child welfare and mental problems. *[Article copies available for a fee from The Haworth Document Delivery Service: 1-800-HAWORTH. E-mail address: <docdelivery@haworthpress.com> Website: <http://www.HaworthPress.com>* © 2004 by The Haworth Press, Inc. All rights reserved.]*

KEYWORDS. Stress reactions, coping, resilience in children, mentally-ill parents, social support, multiprofessional cooperation, psychoeducative methods

INTRODUCTION

The growth of open psychiatric care has increased the time that seriously mentally ill parents spend with their children. Many children also live with their single parent. In order to save children from the problems of adults, children of mentally ill parents are often left outside the care of their parents and without any support from adults.

The onset of the serious mental illness of the parent can be a dramatic life event, which may cause stress reactions both to children and adults and change the everyday life of the family in many ways. There are also quite a few children who are in families with one or both parents having mental health problems. Serious mental illnesses are always challenging for multiprofessional network and one of the reasons for child protection and the placement of children outside home.

After having encountered some children of mentally ill parents in the street at night time, Swedish social welfare workers (Skerfving 1999) asked how psychiatric care recognises the needs of these children. Their question led to a research project. This was due to the fact that in the Nordic countries, as well as in many other countries, there is a lack of information concerning the lives of children in a family with a mentally ill parent. Plenty of studies have been made on the children at risk of mental illness, e.g., schizophrenia or depression, but only a few studies are concerned with the life conditions, experiences, and needs of children living with a parent with a serious mental illness.

Parents with severe mental disorders may have difficulties providing physical and emotional care or may fail to show consistency of care (Masten, Best & Garmezy, 1990). Dunn's retrospective data (1993), based on the interviews of nine adults reared by mothers diagnosed with psychosis, revealed abuse and isolation, guilt and loyalty, social support, resilience and coping as well as grievances concerning mental health services.

There is also a dearth of literature on child carers. Based on different British sources of information, Blyth and Milner (1997, 59-73) summarize the central features and characteristics of the phenomenon 'young carer,' as well as the possible influence this thing can have on the child's development. A definition could be that a young carer is a child or a young person under the age of eighteen who carries out significant caring tasks and assumes such responsibility for another person that would normally be assumed by an adult. It has been estimated that nearly half of all young carers are living with and caring for a mentally ill relative or an alcoholic or drug addict. Young carers usually care for their parents, or occasionally siblings.

Aldridge and Becker (1995) suggest that for many children, caring for others can imply some sort of covert punishment by family, friends, and caring professions. They have found that young carers' lives both as carers and as children are fraught with anxiety, stress and uncertainty. Young carers may, however, derive from other people also positive feedback concerning their caring relationship and maturity (Blyth & Milner, 1997).

There is a need of a study examining subjective experiences of children caring for their mentally ill parents, and the impact of caring on the young person's coping, life style, and growth. Too little is known how the public services respond and how they should respond to the needs of young carers for their mentally ill parents. Also the coping and resilience of children who are not carers but are affected by the psychological and emotional distress caused by their parents' severe mental disorder should be examined.

The children have much to tell about the family life with their mentally ill parent and about their own coping and resilience in challenging circumstances. The narratives are mainly told by adult children of mentally ill parents; younger children have seldom been subjects. The experiences of small children should be heard too. For child interviews special skills are needed, and the ethical points of view must be taken into careful consideration (Andersson, 1998).

AIMS AND PROBLEMS

Our aim was to get information about the personal experiences of younger and older children of seriously mentally ill parents. The questions were:

1. How do the children experience the mental illness and parenthood of their parent?
2. What kind of stress reactions do the children have?
3. How do children cope with daily situations?
4. What is the resilience of these children in the long run?
5. What kind of informal and professional help do the children of mentally ill parents need and get?

SUBJECTS AND MATERIALS

The first sample is based on the data collected in the writing competition arranged by the Central Federation of Child Welfare on the theme 'How my life changed after a member of my family became mentally ill' (Peltoniemi, 1996). The narratives tell about the life of 17 children, six of whom lived with a mentally ill father and eleven with a mentally ill mother. All seventeen texts analysed here were written by women. The youngest of the writers was fifteen, and the oldest writers were living their late adulthood. Fifteen of the writers had lived in a nuclear family with two parents, and two of the writers lived with a single mother. Four of the stories also described the experiences of people who continued to take care of their mentally ill mother/father in her/his own family.

Nearly all of the mentally ill parents, had been in psychiatric inpatient care. The diagnoses mentioned included psychosis and serious depression. Four of the writers had experienced the suicide of a family member. Two respondents witnessed their parents' divorce in their childhood.

The data were analysed by means of qualitative computer program Nud*ist which is based on grounded theory (Strauss & Corbin, 1990, 23). The grounded theory is data-based. The themes dealt with the experiences and feelings of the children at the time of the onset of the parent's mental illness, as well as family roles and parenthood, coping strategies and resilience, social support and professional help.

The narrators very vividly described their experiences, coping skills, the support they received, parenthood, and the roles played by the other members of the family. One cannot definitely base one's assumptions on these narratives, or the exact source of these matters, nor can one assume which of these factors have resulted from the parents' illnesses. It can be noted, however, that the experiences of all the narrators were very similar.

The second sample comprises thematic interviews given by six children, aged between 9 and 11 years. The professionals helped in finding the families with one mentally ill parent and informed them about the study procedures. The children belonged to five families, two of them to the same family. Five of the children had a manic depressive mother and one had a mentally ill stepfather. The children were interviewed at the rehabilitation camp or at home. The interviewer carefully learned to know the children and succeeded in forming a good rapport with them. The children also had permission for interviews from their parents.

The main themes were family and parenthood, mental illness of parent, fears and worries, the stress reactions, and coping with daily life. Also social support from one's siblings, parents, and people outside the family were considered.

The data were gathered by the thematic interviews, which were 25-75 minutes long. The children found it difficult to tell about their life. The difficulty of the topic was reflected in restless non-verbal communication of some of the children. The interviews were tape recorded and transcribed, and classified into categories on the basis of grounded theory.

RESULTS

Children's Experiences of Their Parents' Serious Mental Problems

The adult children of a mentally ill parent were usually unprepared for the changes in their parents when these started to suffer from a serious mental illness. Two of the writers were born to a mentally ill mother. One of them wrote that her mother had always been different from the other children's mothers and that the writer got used to it. She could not know whether her mother's unusual behaviour was due to her mother's illness, but she had received some information of her mother's mental problems from other family members and peers.

The mentally ill mother or father often changed into a totally different person. One writer expressed that the most difficult thing for the people close to the mentally ill was their inability to share his/her delusion world. Two of the ill parents became very quarrelsome, violent, and frightening, and their children lost their sense of security and well-being. One father committed suicide, killing also his wife.

The younger children told that they were not informed about the illness of their parent. They demanded to know more. They were able to make very detailed observations and vividly described how the parent looks like and what (s)he does or does not do when in poor condition.

They often described the passivity of the adult as tiredness. They also observed the emotions of the parents and expressed their relief when the parent was able to better participate in everyday life of the family and to be interested in the child's personal matters (see Figure 1).

The younger children, however, felt rather safe at home. They were allowed to socialise with their peers and also felt at certain times better to be invisible–not to be in the way of the sick parent who lacked energy.

Excerpt from a spontaneous dialogue during the interview:

> C: What did mother do? I wonder . . . if she fell asleep. She usually sleeps all days.
>
> I: Well, yes . . .
>
> C: And she nearly always wakes up at night when the others go to bed . . .
>
> I: Yes, she sleeps at daytime.
>
> C: And she sleeps at night as well. She eats and falls asleep again.

The older respondents wrote that the family life had to be lived on the conditions of the sick parent who often isolated from friends, acquaintances, and relatives. Half of the families socialised very little outside home. Need of information was very common, and the nature of the parent's illness was not explained to the children.

Children's Responsibilities in Families with a Mentally Ill Parent

The serious mental illness of a parent changed the roles and responsibilities of other family members as well as those of parenthood itself. Nearly all writers mentioned that the sick parent lost his/her role as the carer for the family. The sickness weakened the strength of the parent and left him/her buried in his/her private world.

In most cases the person who took the responsibility was not the spouse. If the mother was mentally ill, the healthy father often worked intensively and left everyday chores to children or (in two cases) to grandparents. Three fathers drank heavily, and two left their family after a divorce.

The wives of mentally ill husbands tried to sustain the family, but children had to take responsibilities as well despite their youth. They

FIGURE 1. Mental Illness of a parent as described by a child

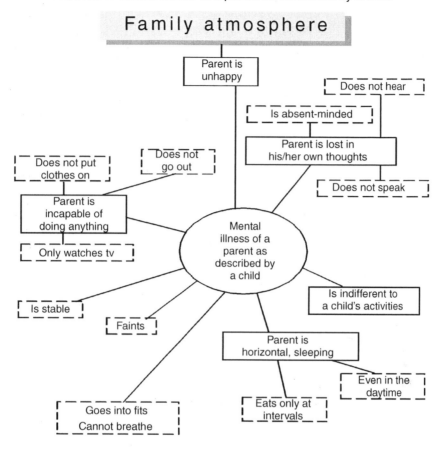

did every chore and took care of their younger sisters and brothers. In many cases they also were worried about the poor financial situation of the family. One of the writers felt that she "lost her mother and received a sick relative instead." One child of a mentally ill mother described that she had become "the mother of her mother." Two writers continue taking care for their mentally ill parents in their own family.

The younger children did not tell about their carer role. One of the children seemed to take care of the younger children in the camp all the time. She felt it was her duty and was abler to concentrate on her own program after getting support from her counsellor.

Stress Reactions of Children with a Mentally Ill Parent

The onset of the illness was sometimes very dramatic, changing the life of the family totally. The children expressed a variety of emotions. One respondent wrote:

> There was suddenly a huge amount of emotions, deep emotions. There are no words to describe the amount of fear and guilt. We only tried to cope somehow. In practice, it meant that everybody kept their emotions inside.

Many types of stress reactions and ways of coping could be found in the stories written by people who had spent their childhood with a mentally ill parent. The parent's mental illness was a shameful secret in many of the families. The children were not allowed to tell their classmates, neighbours, or relatives about things that happened at home. One mother asked her child to tell people that her father was on a business trip when he actually was receiving psychiatric treatment. Some of the children were bullied at school because of the mental problems of the parents. Some writers envied "healthy" families and some expressed their hatred towards the weakness of the sick parent and their dependency on other people (see Figure 2).

The results describing the experiences of the children of mentally ill parents are very similar to those of Dunn's study (1993) "Growing up with a psychotic mother," although the narratives analysed by us dealt with life with mentally ill mothers and fathers.

Indirectly, the texts also showed the loyalty of the children although they did not tell very much about the child's love towards the sick parent. The children felt that helping the parent was their duty. One of the writers became angry at the social worker who asked her to move away from her mentally ill mother. Attachment and consideration can also be found from the writings. One story was about a gentle and jovial father without any power in the family.

The younger children could not describe their emotions, but their body language indicated confusion and nervousness when telling about the mentally ill parent. They also had fears and worries concerning the well-being of their parent. They disliked the visits to the mental hospital. This is clearly revealed in the following dialogue:

I: Has your mother been in a hospital?

C: Yes, in two hospitals.

I: Did you visit her?

C: (hesitant voice)

I: Do you remember what it was like in there?

C: It was not nice. There was a lady . . . who walked around muttering and babbling all the time . . .

I: Yes, it must have been a bit . . .

C: It was not nice when everything looked just awful!

FIGURE 2. Mental illness of a parent as described by an adult child

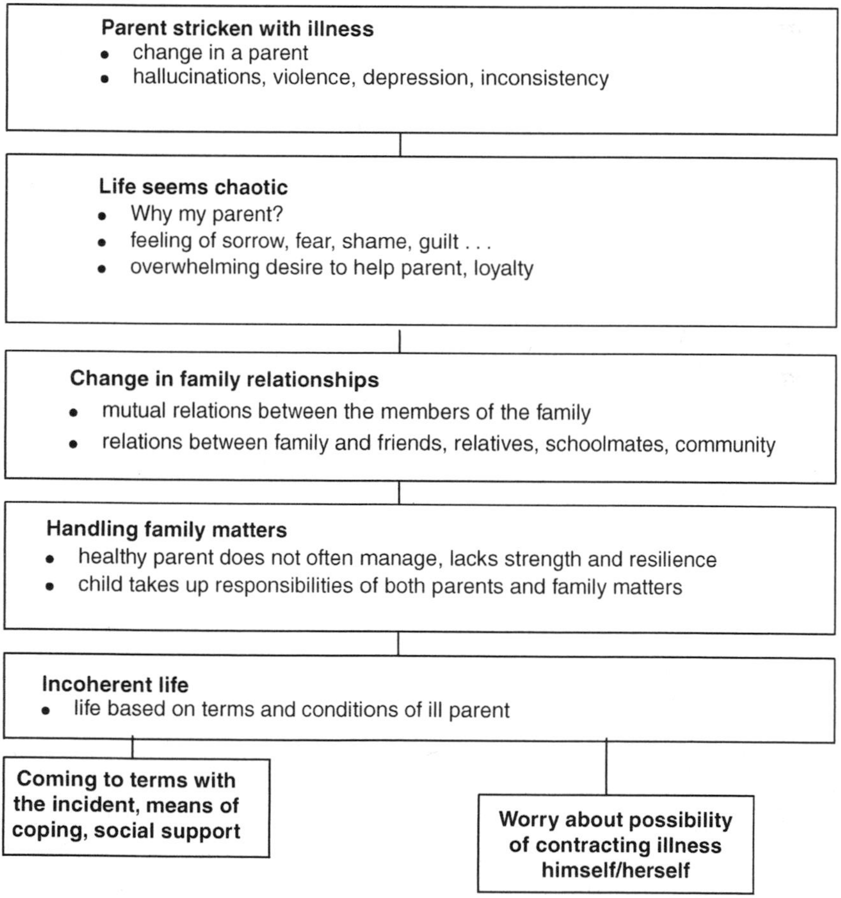

Parent stricken with illness
- change in a parent
- hallucinations, violence, depression, inconsistency

Life seems chaotic
- Why my parent?
- feeling of sorrow, fear, shame, guilt . . .
- overwhelming desire to help parent, loyalty

Change in family relationships
- mutual relations between the members of the family
- relations between family and friends, relatives, schoolmates, community

Handling family matters
- healthy parent does not often manage, lacks strength and resilience
- child takes up responsibilities of both parents and family matters

Incoherent life
- life based on terms and conditions of ill parent

Coming to terms with the incident, means of coping, social support

Worry about possibility of contracting illness himself/herself

Coping and Resilience of the Children of Mentally Ill Parents

Children at risk of psychosocial problems often show varying levels of success across different adjustment domains (Luthar, 1993). Children living with a mentally ill parent may have good practical coping skills, e.g., as for household chores, but they may be lonely and helpless with their rainbow of emotions.

The grown-up children of mentally ill parents estimated that they had, after all, coped rather well. As children they tried to use many kinds of practical and emotional strategies to cope. Their life had been difficult, but they emphasised the importance of learning and inner growth. Some children had a pleasant hobby they could spend time with. They did rather well at school although some writers had periods in their lives when they did not do so well at school and played truant. Some families moved to a different place and had a new start.

All writers had good social support, usually a sister, brother, or friend they could share their experiences with. Family members could understand each other in a situation which outsiders might have found strange. The children sometimes visited other people without telling them about their difficult situation at home. Nevertheless, the children felt that these visits gave them strength and helped them to see more normal life.

Not all writers, however, coped well in the long run. Three of them had mental problems themselves, and one became an alcoholic. The sister of one respondent became an anorectic and the other sister committed suicide.

Most of the younger children seemed to cope reasonably well despite the worries they had. Different types of mental illnesses may affect parenting in various ways. These families had asked for help. The relationship with mother was very close but the relationship with father, stepfather, or mother's boyfriend was often distant. The children succeeded at school and had siblings, pets, peers, and friends. One of the children, however, had a very defensive attitude and started to deny his emotional needs.

On the basis of this and some other studies (e.g., Beardslee & Podorefsky, 1988; Solantaus & Beardslee, 1996), "the resilient child" of a mentally disturbed parent

- is aware of the mental problems of his/her parent
- is able to put his/her thoughts into words and share his/her experiences

- is capable of discerning himself/herself from the emotional experiences of the parent
- does not render himself/herself guilty of the situation
- has another resilient parent or supporting adult who handles everything well
- gets a boost for himself/herself and his/her self-esteem even from beyond the walls of home

Role of Professional Help

Psychologically overwhelming events such as parent's mental illness can be either sudden and unexpected or long-standing and repetitive (Udwin, 1993). Some children are vulnerable and easily develop stress reactions and longstanding problems if they do not have protective factors and processes like social support in their environment. Few writers had received professional help as a child. As adults, the writers emphasised that they would have needed professional help but were not able to ask for it.

One of the reasons for the lack of public services can be the false assumptions social and health care professionals have concerning the availability and quality of support for families. Carers often tend to regard themselves not as carers but simply think that they "take the responsibility they obviously need to take under the circumstances." Parents do not wish to be seen as "failing parents" because they and their children may have fears of negative consequences of identification and a fear of separation (Alridge & Becker, 1993; Blyth & Milner, 1997, 59).

Child welfare legislation in different countries emphasises the best interest of the child in terms that are more or less explicit. In the social welfare system, open care measures for the families of mentally ill parents to assess and support parenting should be developed. The healthy spouses need support to prevent the situation in which they would leave the family. Often there is a need for a child welfare social worker who can help the whole family for a longer period of time and see that the needs of the children are met.

Both young and grown-up children of a seriously mentally ill parent often complained that they did not get any information concerning the illness of their parent. In order to give information and provide possibility to share traumatic experiences with others, pedagogical groups for the children of mental patients have been successfully arranged, e.g., in Sweden and Finland (Skerfving, 1998; Inkinen, 1999).

The effect of five-year long family counselling program (Aronen, 1993) has proven to have positive effects on the mental health of the children in low- and high-risk families. The effect was shown in the ten-year follow up-study. Only two of the subjects of our study received psychotherapy as a child and they were critical of its usefulness. In contrast, Dunn's (1993) study showed that eight of the nine children of mentally ill mothers who started psychotherapy as adults were satisfied with its results. Our opinion is that many of the subjects of our study could have benefited from psychotherapy.

It is time for "invisible children" of mentally ill parents to become visible (Fraiberg, 1974) in social and health care services.

Suggestions for future services:

1. Adult psychiatry should assess the situation of all the family members including children.
2. Meeting places of the children and parents in the mental hospitals must be made peaceful and cosy and children's participation in care negotiations must be developed.
3. Co-operation between child and adult psychiatry and social work, especially child protection services, should be developed. The best interest of the child and the parenting they need should be carefully assessed.
4. Open care child welfare measures should be offered early enough to support the children and the mentally ill and healthy parent. Active cooperation between mental health services, child welfare, day care, school and police are important.
5. Psycho-educational peer groups and–if needed–psychotherapy should be available for children of mentally ill parents.
6. Expertise in helping the children with mentally ill parents should be developed in the education of nurses, GPs and social workers.

CONCLUSIONS

These two small-scale studies reveal that learning to understand the experiences, needs, and coping of children of a mentally ill parent in everyday life is necessary. Giving more professional support to children as well as to their mentally ill and healthy parent may prevent unwanted developmental pathways. More specific research on these questions is needed.

REFERENCES

Aldridge, J. & Becker, S. (1993). Punishing Children for Caring. The Hidden Cost of Young Carers. Children and Society, Vol. 7, Issue 4, pp. 376-387.

Andersson, G. (1998). Barnintervjun som forskiningsmetod. Nordisk Psykologi 1, 18-41.

Beardslee, W.R. & Bodorefsky, M.A. (1988). Resilient Adolescents Whose Parents Have Serious Affective and Other Psychiatric Disorders: Importance of Self-Understanding and Relationships. *American Journal of Psychiatry, 145*(1), 63-69.

Blyth, E. & Millner, J. (1997). Social Work with Children and Youth. The Educational Perspective. Edinburgh Gate: Addison Wesley Longman Limited.

Dunn, B. (1993). Growing up with a Psychotic Mother. A retrospective study. *American Journal of Orthopsychiatry, 63*, 177-189.

Fraiberg, S. (1974). The invisible children. In E. Anthony & C. Koupernik (eds.), The syndrome of the psychologically invulnerable children. New York: John Wiley & Sons.

Inkinen, M. (1999). Lasten ryhmät omaistyön uutena mahdollisuutena. Labyrintti 1, 10-12.

Luthar, S.S. (1993). Annotation: Methodological and Conceptual Issues in Research of Childhood Resilience. *Journal of Child Psychology and Psychiatry, 34*, 41-453.

Masten, A.S., Best, K.M. & Garmezy, N. (1990). Resilience and Development: Contributions from the study of children who overcome adversity. Development and Psychopathology, 2, 425-444.

Peltoniemi, P. (ed.). (1996). Katson rohkeasti takaisin. Psyykkisesti sairaiden omaiset kirjoittavat. Mielenterveyden keskusliitto, Riihimäki.

Skerfving, A. (1998). Föräldrar och barn i den psykiatriska öppenvården. En kartläggning av patienternas föräldrarskap och enheternas rutiner. Rapport. FoU-enheten/psykiatri. Västra Stockholms Sjukvårdsområde.

Solantaus, T. & Beardslee, W. (1996). Interventio lasten psyykkisten häiriöiden ehkäisemiseksi. Duodecim, *112*(16), 1647-1655.

Strauss, A. & Corbin, J. (1990). Basics of Qualitative Research. Grounded Theory Procedure and Techniques. Printed in the USA. Sage Publications.

Udwin, O. (1993). Children's Reactions to Traumatic Events. *Journal of Child Psychology and Psychiatry, 34*, 115-127.

CITIZENSHIP AND PARTICIPATION OF USERS

The Experience of Urban Aboriginals with Health Care Services in Canada: Implications for Social Work Practice

Ron Levin, MSW, RSW
Margot Herbert, MSW, RSW

SUMMARY. This exploratory study investigates the experience of Canadian Urban Aboriginal persons as consumers of health care services. Results highlight significant gaps in the training, skills, and knowledge of health care providers to optimally serve their Aboriginal patients. Also, several programs which are potentially most problematic for Aboriginal patients are identified. The discussion outlines important roles for hospital social workers in improving the care provided to urban Aboriginal patients.

Ron Levin is Associate Professor, University of Calgary, Faculty of Social Work, Edmonton Division, #444, 11044-82 Avenue, Edmonton, AB T6G 0T2, Canada (E-mail: rlevin@ualberta.ca). Margot Herbert is Associate Professor Emerita, University of Calgary, Faculty of Social Work, Edmonton Division, #444, 11044-82 Avenue, Edmonton, AB T6G 0T2, Canada (E-mail: fherbert@ualberta.ca).

[Haworth co-indexing entry note]: "The Experience of Urban Aboriginals with Health Care Services in Canada: Implications for Social Work Practice." Levin, Ron, and Margot Herbert. Co-published simultaneously in *Social Work in Health Care* (The Haworth Social Work Practice Press, an imprint of The Haworth Press, Inc.) Vol. 39, No. 1/2, 2004, pp. 165-179; and: *Social Work Visions from Around the Globe: Citizens, Methods, and Approaches* (ed: Anna Metteri et al.) The Haworth Social Work Practice Press, an imprint of The Haworth Press, Inc., 2004, pp. 165-179. Single or multiple copies of this article are available for a fee from The Haworth Document Delivery Service [1-800-HAWORTH, 9:00 a.m. - 5:00 p.m. (EST). E-mail address: docdelivery@haworthpress.com].

KEYWORDS. Urban Aboriginal consumers, health care services

INTRODUCTION

The Canadian Health Care System

A federal, ten provincial and two territorial governments govern Canadians. According to the provisions of the Canadian constitution (1867), the provinces have jurisdiction for the organization and delivery of health care along with other public services including education and social welfare. There are, however, several populations for whom the federal government retains primary responsibility for delivery of health services. These include members of the armed forces, the R.C.M.P., offshore federal employees, prisoners in federal facilities, and Aboriginal persons who are registered under the Indian Act of Canada. In order to ensure equality of health services to all Canadians, the federal government shares the cost of health care with the provinces. In 1996, the Canada Health and Social Transfer Act, which is the most recent legislation in this area, arranged for the transfer of a "block of funds," consisting of cash payments and "tax points" from the federal government to the provinces. This was to be applied towards hospital and medical insurance, post secondary education and welfare programs. The allocation of resources between these programs was left to the discretion of the provincial governments. However, the Canada Health Act (1984) stipulates the conditions with which provinces must comply to receive cash transfers each year. These conditions include: (a) public administration–the provincial health care insurance plan must be "administered and operated on a non profit basis by a public authority appointed or designated by the government of the province." This provision does not say who actually delivers the health care services; (b) comprehensiveness–the provincial health care insurance plan must " insure all insured health services provided by hospitals, medical practitioners or dentists, and where the law of the province so permits, similar or additional services rendered by other health care practitioners"; (c) universality–to satisfy this criterion the provincial insurance plan must "entitle one hundred percent of the insured persons of the province to the insured health services provided for by the plan on uniform terms and conditions"; (d) portability–this criterion requires that Canadians be covered when traveling within and outside of Canada, at the rate of their home province. Also it stipulates that the provincial plan "must not impose any minimum period of residence in the province, or waiting period in excess of three months before residents of the province are eligible or entitled to insured health services"; and (e) accessibility–this provision requires that the provincial plan "must provide for insured services on uniform terms and conditions and on the basis that does not impede or preclude, either directly or indirectly whether by charges made to insured persons or otherwise, reasonable access to those services by insured persons." Also the province must "provide for reasonable compensation for all insured health services rendered by medical practitioners or dentists" and pay hospitals for the "cost of insured health services." The CHA also sets out penalties if a province allows extra billing by health care providers or sets user fees.

Context

There are approximately 800,000 people in Canada who identify themselves as Aboriginal.[1] About 20 percent live in the seven largest cities in Canada, and another 25 percent live in smaller urban centers (Statistics Canada 1998). Over time, Aboriginal people in Canada have been subjected to systematic colonization and domination. Federal policy historically emphasized assimilation through such means as forcing Aboriginal children to attend residential schools away from their reserves and families, and adoption of Aboriginal children into non-Aboriginal families. It cannot be denied that the experience of oppression continues to affect Aboriginal individuals, families, and communities today. Our limited appreciation of the history, traditions, and values of Aboriginal people, and the impact of these experiences, represent a challenge for those who work with this population. A further challenge is that within the larger population of Aboriginal people there are many different language groups, tribal groups, and geographic settings. As well, it is necessary to distinguish between traditionalists and assimilated Aboriginal people, and those who may have found a way to bridge both the traditional world with modern reality (Morrissette et al., 1993). In spite of these differences, there tends to be a common "world view" among Aboriginal people, characterized by such fundamental beliefs as a connection to the earth which contributes to healing; a holistic view of the universe; a spiritual dimension infusing all aspects of a person's life; a belief that all creatures are linked and mutually interdependent for survival; and that supernatural phenomena constantly affect their lives. This perspective emphasizes harmony, natural laws, and rhythms of nature and sets the context for a group of values that can include, self-determination, a focus on the present, and adherence to traditional healing practices. These dominant characteristics continue to influence the lives of many Aboriginal people.

There is evidence that Aboriginal people are more likely to suffer from hypertension, heart disease, diabetes and other chronic illnesses than their non-Aboriginal counterparts (Shah, Hux, & Zinman 2000), and are therefore disproportionately represented on patient rolls of hospitals and outpatient health services. Although there is research that speaks to the broader socio-economic-cultural determinants of this situation, the actual health care experiences of Aboriginal people in Canada and elsewhere have not been well described (Cheung & Snowdon 1999; Strickland 1999). Since most health care providers are not Aboriginal, there is almost certainly some degree of cultural dissonance, which affects the ways that services are used and experienced by Aboriginal people (Mokuau & Fong 1994; Sanchez & Plawecki 1996; Weaver 1999) and may create barriers for those who seek help with health-related problems.

LITERATURE REVIEW

Mokuau and Fong (1994) suggest that the responsiveness of health services may be measured according to three criteria: availability, accessibility, and acceptability. It is objectively clear that when services are not readily available or accessible, there is concomitant low utilization. As with other human services, barriers associated with availability and accessibility generally correlate with low socio-economic status, which unfortunately is a reality for a huge majority of the Aboriginal population. Less obvious are barriers to utilization that result from health services offered in a way that is culturally unacceptable. When services are not compatible or congruent with cultural values and traditions, they are much less likely to be accessed, even by those who urgently need those services (Mokuau & Fong 1994; Weaver 1999).

Willms, Lange, Bayfield, Beardy, Lindsay, Cole, and Johnson (1992) reported that Aboriginal women, in particular, lacked trust in the health care system. Reasons cited include inexperience of doctors and nurses, lack of communication with patients, cultural insensitivity, and lack of knowledge or understanding of native healing practices. In general, health care providers were perceived to be philosophically and physically distant from their patients. Although this study was largely based on data from small communities, when moved to hospitals in larger centers these same patients reported feeling neglected and denigrated. General distrust of the system was compounded by difficulties in communication and lack of companionship. Gagnon (1989) also described how native patients who were referred to specialists and tertiary hospitals in urban centers were removed from their usual sources of support and understanding and often found themselves with little cultural, linguistic, and organizational understanding of the hospital.

The existence of serious communication problems between native patients and non-native health care providers was also documented in an earlier study of health facilities in a western Canadian city (Waldram & Layman 1989). Interestingly, a subsequent study (Waldram 1990) suggested that in some urban centers, the access issue may be more a function of socio economic status than that of being native. This study also suggested that Aboriginals who were most closely affiliated with their Aboriginal roots were more likely to access available health services. This may explain some of the problems of the urban Aboriginal population, many of whom are less grounded in cultural traditions than their rural counterparts.

Shah and Farkus (1985) described the general poor health of Aboriginal people in Canadian cities as a major challenge to the health care system. Their research cited difficulties in communication and unavailability of culturally sensitive health care services as major barriers to good health care. Shestowsky (1995) identified structural and attitudinal barriers as two major shortfalls in meeting the needs of Aboriginal people living in cities. In addition to a lack of information and programs, results pointed to problems in the areas of communication, provision of cultural services, and stereotyping on the part of providers within the health system. The problems faced by urban Aboriginals seeking health care services were also cited in a report sponsored by Alberta Health (Strengthening the Circle 1990). For elders, in particular, communication problems were prominent when seeking medical attention in hospitals or health centers. Other barriers had to do with lack of familiarity with hospital and medical practices; failure of health care staff to explain things; fear of doctors and other white people in authority; unfamiliar food; a feeling that no one was listening to them; and insensitive treatment.

A review of Aboriginal populations in other countries reveals commonalities in health care experiences with their Canadian counterparts. Both Australian Aborigines and Native Americans are also susceptible to the forms of chronic and stress related illnesses observed in Canadian

Aboriginal people (Lowe & Kerridge 1995). The actual health experiences of Australian and U.S. Aboriginals have not been well documented. What is described, however, are similar barriers to health care services as experienced by Canadian Aboriginals. Yuki (1986) identified problems encountered by the Native American community of Boston, Massachusetts in their contacts with a major hospital. These issues led her and a colleague to spearhead the development of a specialized clinic within the hospital to fill the gap in meeting the health care needs of the Aboriginal population.

Researchers from Australia and North America have called for culturally competent practice when dealing with the health and human service needs of indigenous people (Jackson & Ward 1999; Paterson 1997; Weaver 1998). Several efforts towards meeting the needs of urban Aboriginals were described. For example, in the U.S. the federal division of Indian Health Services employs specially trained Native community health representatives to act as liaisons between Native American communities and the health care system (Dubray & Sanders 1999). A very recent report of a community consultation on the state of urban Aboriginals in Edmonton, Canada found that most Aboriginals who move from rural to urban centers seem to do so for economic reasons. However, the rate of poverty and unemployment they experience seems to indicate that hopes for a better life in the city rarely materialize.

> Significant social problems continue to plague a substantial number of urban Aboriginal people, particularly women and youth. High rates of single parent families, difficulty entering the labour market, inadequate housing and inadequate health care remain problems for many Aboriginal people. (The Edmonton Urban Aboriginal Initiative, 1999, p. 70)

The Edmonton study pointed out that although approximately half of the Aboriginal people in Canada live in urban areas, relatively little research has been done relating to the health needs of this population.

METHOD

Seven key respondents were identified based on recommendations provided by informants with professional and personal knowledge of Aboriginal issues. The criteria for selection of key respondents were that each: (a) held a position which required frequent and broad interaction with urban Aboriginals, (b) possessed a comprehensive understanding of Aboriginal issues as well as the health care system, and (c) was able to clearly articulate his/her views. Six respondents were females and one male. Five were Aboriginal. Respondents included health professionals, administrators of Aboriginal health programs and directors of large inner-city health and social service agencies. We telephoned all key respondents to explain the project and to invite their participation. All agreed to allow the interviews to be tape-recorded. We then faxed the questionnaire together with a covering letter to each respondent several days before the interview. These letters confirmed the purpose of the project, the method, and time and date of appointment. Interviews were between 1-1/2 to two hours in length.

The questionnaire consisted of six open-ended questions. Three questions focused on the knowledge, skills, and attitudes of health professionals, two inquired about hospital programs and health services, and the final question asked the respondent to suggest changes which would make the health system more user friendly for urban Aboriginals. We utilized a grounded theory approach in which we incorporated input from one interview into the next, in order to obtain a final picture, which was as comprehensive as possible. After all interviews were completed, the audiotapes were reviewed, and responses were summarized and grouped into themes.

RESULTS

Knowledge

All respondents acknowledged that health care professionals possess the requisite technical knowledge to treat patients. However, they all indicated that there are profound difficulties in delivering treatment effectively to urban Aboriginals. According to one respondent, "professionals have scientific knowledge but not Aboriginal wisdom. Professionals are focused on scientific measurement but they can only measure twenty-five percent of the picture. They can't measure love, spirit, or emotion." Respondents asserted that the Aboriginal belief system emphasizes wholeness and the interconnection between mind, body, emotion, and spirit while western medicine reduces people to a collection of organs or diseases. Aboriginal spirituality is manifested in rituals such as the pipe ceremony, praying, smudging, circles, and sweats that are incongruent with highly secular western medicine. Three of the respondents indicated that many health professionals are respectful and motivated to learn but lacked training and sufficient insight.

There was significant agreement concerning the role of traditional culture in the lives of urban Aboriginals, particularly those who spend most of their time in the city. Some respondents insisted that most urban Aboriginal persons visit their home communities often and thus continue to be tuned in to their culture. Even those who visit infrequently are "seeking cultural wisdom and yearn to come to the well." However, several respondents pointed out that it is important not to assume that all Aboriginal people are the same. There are often differences in adherence to spiritual beliefs and practices, religious affiliation, kinship and interpersonal relationships, and lifestyle. These differences are based on various factors including personal life experience, socioeconomic status, education, and experience with non-Aboriginals.

Another gap in the knowledge of health care professionals identified by four respondents related to an understanding of the culture of poverty that is the lived reality of many urban Aboriginals. Health care treatment is often premised on having a place to live, food, financial resources, and expectations by health professionals of patient compliance are based on those assumptions. Another lived experience for many urban Aboriginals is growing up in institutional care. Several respondents also indicated that lack of knowledge on the part of health care professionals concerning traditional Aboriginal lifestyle is problematic, particularly when treating elderly urban Aboriginals and persons who spend a lot of time on their home reserves. Differences in diet, pace of life, air and water quality can all contribute to a sense of alienation.

Skills

All respondents agreed that health care professionals have the requisite technical competence but most do not possess the particular skills necessary to care for urban Aboriginal patients effectively. Primary among the skill deficits identified was communication and rapport building. Most often stressed by the respondents was the importance of listening. Aboriginals, particularly the elderly and inner city residents, are customarily not assertive in communication style so the listener must be patient and attentive to the message. This rarely happens in the hectic and fast paced health care environment. One respondent related the example of a diabetic man who refused to seek treatment because he felt that the health professionals had not listened to him. Another indicated that urban Aboriginals who were raised in Aboriginal communities often think in their first language even if not currently fluent in that language. Aboriginal languages often contain nuances not easily translatable into English. This posed difficulties when an Aboriginal patient had to absorb complex information and respond to health professionals in English, particularly when that Aboriginal person was in distress or affected by medications or alcohol. As a result, many Aboriginals in such situations felt humiliated and ridiculed. In a similar vein, another respondent asserted that health care providers usually do not have the skills to appropriately frame their questions, deal with spiritual issues, or approach an Aboriginal elder.

Attitudes and Values

All respondents asserted that health professionals lack the requisite attitudes and values to effectively serve Aboriginal consumers. The predominant scientific view has a different conceptualization of illness, a different orientation to time, and does not acknowledge the "sacred" (spirituality). Aboriginal attitudes and values as modeled by elders are more balanced in mind, body, emotions, and spirit. Also, the expert stance taken by most health professionals in dealing with patients contradicts the expectations of equality and mutual respect held by Aboriginal consumers.

Six respondents indicated that urban Aboriginals often experience discrimination and racism from health care providers. This stems, in part, from systemic discrimination imposed on Aboriginals and is compounded by policies and practices of health care institutions and providers. Ignorance of Aboriginal culture and traditions are also key factors. All respondents indicated that cross-cultural training can be crucial in changing this situation. However, several questioned whether such training could change basic attitudes. One respondent indicated that cross-cultural training (particularly Aboriginal specific content) is often absent from the education of health care providers and when present, offers only generalities and stereotypes. Such training rarely addresses urban Aboriginal realities defined by racism and poverty, nor the complex interplay between Aboriginal culture and the culture of poverty.

Problematic Services/Programs

Six respondents cited obstetrics/gynecology as a program that is most problematic for urban Aboriginals. One indicated that younger women often are uncomfortable with male physicians and when they are pregnant often do not consult a physician until the day they deliver. These women often worry that the doctor will be judgmental about their age and lifestyle. All agreed that another concern is the perceived possibility of intervention by child welfare authorities. While this concern is particularly strong for under-age women, it also felt by others who have a history of child welfare involvement and/or are single, without income. Another stated that grandparents might be afraid of losing grandchildren because the child welfare system considers them too old to provide appropriate care.

Five respondents indicated that emergency departments also pose problems. Aboriginal persons who tend not to see a physician until they are in severe pain use these departments more often. These respondents asserted that Aboriginals are often the victims of discrimination, citing numerous anecdotal accounts of being passed over in favour of less ill non-Aboriginals. Because many Aboriginals tend not to be assertive, they will leave before they are treated, even if acutely ill. These people will then often use non-prescription remedies or will borrow prescribed medications from friends. One respondent also cited problems with psychiatric services. Since there is little access to services in rural settings, Aboriginals use the urban mental health system, which they often experience as impersonal and discriminatory.

Health Care Settings

None of the respondents identified the health care setting (whether physician's office, community clinic, or hospital) as particularly responsive to the experience of Aboriginal consumers. Several expressed the view that all settings create fear and lack of trust on the part of Aboriginals who often experience discrimination and stigmatizing behavior. This is particularly true if the person is "not attractive" (defined by the respondent as possessing very pronounced Aboriginal features), is not well dressed, or behaves differently from non-Aboriginals. This situation is exacerbated by the fact that the entire health care system is underfunded and therefore professionals are too stretched to provide individualized care and attention. This is compounded by the fact that there are very few Aboriginal health professionals. Another aggravating factor is that a significant number of urban Aboriginal people lack supportive friends and family who can assist with childcare or transportation. Another issue mentioned by respondents had to do with the problem of keeping appointments scheduled months in advance since inner city Aboriginals tend to change residences frequently.

Recommended Changes

All respondents cited the importance of increasing the number of Aboriginal health care professionals and decision-makers. However, several identified barriers to this objective including lack of emphasis on science for Aboriginal students, lack of designated spots for Aboriginals in training programs, and lack of sensitivity to Aboriginal culture on the part of advanced education institutions.

Several respondents expressed the need for urban-based Aboriginal health centers with appropriate child care facilities and transportation. Others identified the need for staffing medi-centers and inner city agencies with nurse practitioners to reduce the use of hospital emergency departments. In addition, several respondents suggested outreach centers within emergency departments and the need for family residences to bolster kinship ties between urban Aboriginals and non-urban family members. The importance of expanded recognition and utilization of Aboriginal medicine as an adjunct to western treatment was also emphasized. Several respondents did cite some recent positive developments in specific hospitals. These included the establishment of native liaison positions, "gathering rooms" for patients and families, and acceptance of traditional ceremonies and foods.

DISCUSSION

Given the relatively small number of respondents in this study, results must be seen as preliminary and treated with caution. Nevertheless, it is clear that the experience of many Aboriginal people with the urban health care system is affected by various degrees of cultural insensitivity. The remedy, however, is more complex than simply exposing health care providers to courses on cultural sensitivity.

A basic problem is the tendency for well-educated health care providers to bring "expert" solutions to problems. This sort of problem solving, while sometimes necessary and helpful, needs to be tempered with sensitivity to a very different perception of knowledge than the one that comes from western education. In addition to requiring knowledge about "Aboriginal" behavior, those who provide service to this population need to develop communication skills which result in building rapport, and perhaps most importantly, understanding the perspective of those who see the world quite differently from most non-Aboriginal people. Clearly Aboriginal people experience overt racism, as well as subtle slights that are interpreted as racially motivated. Unfortunately, many health care providers have encountered Aboriginal people only when they are in the most difficult situations and are most vulnerable. As a result, negative stereotypes have become firm attitudes. Others, who have actually worked in Aboriginal communities, may have had the opportunity to know many healthy and happy Aboriginal people, so will bring a somewhat different perspective.

Most persons who live in chronic poverty, Aboriginals and non-Aboriginals, lack sufficient access to the health care system. Many access problems are clearly the result of a system that is generally under resourced. The results of this study indicate, however, that being Aboriginal may create additional problems. There is a complex interplay between the state of poverty and being Aboriginal that is not immediately understood by many non-Aboriginal helpers. Health care providers in a variety of settings are familiar with situations such as the Aboriginal woman who is trying to provide food, clothing, and shelter for her children on an extremely limited income, and confesses that the reason she has not been able to manage is that several family members are staying with her, eating scarce food, and generally disrupting her day-to-day life. Most health care providers would respond to that situation by encouraging this woman (in the name of client empowerment) to get rid of these unwelcome visitors. Often not understood are the cultural norms around this sort of "visiting" which make it impossible for an Aboriginal person to refuse to share with a friend or family member, and asking someone to leave her house would be unacceptable. The cultural norm of visiting is also often evidenced by the number of people who fill the hospital room of a sick friend or relative, sometimes to the annoyance of staff.

Longer than usual waiting time in emergency departments, failure of staff to communicate needed information, and disrespectful attitudes of some health care personnel are clearly experienced as racial bias. Groups that bring particular problems are young Aboriginal women, mothers of young children, and those Aboriginal women for whom seeking medical care from a male doctor is exceedingly difficult and traumatic due to the terrible legacy of authoritarianism and abuse that is so prominent in Aboriginal history.

RECOMMENDATIONS

The findings of this exploratory study are particularly relevant for social workers who have a professional obligation to ensure that consumers receive health services in a manner that is respectful and appropriate. In implementing this responsibility, social workers can bolster and enhance their contributions to the health care team as well as their employing organization. Hospital social workers can assume important and useful roles where Aboriginal populations are major users of health facilities. Specific interventions for social workers in health care to consider include the following:

- There are structural impediments for many Aboriginal patients having to do with lack of congruence between levels of government and subsequent confusion among health care providers regarding reimbursement for services. Lack of childcare in health facilities and long delays in accessing specialist care create additional barriers. Hospital social workers should become knowledgeable about these issues in order to fulfill their responsibilities as informed advocates for their Aboriginal clients.
- Social workers who work with Aboriginal clients must understand their worldview, and be sensitive to nuances related to culture, education, and ways of communicating, as well as the possibility that the social workers' own life experiences will affect the way they view this population. To achieve this, social work directors should ensure that their staff has appropriate training from knowledgeable and expert trainers.
- Social work staff and directors should interpret the special needs of Aboriginal patients to other health care providers, and facilitate training in cultural sensitivity for all members of the health care team.
- Directors should encourage and support hiring Aboriginal social workers and native liaison workers, and include the liaison workers as part of the social work department. This must be done with the awareness that the hospital bureaucracy may be a painful reminder for Aboriginal staff of the oppression that they have already experienced from hierarchically structured mainstream organizations.
- Social workers in Obstetrics and Gynecology should be attuned to the special concerns of young Aboriginal mothers, and liaise with local child protection agency and public health units to ensure that

these women receive support and are not alienated from the systems that can provide needed assistance. Understanding the reluctance of some Aboriginal women to be seen by a male doctor is also crucial.

- Social workers in emergency departments usually encounter the largest number of Aboriginal patients, and have a special responsibility to understand cultural norms, including the culture of poverty, and interpret those norms to other staff.

CONCLUSION

At a time when hospital social workers are attempting to create new roles and to acquire skills that will reinforce their usefulness in the hospital, there would be enormous "added value" if social workers could lead the way in bridging this very real gap in service for Aboriginal consumers. There is also a message here for those who teach or provide field supervision for social work students, regarding the importance of genuine and skilled cross-cultural practice. Clearly more research is needed in order to better describe and understand this complex issue, so the health care system becomes more available, accessible, and acceptable to urban Aboriginal people.

NOTE

1. First Nations, Metis and Inuit.

REFERENCES

Alberta Health Care (1990). Strengthening the Circle.
Cheung, F. K. & Snowden, L. R. (1990). Community mental health and ethnicity minority populations. *Community Mental Health Journal, 26* (3), 277-291.
Dubray, W. & Sanders, A. (1999). Interactions between American Indian ethnicity and health care. *Journal of Health and Social Policy, 10* (4), 67-84.
Edmonton Urban Aboriginal Initiative (1999).
Gangon, Y. (1989), Physician's attitudes toward collaboration with traditional healers. *Native Studies Review, 5* (1), 175-185.
Government of Canada. Canada Health Act. (R.S. 1985 c. C-6).
Herbert, M. & Levin, R. (1995). The advocacy role in hospital social work. *Social Work in Health Care, 22* (3), 71-83.

Jackson, L. R. & Ward, J. E. (1999). Aboriginal health: Why is reconciliation necessary? *Medical Journal of Australia, 170* (9), 437-40.

Lowe, M. & Kerridge, I. H. (1995). 'These sorts of people don't do very well': Race and allocation of health care resources. *Journal of Medical Ethics, 21* (6), 356-60.

Mokaua, N. & Fong, R. (1994). Assessing the responsiveness of health services to ethnic minorities of colour. *Social Work in Health Care, 20* (2), 23-33.

Morrissette, V., McKenzie, B., & Morrisette, L. (1993). Towards an Aboriginal model of social work practice. *Canadian Social Work Review,* 10 (1), 91-108.

Paterson, J. M. (1997). Meeting the needs of Native American families and their children with chronic health conditions. *Families, Systems and Health,* 15 (3), 237-41.

Sanchez, T. R. & Plawecki, J. A. (1996). The delivery of culturally sensitive health care to native Americans. *Journal of Holistic Nursing, 14* (4), 295-307.

Shah, C. & Farkas, C. (1985). The health of Indians in Canadian cities: A challenge to the health care system. *Canadian Medical Association Journal, 133,* 859-863.

Shah, B. R., Hux, J. E., & Zinman. (2000), Increasing rates of ischemic heart disease in the native population of Ontario, Canada. *Archives of Internal Medicine, 2000, 160,* 1862-66.

Shestowsky, B. (1995). Health-related concerns of Canadian Aboriginal people residing in urban areas. *International Nursing Review, 42* (1), 23-6.

Statistics Canada. 1996 Census: Aboriginal data. Ottawa, Canada.

Strickland, R. N. (1999). The importance of qualitative research in addressing cultural relevance: Experience from research with Pacific and Northwest Indian women. *Health Care for Women International, 20* (5), 517-25.

Waldram, J. & Layman, H. (1989). Health care in Saskatoon's inner city: A comparative study of native and non-native utilization patterns. Institute of Urban Studies, Winnipeg, Manitoba.

Waldram, J. (1990). Physician utilization and urban native people in Saskatoon, Canada. *Social Science Medicine, 30* (5), 579-589.

Weaver, H. N. (1998). Indigenous people in a multicultural society: Unique issues for human services. *Social Work, 43* (3), 203-11.

Weaver, H. (1999). Indigenous people and the social work profession: Defining culturally competent services. *Social Work, 44* (3), 217-225.

Willms, D., Lange, P., Bayfield, D., Beardy, M., Lindsay, E. A., Cole, D., & Johnson, N. (1992). A lament by women for the people, the land [Nishnawbi-Aski Nation]: An experience of loss. *Canadian Journal of Public Health, 83* (5), 331-334.

Yukl, T. (1986). Cultural responsiveness and social work practice: An Indian clinic's success. *Health and Social Work, 11* (3), 223-9.

Participation and Citizenship of Elderly Persons: User Experiences from Finland

Heli Valokivi, MScSocSc

SUMMARY. In the article the participation of the aged users and their relatives in a local health care and social service system will be discussed. How is their citizenship defined at the grass roots level? The research data were gathered during a case management project of the action research type in a Finnish rural municipality. The data of this study consist of 13 theme interviews: five elderly persons as care receivers and eight caregivers. The research approach is a dialogue between data based analysis and conceptual reasoning.

Citizenship rights and obligations and participation should be defined flexibly and individually in the context of the local health care and social services. In the research data the elderly persons and their caregivers described participation in multiple ways. The modes of participation vary from passive and active disengagement from the process to contacting, negotiating, cooperating, and demanding. *[Article copies available for a fee from The Haworth Document Delivery Service: 1-800-HAWORTH. E-mail address: <docdelivery@haworthpress.com> Website: <http://www.HaworthPress.com> © 2004 by The Haworth Press, Inc. All rights reserved.]*

Heli Valokivi is Research Fellow, Department of Social Policy and Social Work, FIN-33014 University of Tampere, Finland (E-mail: heli.valokivi@uta.fi).

[Haworth co-indexing entry note]: "Participation and Citizenship of Elderly Persons: User Experiences from Finland." Valokivi, Heli. Co-published simultaneously in *Social Work in Health Care* (The Haworth Social Work Practice Press, an imprint of The Haworth Press, Inc.) Vol. 39, No. 1/2, 2004, pp. 181-207; and: *Social Work Visions from Around the Globe: Citizens, Methods, and Approaches* (ed: Anna Metteri et al.) The Haworth Social Work Practice Press, an imprint of The Haworth Press, Inc., 2004, pp. 181-207. Single or multiple copies of this article are available for a fee from The Haworth Document Delivery Service [1-800-HAWORTH, 9:00 a.m. - 5:00 p.m. (EST). E-mail address: docdelivery@haworthpress.com].

Digital Object Identifier: 10.1300/J010v39n01_12

KEYWORDS. Elderly, health care and social services, participation, citizenship

Many research projects have pointed out the difficulties of elderly people and their relatives in coping with the complicated health care and social service system (Baldock 1997, 76; Glendinning 1998, 137-138). Client-centred and flexible services are often the aim of an individual worker, but the practice is often fragmented and inconvenient from the client's point of view (Ala-Nikkola & Sipilä 1996). The service system in Finland produces more and more specialised and elaborate services, but at the same time the service user is quite confused and often lacks information about the options (Lehto 2000, 35). The person in need may be marginalised onto the edge of the service system or outside it. Her/his full citizenship may be questioned although her/his formal membership status remains unchanged. In this article I will discuss the position of aged clients and their relatives in the local health care and social service system through the concept of citizenship. I examine possibilities and forms of participation, influencing and implementation of citizenship at the grass-roots level. What does user involvement look like from the service user's point of view?

FINNISH HEALTH CARE AND SOCIAL SERVICE SYSTEM

The Finnish welfare state developed into a Scandinavian social service state during the 1970s and 1980s (Alestalo 1994, 73; Nygren et al., 1997, 16-17). This means that the state and the municipalities are responsible for arranging and producing the health care and social services. The services are produced with public tax money for all citizens either free of charge or against a moderate fee. The municipalities are the main producers of the health care and social services (Anttonen & Sipilä 1996, 96). The reform of the state subsidy system and the implementation of the block grant model in 1993 increased municipal (local) responsibility in decision-making processes. The money received as state subsidy is no longer earmarked to certain purposes, but municipalities can decide independently on how to allocate it (Uusitalo & Konttinen 1995, 5; Sipilä & Anttonen 1994, 52-53).

In the 1990s Finland experienced a deep economic depression with the result that the Finnish welfare state has changed somewhat (Martimo 1998, 67). Public funding has diminished and emphasis has moved from universality to selectivity. In the health care and social services, means testing and differences between local systems have increased (Lehto & Blomster 2000, 173; Martimo 1998, 69-72). The thought patterns and policies adopted during the regression years have remained (Vaarama et al., 2000, 76-84). Especially care services for the elderly are determined according to the existing supply and individual needs-assessments are strictly professionally led (Kröger 2003, 32). There has been a major shift towards weakened universalism on social care services for elderly people (Kröger 2003; Lehto 1998).

The public sector produces both institutional and community-based services in Finland. In public opinion it is considered almost self-evident that the home help services and homes for the elderly are funded and run by the public sector. Traditionally, the emphasis in the care of the elderly has very much lain on the institutional sector. Since the late 1980s, one of the central aspirations in developing the service system has been to decrease institutional care and to support the possibility of living at home as long as possible by improving the community-based services, which includes, for example, support to informal caregivers (Lehto & Blomster 2000, 162). According to the most optimistic views, Finland is not dependent on the unpaid care work by women because the public sector takes part in the care of the elderly (Simonen 1993). The public service system has supported women's full-time participation in the working life (Kiiski 1993, 16-19). Children are not responsible for the maintenance of their parents, and daughters and daughters-in-law are not publicly considered natural caregivers (Julkunen 1993, 344). Despite this, services have always been produced mostly by the informal sector, spouses, and children (Vanhusbarometri 1999, 50), but this has remained more or less invisible. The informal caregivers have in many cases had to assume the role of supplementing the public services (Anttonen & Sipilä 2000, 175; Julkunen 1993, 344). Since the 1990s informal care by relatives, neighbours, and the voluntary sector has been more systematically included as a part of the service system (Lehto 2000, 34).

The functioning of the Finnish welfare state has been fairly secure and efficient, but there are difficulties in co-ordinating the services and the benefits, due to difficulties in communication and co-operation between the professions and the agencies (Lehto 2000, 33; see also Noro et al., 1992). Fragmented and specialised services operate from different points of departure, and no one is responsible for the entity of the services needed in individual cases, so that the user may receive inappropriate services (Kraan et al., 1991, 77-78; Baldock 1993). Means testing in each domain, especially in the provision of social services has increased (Anttonen & Sipilä 2000, 175). From the citizens' point of view, the care and services received may be random, fragmented, or non-existent.

CITIZENSHIP OF THE AGED IN THE SERVICE SYSTEM

One of the classical analyses of citizenship is written by T. H. Marshall (1950/1992). He defines citizenship as a full membership in the community. It includes three types of rights: civil, political, and social rights which have been considered as condition of citizenship. According to Ian Culpitt (1992, 6), the theory of citizenship was grounded in the primacy of the practical politics of universal social obligations and rights. Criticism has increased because the active expectations of citizenship have been combined with the passive expectations of welfare entitlements. Bill Jordan (1997, 262) points out that "in emphasising the demands of active citizenship, theorists are (usually unintentionally) strengthening the case of various kinds of exclusion."

Citizenship has also been defined in other ways. David Phillips and Yitzhak Berman (2001, 22) formulate three strands of definitions of citizenship: (1) liberal or individualistic citizenship based on rights to membership via formal status; (2) republican or communitarian citizenship where membership is achieved by taking an active participatory role in a self-determining community; and (3) libertarian citizenship based on the demand of consumers for publicly provided goods. Multilevel, that is local, national, and transnational citizenship rights and obligations do not exist in separate spheres; rather, there is interplay between them. Citizenship itself becomes fragile. In contrast to Marshall's initial statement, we have to consider citizenship more as a process and less as a status (Roth 2000, 26-27). Citizenship is one of the core concepts to consider citizen affiliation with different services.

In a welfare state citizens and the state have a specific, though varying, relation. Citizenship is connected with the implementation of solidarity, equality, and equity. It is believed that these are achieved through social policy benefits and services. The benefits and services differ from each other along a continuum of entitlement and eventuality. Established practice, e.g., the discretionary powers of officials, varies according to this continuum for each benefit and service (Sihvo 1991, 52). On the other hand the criticism has been voiced that the considerable responsibility of the state makes citizens and communities passive (see, e.g., Anttonen & Sipilä 2000, 16).

According to Paul Higgs (1995, 544) the concept of citizenship affiliation with old age has to be based on the notions of both public activism and a public sphere in which to act. Citizenship is also linked with everyday participation. In this perspective, dealing with the health care and social service system is connected to the citizen's rights and the implementation of citizenship. The service system may support the equal participation of individuals as citizens (Hoggett & Martin 1994, 108), or it may fracture citizenship (Hernes 1988a, 200). As citizens, aged clients and caregivers negotiate their rights and the content and delivery of services (Hernes 1988b, 207).

Do the services support the implementation of citizenship or are they an obstacle to it? The notion of citizenship has been brought up as a source of renewal for the welfare state. This has to do with developing a new 'social contract' between citizens and the state in the development and delivery of services. The role of the state has changed from the service provider more to funding agent, contractor, regulator, and evaluator (Camilleri 1999, 34). The services are targeted and selected accurately and closely (Anttonen & Sipilä 2000, 176; Vaarama et al., 2000, 84, 97). The recipients are often subjected to these services instead of having their voices heard within the service system. The dominant managerial discourse on care constrains the elderly people's sense of their possibilities (Aronson 1999, 50).

The structured dependency of older people results from a lack of resources, which in turn prevents participation in society. Lack of participation in society leads to the exclusion and marginalisation of older people. An irony of the citizenship approach is that in trying to overcome structured dependency, many proposals end up homogenising all older people into an undifferentiated group who need to be made equal. In reality citizens are encouraged to take greater personal responsibility for their life situation and needs. However, as those needing health care and social services will discover, at this point they are transformed from consumers into objects of consumption (Higgs 1995, 537-548). Capacity and the recognition of individuality are resources to enforce full citizenship.

The notion of citizenship is linked with the discussion of the quality of life (Phillips & Berman 2001, 22). Social quality is the extent to which citizens are able to participate in the social and economic life of their communities under conditions which enhance their well-being and individual potential (Beck et al., 1997, 3). Community citizenship refers to the possession by members of a community of social and cultural (lesser civil and political) rights and responsibilities as a distinct element of their national citizenship rights. The maintenance of community citizenship rights is conditional upon the community's social quality (Phillips & Berman 2001, 24-25). David Phillips and Yitzhak Berman (2001, 18) list four continuums of social quality: (1) social-economic security/insecurity, (2) social inclusion/exclusion, (3) social cohesion/anomie, and (4) empowerment/disempowerment. The first refers to the way in which the essential needs of the citizens are met. The second refers to belonging and supportive infrastructures in preventing exclusion. The third concerns the processes which create, defend, and demolish social networks. The fourth concerns enabling people, as citizens, to develop their full potential in order to participate in social, economic, political, and cultural processes.

Legislation, official agendas, the ethical codes of social work, etc., expressly mention the clients' participation, self-determination, and right to information concerning their own case. Nevertheless, the Finnish health care and social service system can be described as organisation- and authority-centred (Lehto & Natunen 2002, 12-13; Valokivi 2002, 27-28). The lack of client participation in the procedure and decision-making on their own case is often evident (see Metteri 2003a; Metteri 2003b). Aged persons who need health and social care services are often infirm, and their energy level and functional ability are lowered. Their participation is considered through need fulfilment, security and support networks. Their life situations, daily lives and needs act as constraints for their participation. These are people who will not come out in the street to voice their demands, at least not in person. Another problematic point is the lack of information. Information concerning the health care and social service system is fragmented. However, information is the condition to participation in planning, discussing options and making decisions. There is a need for interpreters and arbitrators between the client's needs and life situation and the health care and social service system and its norms (see, e.g., Aronson 1999, 49-51; Holosko & Feit 1996).

DATA AND METHOD OF THE STUDY

The research data were gathered during a case management (1995-96) project of the action research type, in which the workers built up individual and needs-based service packages in co-operation with clients, their relatives, and the service network. The data for this article were gathered during the first phase of the project, before the implementation of the case management method (see Ala-Nikkola & Valokivi 1997). The target group were the elderly in a rural municipality of approximately 10,000 inhabitants. In the Finnish context such a municipality is considered middle sized.

In this article I will analyse and discuss semi-structured interviews with the aged persons and their relatives. The data and the interviewees were chosen to illustrate the complex involvement of the service users in the context of outpatient services. Within the non-institutional care the aged citizens have possibilities to participate, and there are options in the services. I look at the encounters with health care and social services as experienced and described by the aged clients and the informal caregivers. Their stories contain comments and evaluations of places, professionals, and service practices (Morgan 2000, 209). The research questions are: What do the elderly and their caregivers tell about encounters with the local health care and social service system? What kind of services do they receive and how did service use begin? How can they participate in and influence the services? How is their citizenship defined and how do they define it at the grass roots level, in the local health care and social service system?

The data used in this study consist of 13 semi-structured interviews; five elderly persons as care recipients (in one interview, the interviewee's son was present) and eight caregivers of whom four were wives (in one interview, the spouse was present), two daughters and one daughter-in-law, and one volunteer neighbour. The interview themes were Everyday life, Services, Changes in services, Experiences with the different places of the service system, Needs, Hopes, and Advocate or Case Manager. The elderly, who were cared for at home, needed help in their everyday activities, from preparing meals and washing up to getting into bed. Five of them lived alone in an apartment, and eight lived with their spouse or another relative. Their ages varied from 80 to 94 years. All the wife caregivers were also aged.

The position and participation possibilities of the aged persons and their caregivers are in the focus of this study. The analysis looks for descriptions of encounters with the health care and social service system, of experiences with different service providers and of the individual service paths. Are the users partners or bystanders, actors or objects? The research looks for the forms of participation and influencing which Shemmings (1995, 43) have called participatory practices, and for the limits and possibilities of participation and collaboration. The research approach is a dialogue between a data-based analysis and a conceptual reasoning (Eskola & Suoranta 1998, 83; see also Sherman & Reid 1994). The implementation of the qualitative analysis emphasises the voice of the service users (Gordon et al., 2000, 204-208; McLean Taylor et al., 1995, 27-33).

In the first phase of the empirical analysis, the interview data were read as an entity. After becoming acquainted with the data, the researcher formulated questions from the data for a more detailed reading: How did the service use begin? What kind of encounters have the interviewees had with the local health care and social service system? How do they participate in negotiating, planning and decision-making? Are they active actors or do they withdraw? The data were coded according to these questions. Asking such questions allows an observation of the differences and similarities between individuals, roles and positions. By doing this, the use of the active and the passive voice could be reviewed. The researcher then generated data categories and concepts from and with the data, using coding as a means of achieving this (Coffey & Atkinson 1996, 26-27, 46-47). After coding and formulating analytical data categories and concepts from the data, the analysis looked for the voice of the aged speaking and acting or withdrawing in the descriptions (Rogers et al., 1994, 10). When is the speaker an active actor and doer, and when a passive object? Adopting a bottom-up approach, the researcher sought the grass-root level citizenship, its forms and conditions. The final focus of the analysis was to clarify differences in the modes of participation.

HOW DID THE USE OF THE SERVICES BEGIN?

In this section the interviewees' descriptions of how the use of the services started will be reviewed. How does one begin to use the services? Who takes an active role? What is the process of contacting the local health care and social service system like? In the data there are four perspectives into the beginning of the services. These analytical categories are: personal initiative, activity of relatives, drifting and disagreement.

Personal Initiative and Need for Help

As one grows older, it is sometimes difficult to realise the increasing need for help in everyday life. Asking for help is not a simple matter, as is described by the aged man in the first extract.

Extract 1[1]

M: And then, well see, once again this is how I am I need help in every-thing as I couldn't do a thing for myself. It's a difficult thing, always having to ask some outsider and well, the home, home helper and them.

(Aged man 1, I, 3)

The need for help may be hard to recognise and admit, and it may be difficult to ask for help. Where to ask? Who to contact? What are the al-ternatives? And who will provide the service? The health care and social service system is often unfamiliar and complicated. Service providers are not among the people one knows. This perspective has to do with the ba-sic everyday needs and social security. The interviewee says that he needs help in order to manage. To get the help he needs in daily life, the aged person must ask for it from an outsider, an unknown person, when his own social network offers no help or there is no network. In relation to the system, the interviewee is distant and quite powerless, not a member nor a real consumer.

Activity of Friends or Relatives

In many cases a vigilant relative or neighbour is the first one to realise the need for help and services. The elderly themselves may often be com-paratively passive, mostly due to their weakened or limited capacity. In the next extract the relative is active in arranging the services needed.

Extract 2

F: Well it was my elder son who began to arrange for it [the home help], because, because I just told them that once out of the hospi-tal, or whatever, I can't come back home. That who's going to look after me there, I will always need someone to be there, at home.

(Aged woman 1, II, 16)

This interviewee was hesitant about being sent home at discharge and she admitted the need for help. The aged woman was active in making an assessment of her need and authorised her family member to seek for it. Her social network was there to support her and act on her behalf. The aged person may also reject the thought of service. In such a case the relative or informal caregiver may experience pressure from both directions. S/he assesses and sees the need for service, but the aged person her/himself is against the offered service and may refuse it. Finding out about the possibilities and discussing these with the aged person may be arduous. In such a case the caregiver or the relative has to negotiate with the aged person, other relatives or friends and the service providers.

Sometimes the actions taken do not lead to the desired outcome from the user's point of view (neither the care recipient's nor the caregiver's), as can be seen in the next extract told by a daughter-in-law caregiver. She describes the care negotiations and arrangements during her and her husband's absence.

Extract 3

F: We'd have employed someone ourselves, I asked about it, but I phoned the social services office, might even have been Matti [director of social services] or whoever it was, anyway the office, like to find out whether the local authority could pay part of the salary. And with Maija [manager of home], I actually spoke to several people, anyway Maija said that in fact it'll be a short-term placement which is the option available here. See the difficulty at that time was that Taimi [mother-in-law] refused to come here [home for the elderly]. So that was why we came up with this idea of employing someone ourselves. That would have been best for Taimi.

(Daughter-in-law, IV, 11)

In this extract the service offered does not meet the expressed need. The aged Taimi and her relatives prefer to arrange help at home while the relatives are away on holiday. After finding out about the alternatives, they "came up with this idea of employing someone" to meet their service need. The health care and social service system offers only short-term institutional care. The interviewee knows the two managers of the local social service system so well that she calls them by their first name. Despite this familiarity and active contacts, the daughter-in-law is unable to arrange the service which the family would prefer, and their suggestion is bypassed. The interviewee seeks for support and a solution which would ensure the needed care for her aged mother-in-law and would allow her to carry out her full participation in her social network. The service system does not offer a user-led solution. The users are objects of ready-made services. The system places the applicants before a 'take it or leave it' situation. Genuine options are not offered. A certain extent of social security is provided, but other dimensions of the quality of life are bypassed.

Drifting into the Use of Services

A number of aged persons describe the beginning of service use as drifting into it. Without being active themselves, they have things happen to them, as is described by the aged lady in the next extract.

Extract 4

R: Do you remember when the home helpers began to visit you?

F: I suppose they've been coming for about two years.

R: About two years. Did you yourself find out about them at that time, or was there someone who helped you to contact them?

F: No, they just came to see me and realised that I need help.

R: Was it you yourself who contacted the home help agency, or was it someone, maybe if you have relatives, I mean do they look after these things at all?

F: Well in fact I don't know who had told them. They just came to see me and I can't remember any of the. To see me.

R: Well how did you feel when they came and said you could start using this service?

F: Of course it was nice, but if I only could I would do for myself, then I wouldn't have to wait for someone else.

(Aged woman 2, III, 2)

Coping independently would be the most desirable circumstance for the interviewee. When this is no longer possible, someone has contacted the home help agency, though she does not know or remember who it was. This is quite understandable for an aged person in need of help with her everyday coping. The interviewee describes how "they just came," meaning the home help advisors. The aged woman is an object for the decision-making process and services. She withdraws from participation, and other actors intervene on her behalf. The need for help entails dependency on others and on the system and loss of one's personal freedom of activity. With help and assurance from others, her basic needs are met.

Disagreeing and Dissatisfactory Initiation

In some cases the service offered does not meet the need or the expressed expectation of the aged person or the caregiver. The aged man in the next extract was visited daily by home helpers after his discharge from the hospital, but they could not spend much time in one place. The time spent with him was not satisfactory, according to his son.

Extract 5

M: Well first of all contact with the relatives, I seem to remember we always contacted them, both the central hospital and the health care centre. It's very seldom that they've contacted us for any reason. And er, in my opinion, when you asked about the preparation, the preparation was no good at all. The health care centre didn't prepare the matter in any way, and then, the home help service, well that leaves so much to be desired that it would take me two days to list it all.

R: So in other words, they made one visit a day.

M: One visit a day, and it's as father already mentioned, that they were in a hurry and almost only came to the door to ask if he needs anything from the shop and then practically left.

(Son, V, 2)

In this case the aged man and his son are dissatisfied with the preparation for and content of the service. The son criticises the service system for having failed to contact, inform, and negotiate with them. Another reason for criticism is that the service did not meet the need expressed by the aged man and his relatives. He did not need help with shopping, but something else. The well-being and social quality aspects of the aged man's life situation are not responded satisfactorily. Further on, the father and son adopt the role of a consumer (see Extract 11).

In all cases the initial phases were characterised by a relatively strong orientation to the system. The workers act as gatekeepers of a stable choice of services (cf. Cnaan 1994, 547). The constraints for the activity are rigid. The needs expressed by the aged persons, their caregivers and their family members are filtered through the constraints posed by the system, with the result that some of the needs will be met, while certain needs and citizens are left without support or services. Do services increase or decrease one's citizenship? At any rate, the descriptions of participation are not equal among themselves. Services to which entitlement is achieved through formal status are offered, and from the consumer angle, 'take it or leave it' choices are offered, but the participatory dimension remains insignificant.

PARTICIPATION IN THE SERVICES

In this section I will bring up modes of participation as described by the interviewees and analysed and conceptualised from the data. The modes of participation in negotiation and decisions concerning the services and their form and intensity can vary from (1) passive disengagement from the process to (2) contacting, (3) negotiating and co-operating, (4) demanding, and finally to (5) active disengagement.

Passive Disengagement

The first mode of participation is to withdraw passively. People in need of services may disengage from the services because of a lack of capacity or will to take part in planning and decision-making. In the next extract the aged wife caregiver adopts a distant role.

Extract 6

R: So what about when he [husband] was discharged, were you there to discuss it with the doctor on the ward?

F: No, no I wasn't.

R: Did they contact you by the phone?

F: No, they didn't phone, it's that they just decide these things.

(Wife caregiver 1, VIII, 9)

The wife caregiver tells that on the husband's discharge from hospital she has not been in contact with the institution or vice versa, although her own health is weak. She is acting very passively. She is satisfied with the "decision" made by the service provider and takes it for granted. She is an object for the system. She finds no way of intervening and makes no effort to do so. Neither the needs of the aged caregiver nor her possibilities to take care of the husband's needs are verbalised. No one finds out whether help is needed at home. The aged couple is outside all aspects of social quality. Their citizenship can be described almost non existent.

Contacting

The second mode of participation is that the aged person contacts a service provider, but does not assume an active role during subsequent events. In many cases an aged person contacts the service provider to inform over questions concerning everyday situations.

Extract 7

R: How is it, has the home help advisor ever visited you at home?

M: Oh yes, she has. Once for example she came when, she came, happened so, a bit before, didn't come, no one had been sent, the home helper never came one day, to cook my meal. So I thought that well, I suppose I must phone them since no one's here to cook my meal and then she said, she answered that there must have been some mix-up, that no one's been sent to visit me, and she came herself then.

(Aged man 2, VI, 10)

The aged man receives home help regularly. In an unexpected situation he phones the home help advisor. The advisor arranges help for that day by making the visit herself. Here the aged man makes an contact with the service provider, acting as an informant. He has no other demands or complaints. After the first contact the service provider sorts the matter out and the aged man has no further active role. The responsibility and organisation are assumed by the worker. This episode can be defined through consumerism, where an existing agreement breaks down and the situation is resolved once a contact has been made.

Negotiating and Cooperating

The third mode of participation is to negotiate and cooperate with service providers.

Extract 8

R: Oh yes, about discharge situations, do they contact you or do you go and discuss things, or what?

F: Yes, we agree always on it when I go and fetch her, like next Friday when she's [mother] due to be discharged, we will agree on the next date when she's to be admitted. Sort of depending on how well I think I'll cope here.

(Daughter caregiver 2, X, 3-4)

In a situation involving the mother's discharge from short-term institutional care, the daughter negotiates with the service provider. The condition of the daughter caregiver is considered (in contrast to Extract 6). They agree on the date of the next short-term period according to the daughter's level of coping. The daughter is involved in the process of negotiating, planning, and decision-making. She has adopted an active participatory role in encounters with the service system as an actor (cf. communitarian citizenship). The caregiver and the service provider co-operate and are equally active. The caregiver refers to 'we' as a team. The responsibility for arranging the services needed and the complex supporting the caregiver's coping is divided equally.

Demanding

The fourth mode of participation is to present demands in negotiations and decision-making processes. The caregiver herself may be active and demanding:

Extract 9

F: I've never had any difficulties in getting it [short-term placement for husband] whenever I phone them. I suppose they must know that I can't go entirely without breaks.

(Wife caregiver 2, XII, 4)

The interviewee considers that she is entitled to the services which she regards as suitable for her and her husband. It is only a matter of making a phone call. And if necessary, she contacts whoever is needed to achieve the decisions she wants:

Extract 9 continues

F: I have sometimes asked for cleaning help, because the big window is so awkward so I have asked occasionally if they could. I mean it can't be just left swinging open with no one to help.

R: And have you got it, those times?

F: Oh yes, I've got it. And they know that I'll just keep nagging at them until [laughter].

R: Do you have a reputation of getting your way?

F: ( ) I'll go as high up as I need to.

R: Has there ever been a situation when you've had to?

F: Well no, but there was once, this, when they began, see we had the bathtub and, well, I couldn't get into it, I've got hip replacements, I couldn't have climbed into it and Taisto couldn't either, so they installed a shower. And the doors had to be made wider and I went to see the director, this Vihtonen [director of social services], and then it got started.

R: The alteration?

F: Yes. The local authority paid for it, no problem about that.

(Wife caregiver 2, XII, 6)

The interviewee uses very strong I-language ("I've got," "I'll just keep nagging," "I go as high up as I need to"). The counterpart 'they' refers to the service system and the workers there. Unlike the caregiver in the previous extract, this interviewee makes no reference at all to 'us' as a team. If necessary, she is ready to contact the director of the entire social service department, and does so, too. She not only negotiates, but also makes demands. Her expectations on the service providers are definite and unquestioned. She adopts the role of a consumer (cf. libertarian citizenship). The services are instruments for coping well with everyday life and for caring.

In the next extract, a very determined caregiver leaves her mother at the hospital:

Extract 10

F: Actually, I once had to take her there when she got so that she couldn't stand up at all, so I took her to the local hospital and they said they won't admit her. So I said I can't go home with anyone like this that cannot stand up at all, I said I'd fetch her home the next day if that's what it took, as long as you can make sure she won't, that she'll ( ) but they managed it all right, and they didn't take more than a couple of days. But they were not going to admit her and I said there was no chance of my taking her home.

R: And what happened then?

F: Well, what could I do but leave her there.

(Daughter caregiver 1, VII, 4)

The interviewee describes how her mother's condition gets worse, and she is forced to take her mother to the hospital and to leave her there. She is not negotiating, but acting her demand and carrying out her will in a situation where she sees no other alternative. Her voice is heard through her action.

Active Disengagement

In many cases the aged persons and their relatives or caregivers settle for the services offered. In the active disengagement mode of participation, people in need of help may disengage from the (public) service system due to dissatisfaction and a personal decision to do so. In the next extract dissatisfaction with the offered service leads to other arrangements for the necessary help:

Extract 11

M: And the, later, of course father has got a bit weaker over the years, so I mean it is not enough that the home help service simply pop their head in in the morning. We came to the conclusion that he needs more assistance in any case. That was when we decided to do this [to employ a private nurse].

(Son, V, 4)

Because the father needed more help than he received from and could be arranged by the home help agency, they decided to employ a private nurse. 'They' refers either to the aged man, his son and daughter-in-law or to the son and daughter-in-law. They withdraw from the public service system, and they are dissatisfied with the contribution of the service system. They justify their expectation by their entitlement. As citizens and consumers they decide to stop using and buying the public home help service and to buy the necessary service elsewhere, although the new arrangement is much more expensive for them. They decide to empower themselves by adopting the strong role of a consumer.

Some of the aged interviewees point out that they have done their part in their deal with the state, and they demand the state and the service system to take care of their part. They justify their expectations by saying that they have paid their taxes and helped build up the community. They may be disappointed with the lack of consideration and attention shown by the municipality. In such cases the interviewees describe the situation practically as a contract between themselves as citizens and the municipality (cf. liberal citizenship).

ADVOCATES

The aged persons may have limitations; they may lack the capacity, information, aspiration, etc., for making an initiative, negotiating and demanding the support and services needed (cf. Rose & Black 1985). Who act as the advocates for such persons? In the interviews both relatives or friends and workers within the local health care and social service system are described as advocates for individual aged persons and in certain situations. In the next extract the aged man's informal support network includes two advocates:

Extract 12

R: How about a situation where you need more help or, who can you contact?

M: Well yes, generally the person who's run my errands, has seen to my medications and has fetched them and everything is Riitta Vuori [volunteer, neighbour]. Then there's my sister's son, the younger one, Martti he's called, who lives in the Main Village, he's also helped some. He even visits me every Sunday morning and, sort of protection. Well the other children have also visited, my sister's children, but not as often as Martti has.

(Aged man 2, VI, 8-9)

The interviewee's most important caregiver and advocate is the lady next door. She takes care of matters related to his everyday care and visits him on a daily basis. She is the first person whom he contacts concerning the need for help and any changes in it. The important role of the volunteer neighbour is interesting because the man is also visited daily by home helpers. Another advocate is a relative of his. Their contact is more intermittent, but it is described as a protection and security. The aged man's own role is quite passive and withdrawn.

In the next two extracts the advocates are from the formal service system. The aged person describes and seeks allies within the service system. The advocate may be from the social services or from the health sector.

Extract 13

R: Well, what about if, if you need to make changes, what if you come to the conclusion that something about the services ought to be rearranged or something, who would you contact?

M: Well it's been through Maija [manager of home for the elderly].

R: Through, Maija.

M: Through Maija, and I've actually already spoken to her. Yes, she's such a good person and really good at her job. So yes, I can talk to her about whatever it is and sort out all papers and so.

(Aged man 1, I, 28, 34)

The manager of the home for the elderly is the advocate for this aged man. He describes elsewhere how the manager has previously arranged a rehabilitation period for him. He trusts the manager because of the earlier experience, but the trust is also based on the fact that the manager is a good person and suited for her work. The interviewee describes encounters with the manager as consisting of discussion, and he has an active role in negotiating issues with her. They have a cooperative relationship (cf. communitarian citizenship). In the second case the advocate is from the health care sector:

> Extract 14
>
> F: So this, yesterday this doctor, she saw I was not well and she said, well what if ( ) they won't discharge Esa [husband] yet I mean at all, even today, because I was so ill.
>
> R: Oh yes, that was yesterday when you went to see the doctor?
>
> F: And then she called this Nieminen to ask
>
> R: The ward doctor?
>
> F: Yes, to ask what's to be done, that she has a patient who is so ill that she can't possibly care for anyone. That it's enough if she manages to look after herself.
>
> R: Right, so what happened then?
>
> F: Well he, he wrote a note about it
>
> R: Yes, that he could be admitted earlier there [on the ward]
>
> F: Yes, that he could go in earlier.
>
> (Wife caregiver 1, VIII, 4)

In this extract the doctor of the wife caregiver negotiates by phone with the manager of the ward on which her husband is treated. The wife caregiver is in bad health herself, so her doctor recommends that the short-term institutional care arranged for her husband should start earlier, and this is in fact arranged. Compared to the previous extract, this describes more formal act of advocacy even though both advocates are from inside the service system. Within the encounter with the doctor the interviewee has a passive role. The doctor of the wife caregiver assumes the responsibility of arranging the short-term period on the basis of the wife caregiver's level of coping.

An aged person may cede some or all of her/his rights as a citizen–perhaps the right of speech and the responsibility for actions to either a family member or friend, or to a worker in the health care and social service system. Some aged persons retain their active role, while others assume the passive role of 'recipient.' Workers as advocates know the service system and the service network. Relatives and friends are usually very devoted to their close one. If a relative or a friend acts as an advocate for an aged person, co-operation between workers and the advocate is essential (Kraan et al. 1991, 186-187; cf. Cnaan 1994, 544).

DISCUSSION

If a person's functional ability or will to participate are lowered, how can their citizenship be realised? The role of an active citizen is not the only way to realise one's citizenship. However, the inclusion of citizens whose functional ability or willingness are lowered requires that the system and the workers in it have a sensitive ear. The risk of objectifying and by-passing the citizen is always present. One answer is to consider citizenship as a cooperative phenomenon, where individual needs are taken into account and citizens are helped to reach social quality and participation according to their ability and will. This cooperative citizenship as a process consists of all three strands of definitions of citizenship: liberal, communitarian, and libertarian (cf. Phillips & Berman 2001).

In my research data the interviewees' descriptions of encounters with the local health care and social service system contain different definitions of citizenship and implementation of social quality. Within the encounters, the professionals may support the notion of citizenship, or they may regard the service users as objects of the system. What consequences should this have for the current work practices of the service system?

As John Baldock (1993, 3) has formulated it, "no one is likely to oppose the principle of participation in home care. Everyone is in favour of the idea that frail old people and their carers should be able to express their needs and play a part in the planning of their care." He defines two different models of achieving participation. The first is the managed home care model which is profession-led, and the second is the laissez-faire model which is user- and consumer-led. Both models recognise a right for users to participate in the design and production of their care. How people are assessed for care and how that care is organised is related to user participation. According to my data both models are needed in practice.

As consumers or users, citizens participate by making choices between services, by enhancing the content and degree of services, and by facilitating consumer rights. The truth of this statement can be questioned. Does the consumer or user want to develop the services? (Niiranen 1998, 328). They may be satisfied with 'good enough' services. Vuokko Niiranen (1998, 329) formulates two aspects of participation: individual and communal. In the individual aspect the citizen is a user of services and s/he has a consumer's rights to make choices. In communal participation the citizen is a member of her/his community and a committed partner. The consumer participates and criticises the service system from the outside and exits it when there is disagreement (cf. Extract 11). A member participates and criticises from the inside and uses his/her voice while negotiating and demanding (cf. Extracts 8 and 9).

In the context of the local health care and social services, citizenship rights and obligations and participation should be defined flexibly and individually. In my research data the aged persons and their caregivers described participation in multiple ways. The modes of participation varied from passive and active disengagement from the process and contacting to negotiating and co-operating or demanding. In passive disengagement the citizen withdraws passively, and in active disengagement s/he withdraws due to deciding actively to do so. In the mode of contacting, the citizen informs the service system without intending to assume an active role in the future. In negotiating and cooperating the citizen is involved in the planning and decision-making processes. In the demanding mode the citizen presents demands in encounters with service providers. The aged persons and their caregivers had actively chosen their mode of participation or had been driven into one. This brings up several questions and perspectives to be considered by the local health care and social service system. Given that the system needs to be open and recognise different modes of participation, questions related to these aspects should be asked during encounters with individual citizens: Is the client's mode of participation desired and helpful or detrimental? How can a helpful mode be achieved and supported? What are the individual needs and how can the service system fulfil them?

Most of the interviewees were frail aged people, regardless of whether they were care recipients or caregivers. Their individual life situation varied according to capacity, resources and health. Still, they exhibited multiple modes of participation. Their individual needs were satisfied by the local health care and social service system to a varying degree. Encounters with the service system should be defined from the bottom up, starting from the individual's life situation and capacity. Similarly, the implementation of citizenship with the aged persons and their caregivers is a multiform phenomenon. In my research data, different strands of definitions of citizenship could be found in the local context. The citizenship of aged service users may be examined as a process which supports co-operative citizenship.

Relationship and emotions are core concepts in encounters with the elderly (Austin 1996, 168-169). Advocacy work aims to support, encourage and empower the clients, so that they may participate in decision-making concerning their own case (Hugman 1991, 139; see also Rose & Black 1985; Dant & Gearing 1990, 345). A decision-making process which lies close to the client and involves his/her participation is crucial for ensuring a full participation and social quality (Braye & Preston-Shoot 1995, 80).

To ensure client participation in the service process, there should exist an alliance between the client and the worker. Alliance means a mutual commitment to supporting the client's coping and to responding to her/his needs. The client should be truly heard and included in the negotiations and decision-making, according to the aged person's or caregiver's desire to participate or withdraw. Client participation can be achieved contractually. The service user is included as an equal partner in the service process. The aged person may transfer or delegate discretionary or decision-making power to a worker or an informal advocate or keep it under her/his own control. Alliances are based on mutual trust, which is an empowering element in client work. With help from the advocate, the aged person is a more equal partner in making an agreement. Individual participation and control over it are the condition for enforcing the processes of citizenship rights and obligations.

NOTE

1. All the names of persons, places and institutions have been changed. F is female interviewee, M is male interviewee, and R is researcher; [author's comment], (blurry word) and . . . means interview continues from a later part.

REFERENCES

Ala-Nikkola, M., & Sipilä, J. (1996) Yksilökohtainen palveluohjaus (case management)–uusi ratkaisu palvelujen yhteensovittamisen ikuisiin ongelmiin [Case Management–a new solution for the eternal problems of co-ordinating services]. In A. Metteri (ed.) Moniammatillisuus ja sosiaalityö. Sosiaalityön vuosikirja 1996. [Interprofessional Collaboration and Social Work. Yearbook of Social Work 1996] Helsinki: Edita & Sosiaalityöntekijäin Liitto, 16-31.

Ala-Nikkola, M., & Valokivi, H. (1997) Yksilökohtainen palveluohjaus käytäntönä. Loppuraportti sosiaali-ja terveydenhuollon palvelujärjestelmää ja yksilökohtaista palveluohjausta (case management) koskeneesta tutkimuksesta Hämeenkyrössä ja Tampereella [Case Management as a Practice. Final Report of the Study on the Service System and Case Management at Hämeenkyrö and in Tampere]. Jyväskylä: STAKES raportteja 215.

Alestalo, M. (1994) Finland: The Welfare State at the Crossroads. In N. Ploug & J. Kvist (eds.) Recent Trends in Cash Benefits in Europe. Copenhagen: The Danish National Institute of Social Research, 73-84.

Anttonen, A., & Sipilä, J. (2000) Suomalaista sosiaalipolitiikkaa [Finnish Social Policy]. Tampere: Vastapaino.

Anttonen, A., & Sipilä, J. (1996) European Social Care Services: Is It Possible to Identify Models? Journal of European Social Policy 6 (2), 87-100.

Aronson, J. (1999) Conflicting Images of Older People Receiving Care. In S. M. Neysmith (ed.) Critical issues for future social work practice with ageing persons. New York: Columbia University Press, 47-70.

Austin, C. D. (1996) Case Management Practice with the Elderly. In M. J. Holosko & M. D. Feit (eds.) Social Work Practice with the Elderly. Toronto: Canadian Scholars' Press, 151-175.

Baldock, J. (1997) Social Care In Old Age: More Than a Funding Problem. Social Policy Administration 31 (1) March 1997, 73-89.

Baldock, J. (1993) Participation in Home-based care. Paper in Innovation and Participation in Care of the Elderly–Italy meets Europe. Rome May 20-22, 1993.

Beck, W., van der Maeson, L., & Walker, A. (1997) Introduction. In W. Beck, L. van der Maeson & A. Walker (eds.) The Social Quality of Europe. Hague, Netherlands: Kluwer Law International, 1-13.

Braye, S., & Preston-Shoot, M. (1995) Empowering Practice in Social Care. Buckingham: Open University Press.

Camilleri, P. (1999) Social work and its search for meaning: Theories, narratives and practices. In B. Pease & J. Fook (eds.) Transforming social work practice. London: Routledge, 25-39.

Cnaan, R. A. (1994) The New American Social Work Gospel: Case Management of the Chronically Mentally Ill. British Journal of Social Work 24 (5), 533-557.

Coffey, A., & Atkinson, P. (1996) Making Sense of Qualitative Data. Thousand Oaks: SAGE Publications.

Culpitt, I. (1992) Welfare and Citizenship. Beyond the Crisis of the Welfare State? Guildford, Surrey: SAGE Publications.

Dant, T., & Gearing, B. (1990) Keyworkers for Elderly People in the Community: Case Managers and Care Co-ordinators. Journal of Social Policy 19 (3) July 1990, 331-360.

Eskola, J., & Suoranta, J. (1998) Johdatus laadulliseen tutkimukseen [Introduction to Qualitative Research]. Tampere: Vastapaino.

Glendinning, C. (1998) Conclusions: Learning from abroad. In C. Glendinning (ed.) Rights and Realities. Comparing new developments in long-term care for older people. Bristol: The Policy Press, 127-142.

Gordon, T., Holland, J., & Lahelma, E. (2000) Making Spaces: Citizenship and Difference in Schools. Chippenham, Wiltshire: Macmillan Press ltd.

Hernes, H. M. (1988a) Scandinavian Citizenship. Acta Sociologica 31 (3), 199-215.

Hernes, H. M. (1988b) The Welfare State Citizenship of Scandinavian Women. In K. B. Jones and A. G. Jónasdóttir (eds.) The Political Interests of Gender. Oxford: SAGE Publications.

Higgs, P. (1995) Citizenship and Old Age: The End of the Road? Ageing and Society 15: 535-550.

Hoggett, P., & Martin, L. (1994) Consumer-Oriented Action in the Public Services. Working Paper No.WP/94/23/EN European Foundation for the Improvement of Living and Working Conditions.

Holosko, M. J., & Feit, M. D. (eds.) (1996) Social Work Practice with the Elderly. Toronto: Canadian Scholars' Press.

Hugman, R. (1991) Power in Caring Professions. Houndmills: Macmillan.

Jordan, B. (1997) Citizenship, association and immigration: Theoretical Issues. In M. Roche & R. van Berkel (eds.) European Citizenship and Social Exclusion, Ashgate: Aldershot, 261-272.

Julkunen, R. (1993) Sosiaalipolitiikkamalli, sukupuoli ja hoivatyö [The Model of Social Policy, Gender and Caregiving Work]. In O. Riihinen (ed.) Sosiaalipolitiikka 2017 [The Social Policy 2017]. Juva: WSOY.

Kiiski, S. (1993) Naisten työttömyys lisääntyy, mutta nainen pysyy työvoimassa [The Unemployment of Women Is Increasing, But Women Are Staying in the Labour Force]. Hyvinvointikatsaus 3, 16-19.

Kraan, R. et al. (1991) Care for the Elderly. Fankfurt am Main: Campus Verlag; Boulder, Colorado: Westview Press.

Kröger, T. (2003) Universalism in Social Care for Older People in Finland–Weak and Still Getting Weaker. Nordisk Sosialt Arbeid 1, 30-34.

Lehto, J. (2000) Saumaton palveluketju mosaiikkimaisessa järjestelmässä [Seamless Chain of Services in a Mosaic-like System]. In S. Nouko-Juvonen, P. Ruotsalainen & I. Kiikkala (eds.) Hyvinvointivaltion palveluketjut [Service Chains in the Welfare State]. Helsinki: Kustannusosakeyhtiö Tammi.

Lehto, J. (1998) Muuttuuko pohjoismainen sosiaali-ja terveyspalvelumalli? [Does the Scandinavian Health and Social Service Model Change?] Yhteiskuntapolitiikka 63 (5-6), 413-424.

Lehto, J., & Blomster, P. (2000) Talouskriisin jäljet sosiaali-ja terveyspalvelujärjestelmässä [The Traces of Economic Crisis in the Social Services and Health Care System]. In H. Uusitalo, A. Parpo & A. Hakkarainen (eds.) Sosiaali-ja terveydenhuollon palvelukatsaus

2000 [Social Welfare and Health Care Service Review 2000]. Stakes Raportteja 250. Helsinki: Stakes, 161-184.

Lehto, J., & Natunen, K. (2002) Johdanto [Introduction]. In J. Lehto & K. Natunen (eds.) Vastaamme vanhusten hyvinvoinnista. Sosiaali-ja terveyspalvelujärjestelmän sopeuttaminen ikääntyneiden tarpeisiin [We Are Responsible for the Well-being of the Elderly. Adapting the social welfare and health care system to meet the requirements of the elderly]. Helsinki: Suomen Kuntaliitto [the Association of Finnish Local and Regional Authorities], 11-14.

Marshall, T. H., & Bottomore, T. (1950/1992) Citizenship and Social Class. London: Pluto Press.

Martimo, K. (1998) Community Care for Frail Older People in Finland. In C. Glendinning (ed.) Rights and Realities. Comparing new developments in long-term care for older people. Bristol: The Policy Press, 67-81.

McLean Taylor, J., Gilligan, C., & Sullivan, A. M. (1995) Between Voice and Silence. Cambridge, Massachussetts, London, England: Harvard University Press.

Metteri, A. (ed.) (2003a) Asiakkaan ääntä kuunnellen. Kitkakohdista kehittämisehdotuksiin [Listening to the voice of the client. From pitfalls to practice strategy developments]. Helsinki: Edita.

Metteri, A. (ed.) (2003b) Syntyykö luottamusta? Sairastuminen, kansalainen ja palvelujärjestelmä [Sickness and the system: Citizens' needs]. Helsinki: Edita.

Morgan, S. (2000) Three prisoner's stories. Talking back through autobiography. In J. Batsleer & B. Humphries (eds.) Welfare, Exclusion and Political Agency. London & New York: Routledge.

Niiranen, V. (1998) Kuntalaisten asiakkuus ja osallisuus järjestöissä–kooptaatiota, säästöjä, osallisuutta–vai jotain muuta? [Clienthood and Participation of Municipal Residents in Organisations–Co-opting, Savings, Participation–Or Something Else?] Kunnallistieteellinen aikakauskirja 26 (4), 326-336.

Noro, A., Aro, S., & Jylhä, M. (1992) Vanhuksen sairaalasta kotiuttaminen henkilökunnan ja potilaan näkökulmasta. [The Discharge of an Old Person from the Hospital in the Viewpoint of the Personnel and the Patient]. Helsinki: Sosiaali- ja terveyshallituksen raportteja 71.

Nygren, L. et al. (1997) New Policies, New Words–the Service Concept in Scandinavian Social Policy. In J. Sipilä (ed.) Social Care Services: The Key to the Scandinavian Welfare Model. Aldershot: Avebury, 9-26.

Phillips, D., & Berman, Y. (2001) Social quality and community citizenship. European Journal of Social Work 4 (1), 17-28.

Rogers, A. G., Brown, L. M., & Tappan Mark B. (1994) Interpreting Loss in Ego Development in Girls: Regression or Resistance? In A. Lieblich & R. Josselson (eds.) Exploring Identity and Gender. The Narrative Study of Lives. Volume 2. Thousand Oaks, London, New Delhi: SAGE Publications, 1-36.

Rose, S. M., & Black, B. L. (1985) Advocacy and Empowerment: Mental Health Care in the Community. London: Routledge & Kegan Paul.

Roth, R. (2000) Changes of New Local Policies in European Cities-time of Civil Society? In A-L. Matthies, M. Järvelä & D. Ward (eds.) From Social Exclusion to Participation. Laukaa: University of Jyväskylä, Department of Social Sciences and Philosophy, Working Papers no 106, 19-40.

Shemmings, D. & Y. (1995) Defining participative practice in health and welfare. In R. Jack (ed.) Empowerment in Community Care. Bury St Edmunds, Suffolk: Chapman & Hall, 43-58.

Sherman, E., & Reid, W. J. (eds.) (1994) Qualitative Research in Social Work. New York: Columbia University Press.

Sihvo, T. (1991) Kansalaisuus ja sosiaalihuolto [Citizenship and Social Services]. Helsinki: Sosiaali-ja Terveyshallitus, Tutkimuksia 9/1991.

Simonen, L. (1993) A Woman's Place Is Home? Transformations of the Welfare State in the 1990s Finland. In H. Varsa (ed.) Shaping Structural Change in Finland. The Role of Woman. Helsinki: Ministry of Social Affairs and Health. Equality Publications Series B: Reports 2, 137-145.

Sipilä, J., & Anttonen, A. (1994) Finland. In A. Evers, M. Pijl & C. Ungerson (eds.) Payments for Care. A Comparative Overview. Aldershot: Avebury & European Centre Vienna, 51-66.

Uusitalo, H., & Konttinen, M. (1995) Sosiaali-ja terveyspalvelujen kehitys laman vuosina: yhteenvetoa ja tulkintoja. In H. Uusitalo & al Sosiaali ja terveydenhuollon palvelukatsaus [Social Welfare and Health Care Service Review]. Jyväskylä: STAKES Raportteja 173, 1-10.

Vaarama, M., et al. (2000) Vanhusten palvelut. In H. Uusitalo, A. Parpo & A. Hakkarainen (eds.) Sosiaali-ja terveydenhuollon palvelukatsaus 2000 [Social Welfare and Health Care Service Review 2000]. Stakes Raportteja 250, 75-98.

Valokivi, H. (2002) Ikääntynyt kansalainen ja omainen sosiaali-ja terveyspalveluissa johdon kertomana [Aged Citizen and Relative In Health and Social Services Told by Mangement]. In J. Lehto & K. Natunen (eds.) We Are Responsible for the Well-being of the Elderly. Adapting the social welfare and health care system to meet the requirements of the elderly. Helsinki: Suomen Kuntaliitto [the Association of Finnish Local and Regional Authorities], 15-30.

Vanhusbarometri 1998 [Old Age Barometer] (1999) Sosiaali-ja terveysministeriön selvityksiä 1999:3, Helsinki: STM.

Mental Homelessness:
Locked Within, Locked Without

Shuvit Melamed, MSW

Danny Shalit-Kenig, MA

Marc Gelkopf, PhD

Arturo Lerner, MD

Arad Kodesh, MD

SUMMARY. The concept of Mental Homelessness is presented and developed. This paper will provide a historical review of the connection between mental illness and housing and the changing approaches toward institutionalization and de-institutionalization over several centuries. Case illustrations from practice in Israel will be presented to highlight the theme of *home*, or rather the theme of *lacking a home* as an element which may be inherent to a mental illness.

More specifically, the paper argues that homelessness is a *state of mind* of which the actual, physical homelessness may be a manifested re-

Shuvit Melamed, Danny Shalit-Kenig, Marc Gelkopf, Arturo Lerner and Arad Kodesh are affiliated with the Lev HaSharon Mental Health Center, Sackler School of Medicine, Tel-Aviv University.

Address correspondence to: Shuvit Melamed, Lev HaSharon Mental Health Center, P.O. Box 90000, Natanya, 42100, Israel (E-mail: shuvka@hotmail.com).

The authors gratefully wish to acknowledge Sigal Bar-Nir, MA, for her insightful conceptual and editorial remarks.

[Haworth co-indexing entry note]: "Mental Homelessness: Locked Within, Locked Without." Melhamed, Shuvit et al. Co-published simultaneously in *Social Work in Health Care* (The Haworth Social Work Practice Press, an imprint of The Haworth Press, Inc.) Vol. 39, No. 1/2, 2004, pp. 209-223; and: *Social Work Visions from Around the Globe: Citizens, Methods, and Approaches* (ed: Anna Metteri et al.) The Haworth Social Work Practice Press, an imprint of The Haworth Press, Inc., 2004, pp. 209-223. Single or multiple copies of this article are available for a fee from The Haworth Document Delivery Service [1-800-HAWORTH, 9:00 a.m. - 5:00 p.m. (EST). E-mail address: docdelivery@haworthpress.com].

Digital Object Identifier: 10.1300/J010v39n01_13

flection of. If so, even if a mental patient does initially own a home, he or she is at high risk to lose it somehow.

This work is a primary attempt at developing a new idea, stemming originally from the field of mental health, with an attempt to widen its theoretical scope to populations not usually defined as mentally ill. Clinical characteristics are presented, as well as an attempt at a theoretical formulation of this concept permitting the development of therapeutic implications. These are presented in relation to existing psychodynamic concepts and therapeutic approaches related to the phenomenon of homelessness. *[Article copies available for a fee from The Haworth Document Delivery Service: 1-800-HAWORTH. E-mail address: <docdelivery@haworth press.com> Website: <http://www.HaworthPress.com> © 2004 by The Haworth Press, Inc. All rights reserved.]*

KEYWORDS. Home, mental illness, homelessness, psychology of home, mental homelessness, institutionalization, de-institutionalization

. . . The idea of rounding up all the mad and mentally ill to live together under one and the same roof seemed in itself a symptom of madness [. . .] At the end of the seventh day, the fiestas were over. The town at last had a madhouse of its own. *Machado de Assis, O Alienista (translation ours, Melamed et al.)*

MENTAL ILLNESS AND HOMELESSNESS: A CHRONOLOGICAL REVIEW

Common belief has it that the conjunction of psychiatric disorder and homelessness is a contemporary phenomenon; however, historical antecedents are quite numerous, though poorly documented (Timms, 1996). In ancient times and in the Middle Ages, a communal approach to mental illness prevailed; treated or untreated, the local madman (as the proverbial village fool) was part and parcel of his community, as psychiatric institutions proper were yet to be invented.

The Inquisition turned mental patients of all kinds into outcasts, exiled or otherwise isolated, and 'psychiatry' was conceptualized as an instrument in the service of "healthy" society. It was this basic approach that eventually brought about the creation of dedicated psychiatric hospitals, the primary purpose of which was not to cure but to segregate the "ill" from the "healthy." Putting its mental patients away in closed wards or in any other type of isolated living allowed society to feel safe, protected from its own "freaks." It was a variant of other methods of exclusion: "Leprosy disappeared, the leper vanished, or almost, from memory. These structures remained. Often, in these same places, the formulas of exclusion would be repeated, strangely similar two or three centuries later. Poor vagabonds, criminals and 'deranged' minds would take the part played by the leper [. . .] With an altogether new meaning and in a very different culture, the forms would remain–essentially that major form of a rigorous division which is social exclusion but spiritual reintegration [. . .] the *Narrenschiff* . . .–[the ship of fools] conveyed their insane cargo from town to town. Madmen then led an easy wandering existence. The towns drove them outside their limits; they were allowed to wonder in the open countryside, when not entrusted to a group of merchants and pilgrims" (Foucault, 1967, p. 7-8).

It was only later that therapists of all kinds started to become interested in the strange morbidity that had so far been treated only by means of containment and restraining. This was the beginning of the first psychiatric revolution–the medicalization of society's approach to mental illness, heralded by Pinel (ibid., p. 241), who built the first proper psychiatric institutions. "Freaks" were now seen as "patients" and received not confinement or isolation but therapy and treatment. This was the beginning of modern-day institutionalization, the flip-side being that it precluded, or at least severely impaired, patient's chances of reintegrating in the community.

Institutionalization was also greatly influenced by urbanization and its consequent reduction of individual physical space. Close in proximity and thus more evident, mental illness was no longer viewed as just a "lunatic" pattern of behavior but as something to be feared, a societal problem; it became society's task to provide the mentally ill with a shelter, a home. But the high and ever increasing cost of housing, the growing number of mentally ill, the outcry of antipsychiatry against mental institutions and the overall rise in the number of homeless turned the idea of providing a home for those who had to be taken out of their original homes into a financial impossibility (Gerhart, 1990).

This was the financial and social background out of which stemmed, somewhere in the 1960s and under President Kennedy, the notion of deinstitutionalization. It was in fact the beginning of the third psychiatric revolution-that of The Era of Community–in which the treatment of the mentally ill was perceived as belonging to the communal sphere. But since none of the social, organizational, administrative, legal, or financial infrastructures was provided to support the move for deinstitutionalization, its unfortunate result was inadequate care for the mentally ill and an even bigger increase in the number of homeless (ibid.).

History therefore supports the coincidence of mental illness and homelessness. Indeed, this relation is plausible since it is logical to assume that the more deprived and incapacitated–and mentally ill individuals in particular–would find it harder to cope, to have a place of their own, and would require assistance in finding some sort of home.

INSTITUTIONALIZATION AND DE-INSTITUTIONALIZATION

This subject has been increasingly explored and dealt with in the last two decades. The growing public attention to the homeless phenomenon gave rise to a volume of academic literature focusing on the link between homelessness and mental illness. At least one social work publication (Community Mental Health Journal of October 1990) dedicated an entire issue to this particular link. Other publications carried articles that were addressing diverse aspects of this link: the particular needs of the combined mentally ill homeless population (Martin, 1990; Rife, First, Greenle, Miller and Feichter, 1991), clinical implications (Susser, Goldfinger and White, 1990), and social welfare implication (Hoff, Briar, Knighton and Van, 1992; Linhorst, 1992).

The cause-effect of this link was also brought up in several publications (e.g., Belcher and Rife, 1989; Linhorst, 1992; Pam, 1994). Regarding culture as a major determinant of personality and mental health, Pam (1994) discusses "the new schizophrenia," which is in fact a social type of schizophrenia, stemming from the cultural fragmentation of family bonds, rather than by enmeshed, dysfunctional, and a reclusive family ties that is traditionally regarded as a determinant of schizophrenia. Social intervention techniques are discussed in Hoff, Briar, Knighton and Van (1992). However, it is still unclear why the mentally ill would develop homelessness. Belcher and Rife (1989) introduce the Social Breakdown Syndrome (SBS), a chronic social deficit that some individuals with schizophrenic-type disorders often develop; indeed, the concept of SBS could be the missing link between homelessness and schizophrenia.

Various classifications of different "types" of homeless people have been suggested in the literature. Hoff et al. (1992) classifies the homeless as either victims of economic changes, or as victims of failed dc-institutionalization. Arce and Vergare (1984) suggests a threefold distinction: situational, episodic and chronic homelessness (in Gerhart, 1990, p. 29).

However, another classification, functional in essence, seems to arise. Some homeless people–i.e., situational–can be helped; if taken care of–arranged in some kind of housing project and so on–their homelessness problem is likely to be resolved. But there are others who seem to be totally "unhelpable"; giving them the key to a four-wall anything, handing them the solution to the physical problem, simply does not work. Beyond issues of narcissism, ego strengths or cognitive deficiency, beyond the vicissitudes of life and actual dire straits, these patients seem to be homelessness-prone or indeed, chronically homeless. What these people really seem to lack is not a house but a home and, more precisely, an inner home. A place that they can call their own; a locality which has a potential to give them a sense of inner security; a place in the sun that in some degree can give them a mirror of themselves; a place of rest. In these cases, it seems to us that mental illness is not a mere contributing factor to but, indeed, the primal and specific cause of homelessness. We therefore submit that homelessness may be viewed in some cases-the characteristics of which are brought below–as a distinct state of mind, that of *Mental Homelessness,* which gradually infiltrate the individual's behavior and may–or not–manifest as a prime symptom in his or her lifestyle.

CLINICAL VIGNETTES

Although still at a very primary stage of a new idea, as part of our attempt to understand and develop this concept we shall present three cases which seem to us to have recognizable behavioral and emotional characteristics suggestive of Mental Homelessness. These cases will help us to better understand the relevancy of the idea of Mental Homelessness and to help us develop its clinical ramifications.

David[1]

Diagnosed as suffering from schizophrenia and a personality disorder, David–a "hip" looking, smartly dressed, fashionable, angry, get-into-trouble-type man in his thirties–has a record of repeated hospitalizations, the most recent of which lasted almost a year. Handsome, tall, and well groomed, he conveys an erroneous and overrated image of his abilities. His good looks are deceiving;

everyone consequently seems to expect him to get hold of himself: "why don't you do something with your life already." When David met his therapist for the first time–in the corridors of the psychiatric rehabilitation ward where he was hospitalized–he said, in a very agitated tone of voice: "I have nowhere to go and I feel that they want me out of the hospital." David had no direction he felt he wanted to pursue in his life and had nowhere to go. His mother and step-father did not want him at home, nor did they offer to help him in any way. He had been referred to several vocational training programs which he never completed. He also applied to an Israeli non-profit organization managing sheltered work programs and group homes for the mentally disabled, but failed to comply with their rules. David also tried to work outside of the hospital, in sheltered programs offered by his social worker and even in work places he found for himself. In spite of his manifest wish to find work, he never managed to keep a job for more than a week, and even the most elaborate and promising rehabilitation programs offered to him invariably failed. He seemed to have gotten himself into a true catch-22 situation: Without work he could not find a place to live, but with nowhere to live he could not find a job. Not eligible for financial assistance–he had misused money he received in the past–David had turned himself into a persona non grata for most help agencies; to them, he was "burnt."

Getting David to agree to actually attend therapy sessions was no easy task. During many weeks David simply refused to meet with his therapist. Even when he did agree, he still could not commit himself to an ordinary therapeutic setting; he preferred to meet "occasionally," without any fixed day and time. In the first few weeks, his therapist met him "informally"; Some sessions–a more appropriate term would be "encounters"–took place in the corridor. And no matter where the encounters were held, they were almost always about exchanging cooking recipes. A former chef, David took great pride in his knowledge of cooking secrets.

In the first proper session David said, "I have no home." He accepted the suggestion that he was in fact referring not only to an external, but also to an inner home. Other home-related themes that were mentioned, besides cooking and cooking recipes, were "opening a door-closing a door" and "a stable home" (with regard to his ambivalence about keeping a regular therapeutic setting).

The theme of "homelessness" was present throughout David's sessions. In fact, it sometimes served as an indicator to David's rehabilitation effort and readiness. When he spoke of the things he had to do in order to settle in a group home–e.g., claim his disability allowance from

Social Security–or expressed his pain and grief over his homelessness, it was regarded as signs of increased responsibility and self care.

At a certain point, David asked to be accepted to the ward's rehabilitation workshop, a long-term intervention program designed to provide rehabilitating patients with basic work-related skills. Since this was considered a costly and complex intervention, only good prospects–that is, patients who seemed likely to be able to truly benefit from the program–were admitted. With his poor employment record David was not welcome there. Nevertheless, his therapist persuaded the program administrators that David should be accepted, were it only for the sole purpose of providing him, once in his life, with an unconditional experience of success. Against all odds, David seemed to thrive in the program. He not only succeeded in keeping a steady occupational setting for a relatively long period of time but also greatly improved his ability to adhere to external schedules and even developed other working habits. This happy stage, however, did not last long. After six months David quit the workshop, left the hospital and was not seen again.

Jack

Jack is a male patient in his fifties, diagnosed with adjustment disorder, after a long and gradual decline in his marital relationship and economic situation. In the last few years he was hospitalized several times, in psychiatric as well as in a general hospitals.

People who meet Jack in everyday life often mention his preoccupation with issues related to a "home"; for example, when he travels abroad he always carries in his bag some hot green peppers, to give "alien food"–during flights or in foreign restaurants–a familiar taste of home. But in fact Jack has no home.

In the relatively recent past he used to be a successful businessman. He was married, had children, built a home, acquired property and belongings and traveled around the world. But he left his wife and his children, left them all his material belongings, tried in vain to start a new family and got increasingly entangled, taken by what seemed to be a spiraling vicious circle of financial and personal deterioration, until he felt that everything was collapsing "like a house of cards."

Jack's use of the term "house of cards" is far from being incidental. In fact, "house of cards" seems to be a strikingly adequate oxymoron: a "house" (and even more in the Hebrew idiom: a tower)–an architectural structure supposedly having a clear and massive presence and authority–that is made of cards–a flimsy, shaky, unreliable structure unable to withstand any pressure or threat due to its internal basic instability; a structure that is *inherently* unstable and unreliable.

With no higher education, Jack has nevertheless acquired a great deal of "street wisdom," which must have helped him a great deal in his business. He exerts most of his efforts and energy on clinging to people, and especially women, persuading them to take him home with them. Money is not the object here. Although Jack lives on a small social security disability pension, he is quite lavish in his spending and likes to bring expensive presents to everyone he is in contact with. He buys clothes as presents to his lady-friends and he always seems to want to give. He seems to be driven by the need not to be left with anything that belongs to him, to give away everything he owns so that he would not own anything himself. He does not have a permanent address. He is constantly on the move, never settling anywhere and always being thrown away, on his way to somewhere else.

Jack's problem is not a lack of support systems, either. Different Israeli welfare authorities have been unsuccessfully trying to help him find a place to live. There are in fact two female social workers working on his case, and somehow he still has nowhere to live. It seems that what Jack is looking for is not merely a place to live but a home.

Despite many years as a nomad, and although in others areas his capacities seem to be intact, Jack systematically refuses to learn how to cook, and can't even make his own cup of coffee. He explains that "the art of making coffee somehow eludes him . . . "; when it comes to finding solutions to his own way of life, he seems to be in a state of total helplessness.

Both his parents are still alive but Jack hardly ever mentions them. He is not wanted in their home and he has virtually no contact with them–or with his many siblings. He always carries a backpack containing papers and documents, newspaper excerpts and photographs from the time he had a family and owned his own company. The image of a successful man, which he tries to convey, includes bragging about his financial successes and about his fatherhood–although in fact he has hardly maintained any contact with any of his children.

On his last day at the hospital he came in late, breathing hard and carrying grocery bags. He looked like he was coming back home from the market. He brought tomatoes, cucumbers, grapes, soft drinks . . . In the group he described the hospital ward as "an escape hatch," "a haven." He explained: "you showed a personal attitude, you related to every little thing very seriously and respectfully," "you cared." He compared the ward's staff to parental figures: the chief psychiatrist was "a father," the nurse "a mother" and concluded: "if one understands that, one can nurse, suckle and feed on what you can offer him."

Maurice

Maurice, too, seems to be unable to settle down anywhere. But his itinerary is much more widespread, in fact encompassing the entire planet. He was born a wanderer. "I never went to the same school for more than a year, and I don't have any friends left from any school I ever went to. I have traveled so much that there is no language that I truly master." His parents kept moving, looking for the ultimate location, but did not know how to feed, contain, hold, and support their children, and particularly this child, whose development was fraught with difficulties. Maurice's first episode of asthma occurred at birth, and as an infant he suffered not only from asthma but also from digestive, dermatological, and other problems. Maurice does not remember all this but only tells, with a great deal of pain and anger, about the experiences of abandonment he had as a child.

A child with learning and conduct problems, Maurice was thrown away from one place after the other; his parents could not find an educational framework that would suit his needs.

Maurice learned to survive. He has been wandering in the world for many years. He restlessly moves from place to place, trying to start something of his own. He tried to get as far away from his father as he could, and found a place in another continent. He acquired a profession in which he was successful (his profession is not very different from that of his father's). He tried to ignore and repress the pain and almost cut all of his contacts with his family of origin. But in his heart he still yearned for his father. For a while he felt that he was doing OK, but his angry outbursts and temper tantrums became more frequent and more powerful, and he felt he was getting into more and more trouble.

When he finally collapsed he called his parents, who arranged for him to fly back to their home and sought treatment for him. For a while he lived in their home, where they had occasional quibbles and angry outbursts, always followed by a "Returning of the Key" ceremony (or, more accurately, a "Throwing Away of the Key" to his parents' home). Being without a key probably has to do with more than just this particular home where his parents currently live. More than just a sort of concrete behavior–he throws away the key to their home and in fact remains without any key–this act symbolizes Maurice's lack of key to an *inner* home. He throws away the key, concretely as well as emotionally, and returns to his familiar inner experience of homelessness.

Maurice also has many plans in which he always envisages traveling. "Ill go there and then I'll travel here." From his parents' home, he uses the Internet to find occupation around the world. He makes deals and transactions related to his profession, in various relevant workplaces all over the globe. He promises to leave "in February, March and April next year." This search is also indicative of his changing mental state. When he is stressed and in a poor emotional state, he finds several jobs in parallel. When he stabilizes, he hardly looks for work at all.

Although Maurice is an energetic and charismatic professional, he does not succeed in finding work "here." *Prima facia*, there are many good reasons for that. "Here I'm offered insultingly small and miserable sums of money," "here people want to take advantage of me and steal my professional secrets." Although he was self-employed for many years, succeeded in his work and made a good living, when he is here, in his father's turf, he is again a child yearning for his father's attention and care. He cannot succeed without him. He also refuses to even listen to the possibility of receiving support from mental health authorities, and rejects with contempt all attempts to rehabilitate him and help him find work or a place to live. He therefore remains a workless professional, a young, handsome, and talented homeless.

CLINICAL CHARACTERISTICS

The above mentioned three cases as well as other examples are telling of the emotional and behavioral characteristics of Mental Homelessness. As an attempt to conceptualize these narratives into a clinical framework that will allow at some point to be empirically studied, we present a number of clinical characteristics. Although these characteristics concur with the DSM-IV classification of Narcissistic personality disorder, these patients were not necessarily diagnosed as such. We suggest that another common denominator may account for the joint presence of these characteristics in these individuals. These points are further discussed below.

1. *Unexplained inability to find a home:* these patients' inability to find, rent, settle down in, or hold to a home does not seem to be related to the availability of financial *or mental* resources. Highly intelligent and quite capable of handling various tasks in everyday

life, the specific task of finding a place to live and holding to it seems to be an insurmountable challenge for them.

2. *Unawareness to one's homelessness:* although these individuals have neither a home nor a place to live, they are usually unaware to their homelessness. Using the most basic defense mechanisms of denial and projection, they tend to account for their situation by pointing at the circumstances, other people, or just by saying "it happens."

3. *No suffering:* they do not express any experience of mental suffering with regard to the fact that they have no home. Their wish for the inaccessible and unobtainable home is not accompanied by mental pain. When they do experience distress, it seems to be more related to immediate and concrete matters (e.g., no place to put one's belongings for tonight), rather than to more general emotional concerns.

4. *Inability to establish a long-lasting relationship:* personal, professional, geographical or other relationships all seem to be doomed to failure from the start (this applies even to their hospitalization periods, which are often rather short and tend to end abruptly). Another facet of this handicap is the lack of any long-lasting experience of success.

5. *Narcissistic vulnerability:* these patients all seem to have experienced some form of severe abandonment and have a basic experience of rejection.

6. *Flashy self-presentation:* they try to create a successful image of themselves; they are extremely particular in the way they dress or speak (e.g., using pompous language).

7. *The predominance of home-related ideation:* home and home-related words, terms and concepts ooze out of these patients' verbalization and behavior: they frequently mention home or home-related concepts, or engage in home or home-related activities (i.e., cooking, shopping, food).

AN ATTEMPT TO DYNAMIC THEORETICAL CONCEPTUALIZATION

This paper started with a historical view of a special population: homeless people who are also mentally ill. Several cases in our clinical practice–three of which are brought here–suggest that underlying actual homelessness there could exist a particular state of mind. In the following section we shall attempt to explore this concept, as well as some possible clinical applications and explanations of these particular patients' choice of symptom.

The three cases brought here were conspicuous in our clinical work, because of their extremeness and their apparent common traits. First and foremost, their homelessness was more than just mere "placelessness," as they demonstrated a seemingly constant tendency to become homeless. We hypothesize that this is reflective of a weakened or failing inner structure, a state we refer to as Mental Homelessness. We suggest that this notion may serve tentatively as a paradigmatic conceptual model describing at least some aspects of human behavior

Viewed in this light, it is interesting to explore these patients' choice of actual homelessness as chief manifested symptom. Presumably, traumatic situations from childhood, in which the child was not contained, lead the child to create his own solutions, such as the lack of mental pain, common to all these patients. This is a mechanism of self sufficiency (Gerzi, 2000), in which the individual seems to state: "I'm not needy, I can fill my voids all by myself." On a practical level, such an individual creates a golden fantasy (ibid.) for himself, an imaginary wonder-world in which everything is perfect and there is neither pain nor lack or want. For example, by becoming–and remaining–homeless, the individual is put in such a strenuous situation that requires all of his being to be invested in one and only thing–survival. In such conditions there is hardly any mental room left for any other experience. The feeling of neediness is therefore efficiently muffled, obstructed, obliterated. Homelessness would be a highly efficient, though extreme, type of distraction.

Homelessness is also a state of ultimate neediness, accompanied in these patients by a seemingly paradoxical lack of subjective mental pain. The symptom is carefully designed so as to hide but at the same time also point out the huge void, the hole in the psyche. Kohut (1986) explains that "A patient whose self has been damaged [. . .] reactivates the specific needs that had remained unanswered by the specific faulty interactions between the nascent self and the self objects of early life" (p. 177). Winnicott, in "Fear of Breakdown" (1989), writes: " . . . The patient needs to 'remember' [. . .] but it is not possible to remember something that has not yet happened, and this thing of the past has not happened yet because the patient was not there for it to happen to. The only way to 'remember' in this case is for the patient to experience this past thing [. . .] " (p. 92).

One might speculate that the place where mental disorder develops is at one's inner home. This seems to mainly refer to the function of home–containment, holding, mirroring and so on–which is a maternal, self object's function (Kohut, 1986). When a failure occurs in the relations with figures serving as self objects, then the home function–the maternal environment–is impaired, as is the potential for the development of an independent self.[2]

THERAPEUTIC IMPLICATIONS

What is the scope of Mental Homelessness? Is this a new concept? Does it suggest a modified diagnosis? Does it offer a new work methodology? Within what boundaries can it be applied? How does it relate to other concepts? Originally developed in the therapy room, the idea offers a working concept in the field of mental health, and seems to fit well within existing psychodynamic conceptual frameworks. At the same time however, it seems that the idea has a potential to be looked inspiring in other everyday sociological fields as well.

Mentally ill homeless people have always represented a very unique problem for the various help agencies. But as was also described above, the existence of an inner Mental Homelessness has never been taken into consideration and most attempts to deal with this so particularly mixed population therefore focused merely on these clients' concrete problems of everyday life.

The perspective of Mental Homelessness is a descriptive-paradigmatic model that may also affect the therapeutic approach. This approach may lead to increasing the therapeutic leverage towards developing, or/and consolidating the mental home of those whose 'inner sanctuary' has been either absent or seriously incapacitated. The theme of home is familiar, well-known and non-threatening to the patient. The metaphor of homelessness may serve a non-threatening space of dialogue and interpretation, an intermediate domain functioning as a translation space, in which the therapeutic dyad speaks of place but refers to home, and speaks of home but refers to the self.

CONCLUSION AND SUGGESTION
FOR FURTHER DEVELOPMENT

In our efforts to re-create and narrate our patients' personal stories and pathogenesis we found the conceptual framework of inner homelessness to be an efficient tool–even when there was no external manifestation in the form of actual homelessness–one that aided us in our attempts to understand a little better the patient's life history, and most important, his or her everyday experience.

The cases described above illustrate the difference between "home" and "place," or between homelessness and the "mere" lack of place, or "placelessness." There can be no home without a place, and no inner home without an inner place to place it in.

Major territories for future investigation may include the psychodynamics of the perception of space. This will inevitably be related to our perception of the world, the constitution of our inner place and therefore affect the very way in which we conceive of family, community, city, state and country.

These thoughts and observations also stress the need to develop new tools, as we are currently undertaking, for assessing and measuring Mental Homelessness, both in mentally ill populations as well as in the population at large and even in micro and macro societal frameworks such as the workplace or the nation.

The collapse of the old space-related concepts–home, nation–and, on the other hand, the emerging and omnipresent cyberspace, emphasize the importance of investigating the psychological and metaphorical meanings of the concept of place (Harvey, 1986); such investigation is sure to produce new practices, new meanings and new definitions to what humans regard as (their) place and home in the world. Understanding the suggested concept of Mental Homelessness may lead to a further understanding of larger social and societal questions.

NOTES

1. All names and identifying details have been altered.

2. In his explanation of Winnicott's concept of "the capacity to be alone," Ogden (1986) writes: "What is internalized [. . .] is not the mother as an object, but the mother as environment. The premature objectification (discovery of the mother as object), and internalization of the object-mother lead to the establishment of an omnipotent internal-object-mother. This internalization of mother as omnipotent object is quite different from the establishment of the capacity to be alone (the former process is often a defensive substitute for the latter)" (pp. 181-182).

REFERENCES

American Psychiatric Association, (1994) *Diagnostic and Statistical Manual of Mental Disorders,* Fourth Edition. Washington, DC, American Psychiatric Association.

Belcher J.R., & Rife J.C. (1989). Social breakdown syndrome in schizophrenia: Treatment implications. *Social Casework: The Journal of Contemporary Social Work* 70 (10), 611-616.

De Assis, M. (1882). O Alienista, in *Memorias Postumas de Bras Cubas* (Hebrew translation, 1987: Keter Publishing House, Jerusalem).

Foucault, M. (1967). *Madness and Civilization, A History of Insanity in the Age of Reason*, Great Britain: Tavistock Publications, Ltd.

Gerhart, U.C. (1990). *Caring for the chronically mentally ill.* New Jersey: F.E. Peacok Publishers, Inc.

Gerzi, S. (2000). Regashot shel choser u'maatefet ha'ahava/Feelings of lack and envelop of love. A lecture at the *Kenes Kachol Lavan/Blue and White Conference of the Israeli Psychotherapy Association*, Herzelia: Dec. 2000.

Harvey, D. (1996). *Justice, nature and the geography of difference.* Oxford: Blackwell Publishers.

Hoff, M.D., K.H. Briar, K. Knighton & R.A. Van. (1992). To survive and to thrive: Integration services for the homeless mentally ill. *Journal of Sociology and Social Welfare* 19 (4), 235-255.

Kohut, H. & Wolf, E. (1986). The disorders of the self and their treatment: An outline. In Andrew P. Morrison, MD (Ed.) *Essential Papers on Narcissism.* New York University Press. pp. 175-196.

Linhorst, D.M. (1992). A redefinition of the problem of homelessness among persons with a chronic mental illness. *Journal of Sociology & Social Welfare* 19 (4), 43-54.

Martin, M.A. (1990). The homeless mentally ill and community-based care: Changing a mindset. *Community Mental Health Journal* 26 (5), 435-449.

Pam, A. (1994). The new schizophrenia: Diagnosis and dynamics of the homeless mentally ill. *The Journal of Mind and Behavior* 15 (3), 199-222.

Rife, J.C., First, R.J., Greenle, R.W., Miller, L.D. & M.A. Feichter (1991). Case management with homeless mentally ill people. *Health and Social Work* 16 (1), 58-67.

Susser, E., Goldfinger, S.M., & White, A. (1990). Some clinical approaches to the homeless mentally Ill. *Community Mental Health Journal*, 26 (5), 463-480.

Timms, P. (1996). Homelessness and mental illness: A brief history. In Bhugra, Diesh et al. (Ed.). *Homelessness and mental health. Studies in social and community psychiatry.* (pp. 11-25) Cambridge, England UK: Cambridge University Press.

Winnicott, D.W. (1989). Fear of breakdown. In Winnicott, C., Shepherd, R. & Davis, M. (Eds.). *D.W. Winnicott Psycho-Analytic Explorations.* Cambridge, Massachusetts: Harvard University Press. pp 87-95.

PART II

SOCIAL WORK METHODS
IN HEALTH AND MENTAL HEALTH

Introduction:
Part II

Pirkko-Liisa Rauhala, PhD
Anna Metteri, MSocSc, PhD
Teppo Kröger, PhD
Anneli Pohjola, PhD

This special volume is the second part of the three edited proceedings issues of the 3rd International Conference on Social Work in Health and Mental Health held in Tampere, Finland in 2001. In this volume, the focus is on social work methods used and applied in health and mental health.

While starting to discuss methods in social work, two basic perspectives have to be taken into consideration. *First,* in the case of such a subject as social work, the academic discipline and the everyday practice are tightly connected and intertwined with each other–they can neither live nor proceed apart from one another. It implies that research methods and practice methods are close to each other. From the very beginning of social work, the research orientation has been an intrinsic part of social work. What else does a social worker do than try to investigate the social and human reality which she or he is acting in and part of?

Second, while mentioning the word "method," all of the classical repertoire of social work research are included: case analysis, community analysis, macro analysis, evaluation, empirically oriented theorising, etc., and all the variations of these, the whole diversity of tools by which

---

[Haworth co-indexing entry note]: "Introduction: Part II." Rauhala, Pirkko-Lisa et al. Co-published simultaneously in *Social Work in Health Care* (The Haworth Social Work Practice Press, an imprint of The Haworth Press, Inc.) Vol. 39, No. 3/4, 2004, pp. 227-229; and: *Social Work Visions from Around the Globe: Citizens, Methods, and Approaches* (ed: Anna Metteri et al.) The Haworth Social Work Practice Press, an imprint of The Haworth Press, Inc., 2004, pp. 227-229. Single or multiple copies of this article are available for a fee from The Haworth Document Delivery Service [1-800-HAWORTH, 9:00 a.m. - 5:00 p.m. (EST). E-mail address: docdelivery@haworthpress.com].

we try to understand ourselves and our fellow human beings and to recognize the social contexts in which we live, in sickness and in health, in good times and in bad.

In the process of organising the papers into this second volume, such categories for titles as comparative method, evaluating method, case analysis method, networking method, bridge-building method, and innovation as a method, came into our minds. Nevertheless, it became evident that if we try to apply the lists of methods as a typological frame, we are going to lose much of the content of the papers. Another way was to be found in order to highlight the variety of methods used in the reports, but not at the cost of substance. The question of method is: *how* the things were done, and *if* the intended goals were reached or not, and what kind of non-intended consequences appeared. We decided to combine the how-question with the substance fields represented in the papers. Not surprisingly, the methods as such are not the focus of our four subtitles.

Under the first subtitle, we collected papers which underline the diversity of societies. The prominent nominator for diversity in our global era is the ethnic dimension. The complexity of ethnic relations can open up our eyes, so we can better recognize the other dimensions of increasing diversity in contemporary societies too. In research and practice, the need for methods in managing the diversity is obvious, in order to advance mutual understanding and human dignity, as well as to initiate dialogues by which exclusion, conflicts and confrontations can be buffered. The articles collected under this title give a good glimpse into approaches and fields which matter in advancing our knowledge basis of diversity.

In the articles of the second section of this volume, the voice of social workers and service users will be discussed. In many roots of classical social work, the clients and service users have been interpreted as partners in the process where solutions for their troubled life situations are searched for. In the development of service systems, the organisations have often enlarged to such an extent that the individual actors can lose the sense of meaning in the processes concerning themselves. Social workers from all over the globe have reported frustration and powerlessness in organizing their work according to the needs of citizens and in cooperation with the service users; other professionals like lawyers and medical experts do not always without hesitation appreciate the social work expertise as useful for their own practice. On the other hand, social workers quite often work alone in a big organisation, without collegial support. That is why innovative openings are needed to strengthen the co-operation among social workers themselves, with other professionals, and especially with service users. In the papers of this section, some new ideas concerning the mentioned issues are launched.

Empowerment is the number one concept in contemporary social work discussions. We would say that it has always been in the focus, only the word has varied over time. Classical community work emphasized the building of social networks, and the classical case work focused on empowering the person to manage his/her own life. According to our interpretation, in the current discussions both dimensions of classical social work are put into the same setting, and the methods for increasing the inclusion, participation, and affiliation are searched for. In the reports of the third section, the expertise of service users is emphasized: in their own issues they are the most relevant informants and knowledge producers. The empowering practice in social work means acceptance and appreciation of the everyday-life knowledge as equal with professional and academic knowledge; by stating this we do not deny the difference between the mentioned types of knowledge but underline the meaning of unique human experience as the key element for successful practice. Additionally, in this section we also have an example of an innovative intervention study of how to empower citizens, in this case truck drivers themselves, to practice preventive action in order to advance the well-being of the whole community.

The fourth subtitle consists of two reports which are carefully conducted studies of quite special life-cycles and, at the same time, they call for enhancement of individual living chances and for human rights. The two papers of this section deal with extreme, dramatic life events of individual persons. By focusing on very special life-cycles, we can increase our understanding of how the diversity and similarity of human life have to be interpreted in the same context. Social work defends human life, and one method for doing this is to increase the knowledge basis of life-cycle perspective. The understanding of the uniqueness of individual life-cycles provides a firm basis for promoting human rights–the right to have a life-cycle.

Cultural Competence in Psychosocial and Psychiatric Care: A Critical Perspective with Reference to Research and Clinical Experiences in California, US and in Germany

Dagmar Schultz, PhD

SUMMARY. The impact of culture and ethnicity on the diagnosis and treatment of patients with mental disorders has been of growing interest

Dagmar Schultz is Professor, Alice-Salomon-School for Social Work and Social Pedagogics, and Private Lecturer, Free University of Berlin, Germany.

Address correspondence to: Dr. Dagmar Schultz, Alice-Salomon-Fachhochschule für Sozialarbeit und Sozialpädagogik, Alice-Salomon-Platz 5, D-12627 Berlin, Germany (E-mail: dagschultz@aol.com).

[Haworth co-indexing entry note]: "Cultural Competence in Psychosocial and Psychiatric Care: A Critical Perspective with Reference to Research and Clinical Experiences in California, US and in Germany." Shultz, Dagmar. Co-published simultaneously in *Social Work in Health Care* (The Haworth Social Work Practice Press, an imprint of The Haworth Press, Inc.) Vol. 39, No. 3/4, 2004, pp. 231-247; and: *Social Work Visions from Around the Globe: Citizens, Methods, and Approaches* (ed: Anna Metteri et al.) The Haworth Social Work Practice Press, an imprint of The Haworth Press, Inc., 2004, pp. 231-247. Single or multiple copies of this article are available for a fee from The Haworth Document Delivery Service [1-800-HAWORTH, 9:00 a.m. - 5:00 p.m. (EST). E-mail address: docdelivery@haworthpress.com].

and concern to professionals in the United States and also in Germany. This contribution intends to give an overview of key aspects regarding competence in intercultural situations using research and clinical experiences from the United States and from Germany. The issue of racism and discrimination as contributing factors in the development of mental disorders will be critically examined from a US and a German perspective. *[Article copies available for a fee from The Haworth Document Delivery Service: 1-800-HAWORTH. E-mail address: <docdelivery@haworthpress.com> Website: <http://www.HaworthPress.com> © 2004 by The Haworth Press, Inc. All rights reserved.]*

KEYWORDS. Cultural competence, psychiatric care, minorities, racism, mental disorders, psychopharmacology, empowerment of patients

CULTURAL COMPETENCE
AS A PROFESSIONAL QUALIFICATION

"Globalization" is a much cited and used concept for the internationalization of capital, of media and cultural expressions. These times of globalization are also characterized by voluntary and involuntary migration. Most societies are confronted by the challenge of integrating immigrants and refugees as well as members of ethnic minorities who have lived in these countries for generations, but still experience more or less severe discrimination.

Competence in dealing with intercultural situations has been recognized as a professional requirement by industry and business, and they have begun to develop integrative strategies. Professionals in the area of health, psychology and psychiatry also need to acknowledge *competent behavior in intercultural situations as a necessary professional qualification* so as to avoid harmful and costly deficits in qualified and effective care.

In 1999 and 2000, I studied programs of cultural competence and diversity in community mental health care which were established or funded by the state of California focusing on San Francisco and Oakland. Against the background of concepts of cultural competence and experiences of clinical work in California, I am presently doing research in mental health programs of hospitals and community institutions in Berlin, Germany (Schultz, 2002). Cultural competence, intercultural therapy and counseling, transcultural care–these concepts have been discussed during the past years on a theoretical level in Germany, but unfortunately have been put into practice only sporadically in individual institutions or by individual psychologists and psychiatrists without any systemic institutional and state planning. In this contribution, I intend to give an overview of key aspects regarding cultural competence using research and clinical experiences from the United States and from Germany.

The following questions will be addressed:

1. How can we define cultural competence in psychiatric care?
2. What are the necessary qualifications and wherein lie the difficulties and pitfalls of becoming a culturally competent professional?
3. Why is cultural competence necessary and who benefits from it?
4. How can concepts of cultural competence be put into practice?

DEFINITIONS OF CULTURAL COMPETENCE IN PSYCHIATRIC CARE

On a general level, cultural competence signifies the ability "to communicate in an appropriate and successful manner in an unfamiliar cultural environment or with persons from another culture" (Hinz-Rommel, 1996, 20). Basically, intercultural competence means the gradual increase of the ability of social interaction. This involves empathy, respect for and appreciation of the other person, sensitivity, clarity and genuineness in the encounter with a client (Koray, 2000, 23). We can see here that the attitude toward another person, a culturally non-specific aspect, is very important.

In relation to psychiatric care, the American Psychiatric Association formulated its view of cultural competence in a section of its guidelines entitled "Considerations for Sociocultural Diversity":

> The process of psychiatric evaluation must take into consideration, and respect, the diversity of American subcultures and must be sensitive to the patient's *ethnicity, place of birth, gender, age, social class, sexual orientation, and religious/spiritual beliefs.* Respectful evaluation involves an empathic, nonjudgemental attitude toward the patient's explanation of illness, concerns and background. An awareness of one's possible biases or prejudices about patients from different subcultures and an understanding of the limitations of one's knowledge and skills in working with such patients may lead to the identification of situations calling for con-

sultations with a clinician who has expertise concerning a particular subculture. Further, the potential effect of the psychiatrist's sociocultural identity on the attitude and behavior of the patient would be taken into account in forming a diagnostic opinion. (quoted in Lu, 1999a, 13; emphasis by the author)

This definition points out several important aspects:

- Cultural diversity includes gender, social class, sexual orientation and religion/spiritual beliefs. One could add physical disabilities to the list. The focus in the literature and in much of of the practice–except in California–has been on a more conventional restrictive view of cultural diversity equaling ethnic diversity. The advantage of the inclusive view is that it encourages a broader sensitization. In addition, people do combine different identities, for instance, a Black German or a Turkish migrant may be gay and/or belong to a religious minority.
- The definition emphasizes self-reflection, namely the clinician's consciousness

  - of her/his own prejudices,
  - of her/his limitations in knowledge and skills,
  - of the potential effect of her/his own sociocultural identity in the interaction with the patient.

What is not mentioned here is a self-critical view of Western medicine and psychiatry. In other contexts, however, alternative treatments and the services of traditional healers have been included in proposed system standards in the U.S., such as by committees of professionals, experts, and users of four underserved/underrepresented ethnic groups, who formulated standards under the tutelage of the U.S. Department of Health (U.S. Department of Health, 1999).

Culturally competent services can thus be defined as a set of congruent behaviors, knowledge, skills, attitudes and policies that work effectively in cross-cultural situations between a system, agency, or the clinician and the patient/family (Lu, 1999a, 12).

NECESSARY COMPONENTS OF CULTURAL COMPETENCE

There is an increasing awareness of the importance of an individual's identity in terms of race, ethnicity, culture, and class as it relates to treatment for mental illness. This awareness, however, needs to feed into the acknowledgement that a euro-centric approach dominating behavioral health services does not take into account the cultural specific needs of the consumer, but oftentimes serves as a barrier to access and appropriate treatment (Lu, 1999b, 18). Self-reflective integration of bio-psycho-social knowledge is a necessary start for change.

Language Capacities

On the clinical level, one basic standard of cultural competence calls for *language capacities*. Lack of language capacity and not using a qualified interpreter can lead to situations as described in the following examples from Germany:

- A Turkish woman speaks with a Turkish psychologist and tells him that this is the first time in 22 years that she can describe her problems in her mother tongue. Before, she always had to speak through a third person, and frequently her children or relatives were asked to translate.
- In a psychiatric ward a Turkish cleaning woman translates a conversation between a doctor and a patient. The doctor asks her why she stops translating what the patient is saying. She says: "Oh, he is just talking nonsense. He keeps repeating that he is hearing voices."

In at least parts of the United States and in several European countries it is forbidden to use cleaning personnel or relatives as interpreters, which is still common practice in Germany. While it should be a requirement in the training of medical personnel, psychologists and counselors to learn at least one foreign language, there will always be a need for interpreters for certain languages. These interpreters should receive training that gives them sufficient background in psychology and therapy to work as an informed partner with the patient and the psychologist/psychiatrist.

Cultural Knowledge and Sensitivity on a Biological level

Next to language capacities, competence in dealing with intercultural situations involves *cultural knowledge and sensitivity on a biological level*. Ethnic groups vary in the metabolization of certain drugs. Drug metabolizing enzymes called the cytochrome P450 enzyme system and found mostly in the liver are responsible for breaking down medications. Mutation patterns of these enzymes show "dramatic cross-ethnic differences" (Lin, 1999, 60). These differences can also be responsible for how side effects are experienced. Slow metabolizers, found particularly among Southeast Asians and African Americans, maintain higher blood levels of medication and thus require lower doses. Yet African Americans in particular are more likely to be viewed as violent than Caucasians or Asians and often receive excessive doses of psychotropics (Lawson, 1999, 30). Dr. William B. Lawson, Professor of Psychiatry at the University of Indiana, writes: "As a consequence African Americans, who may be suspicious of mental health providers in the first place, may be less tolerant of medication side effects and less invested in medication compliance." He also points out: ". . . African Americans are more likely to get antipsychotic medication irrespective of diagnosis . . . Community surveys consistently show that African Americans who have major depression are only treated half the time. When treatment is provided it can often be punitive" (Lawson, ibid.). Studies further suggest that African Americans may experience more tricyclic antidepressant side effects and are more likely to develop tardive dyskinesia, a serious movement disorder (Lawson, ibid.).

Response to medication is also influenced by environmental factors such as nutrition, smoking, the intake of herbal medicine–factors which are intertwined with social class and with cultural traditions. Clinicians are now developing methods to measure enzyme activity to guide the physician in selecting the right drug and dose. As Michael W. Smith, MD writes: "The best approach is to treat each person as an individual, using information about one's diet, habits, medication and culture as a guide" (Smith, 1999, 16).

Cultural Knowledge on a Psychological Level

Cultural knowledge on a psychological level implies becoming familiar with the perception of death, age, mental illness, with the meaning of hallucinations, contact with the ancestors, etc., in different cultural groups, and being aware of the fact that psychological problems often are somatized, i.e., described by a patient as physical pain. While white Germans may be more likely to express their psychological symptoms, such as anxiety, depression or suicidal tendencies, Turkish migrants or Asian or Hispanic patients may complain of physical pain. An example from Germany: A Turkish woman describes her depression to the doctor as a state of chronic pain, which results in a false diagnosis, in frequent change of doctors and, on account of lacking cultural and linguistic competence of the doctors, in wrong prescriptions and in generating illness instead of healing.

Diagnosis and therapy require a basic knowledge of the cultural traditions of the client and of the social system the traditions are rooted in. Many Turkish people go to a *hodscha,* a traditional healer, also while seeing German medical doctors. Healing traditions based on Black and White magic may play a significant role, and a Western therapist needs to consider whether and how to integrate them in her/his approach. Dietrich F. Koch, psychologist in Xenion, Psychotherapeutic Counseling Center for Politically Persecuted Persons in Berlin, Germany, writes about working with a patient from Bangladesh by practicing Black and White Magic in his sense with him: "I try to make changes within his system, changes that make sense for him at this particular point in time" (Koch, 1998, 152). Since the ability of understanding often is limited for white Western therapists, Koch relates that working with qualified interpreters from the cultural group of the patient can be a tremendous advantage.

Asians may interpret mental illness in the framework of their medical model, which is far more wholistically oriented than Western medicine. The physical body and emotions are seen as an integrated whole, and the goal is for the human body to be in harmony and balance with the forces of the universe in order to maintain both physical and psychological health (Cheung, 1999, 44). This means that the Asian experience "is a full-bodied one, a large world-view which embraces many aspects of living . . . Symptom removal alone is inadequate," writes Walter Owyang, Professor of Psychology and clinical psychologist in describing treatment programs for the Southeast Asian population in San Jose, California which have existed since the '80s (Owyang, 1999, 46).

Religion may play an important role in the interpretation of mental illness (supernatural forces are the cause) or in overcoming illness. Frequently, religious practice is connected with traditional healing such as the use of herbal medicine. Native Americans revive traditions of sharing emotional frustrations with medicine people during a sweat lodge. The Native American Health Center in Oakland, California brings in medicine people from different tribes who do ceremonies for people in hospitals. It engages patients in cultural activities to help repair marginal identities and address issues such as post traumatic stress, grief of generations over the loss of land and life (interview with Janet King, counselor, Feb. 3, 2000).

The Instituto Familiar de la Raza in San Francisco, directed by Dr. Concha Saucelo, combines indigenous traditions of Latinos, Chicanos and Latino Indios such as "sweats,' rites of women, dance groups, etc., with Western therapeutic practices. For some of these contexts, it will be absolutely necessary to have a therapist from the particular cultural group. The Instituto also offers a program of training and supervision for interns who are working on their master degree, their PhD and for post doctoral students.

Social Knowledge and Self-Reflection

Generally, the work needs to be regarded as a continuous process of learning. Learning about other cultures requires first of all a self-reflective stance as addressed in the declaration of the American Psychiatric Association cited above. Dr. Ernie Rodrigues of Cañada College in Redwood City, California states that a conceptual understanding of cross-cultural issues in not enough. "What is truly needed is a compassionate level of relational competence which incorporates an understanding of cross-cultural dynamics . . . to actually be able to speak about those cross-cultural issues which impact the client's experience . . . More typically what seems to occur is a process of avoidance fueled by fear. Under the rubric 'we are all human' is the implication that 'we are all the same' so there is no need to bring uncomfortable issues of race and ethnicity into the relationship" (Rodriguez, 1999, 6). Rodriguez calls for a practical understanding of the concept of worldview which he defines as one's experienced reality:

> We must be able to recognize that we operate from within a worldview and simultaneously be able to be free of our worldview so that we might be able to understand and appreciate the meaning of another's worldview perspective . . . Trying to replace another's reality with our own is a good working definition of oppression. If we are to be oppression sensitive we must work from *within* the person's experience . . . the critical component in effective cross-cultural work is developing a working knowledge of our own worldview, including the biases we bring to our work with others. Only then will compassionate healing be possible. (Rodriguez, 1999, 7)

Knowledge and skills in these areas in combination with self-reflection can prevent false diagnoses which often occur on account of stereotyped views of certain immigrant groups. An example in a text by two psychologists from California:

. . . it is disturbing to see in a report that a shy, monolingual submissive Latina woman is labeled as 'schizoid' personality, because she 'avoids eye contact' when you know that initial shyness and some reserved attitude is 'culturally' normal for many Latina women. (Valencia, 1999, 35)

At the same time, professionals have to be aware that cultures are not static, but in a constant dynamic process of change. This means, for instance, that the psychological problems of a first generation immigrant most likely are different from those of her/his grandchildren. Class issues, race and gender are closely tied with culture-based experiences and need to be taken into consideration. African American lower class persons, e.g., tend to be viewed as violent, Asians as submissive even when the objective data demonstrates the opposite (Lawson, 1999, 30). In short, when calling for cultural competence we need to be aware of the danger of pigeon-holing people by following limited imaginations of certain cultures. The individual and her/his experiences have to be at the center of attention and concern.

On the social level an understanding of the worldview of a client from a discriminated minority requires an awareness of the impact of socio-economic class and of discriminatory experiences, of family and community structures, of gender and generation issues and of the significance of collective memories of oppression and of (potential) support through cultural traditions.

EXPERIENCES OF RACISM AND DISCRIMINATION AND OF WHITE SKIN PRIVILEGE AS FACTORS IN THE INTERACTION OF THERAPISTS AND PATIENTS

While in the United States *research* on the psychological and social effects of racism has also found attention in the field of mental health (see, e.g., Thompson & Neville, 1999), it is significant that in Germany there have been hardly any studies done from this perspective. Jochen Zeiler, Professor of Psychiatry at a Berlin hospital and his colleague Dr. Fuat Zarifoglu, at the time the only Turkish psychiatrist at all of Berlin's hospitals, stated in a paper on "Ethnic discrimination and psychic illness" at the World Congress for Social Psychiatry in Hamburg in 1994:

A series of epidemiological studies of migrant populations have examined how geographic and social mobility and how social disintegration and cultural change influence the manifestation and course of psychic illnesses. Strangely enough, however, discrimination as a psychosocial stress factor has never become the object of psychiatric research . . . And the question is permitted whether science as one of the societal activities dominated by the social majority finds it difficult to devote itself to the central problems of minorities who are largely excluded from the political process of decisionmaking. (see Zeiler & Zarifoglu, 1994, 101)

Acknowledging everyday racism and discrimination, an insecure resident status, economic problems and the lack of a positive vision of the future as possible factors for mental disorders would definitely have consequences for the therapeutic practice. It would require labor intensive cooperation with social services, much more investment in community relations and aftercare, and facing the question how to deal with structural racism as an individual and as an institution. If, for instance, it becomes clear that the psychosis of a migrant woman is directly related to the continuous threat of having to leave the country and her family, this legal insecurity must be ended. Otherwise even the best neuroleptic prophylaxis will not prevent relapses (Zeiler & Zarifoglu, ibid.).

Frequently, social conditions and collective (historical) experiences of minority persons cause mistrust and prevent persons from seeking professional help in situations of mental stress. In a big Berlin hospital in an immigrant district, 50% of the persons being received in the emergency ward are immigrants who are diagnosed with psychic disorders. This indicates that people go to the hospital or to a psychiatric institution only in the state of absolute crisis. Persons without a permanent residence status in Germany also fear to lose their tenuous status if they are registered as a "problem case."

Mistrust of the medical establishment and of psychiatric drugs is widespread among certain minorities and has many reasons:

- For African Americans, the infamous Tuskegee syphilis study in which patients were denied effective treatments in order to study the natural history of syphilis appears to have a lasting effect.
- Fear of false diagnosis: There is considerable evidence that African American patients with mania are more apt to be misdiagnosed as having schizophrenia and receiving antipsychotic medications

(Gray, 1999, 25). In Germany there has not been research on differential treatment of psychiatric patients, but the lack of cultural competence in many institutions suggests that misdiagnoses are taking place.

- Fear of abuse or false application of medications.
- Fear of being even more stigmatized in addition to being marginal already, since the dominant society/culture itself attaches a strong stigma to mental illness.

The white therapist of the dominant group is, therefore, seen as a person of *power*–power on account of white skin privilege and on account of being part of the mental health system. The professional, whether a member of the dominant group or of a minority, has to be conscious of the fact that she/he actually does have power, however little it may be, and that the relationship to a client is a dominance-subordination relationship. The next step can be to use that power in a constructive manner to empower clients. Renée Hatter, pedagogue and psychologist in California, describes this process of transference of power writing about African American counselors. These counselors were inadequately trained and experienced their known powerlessness and marginal position within the mental health system. They demonstrated oppressive behavior toward their African American clients so as to give themselves a sense of power. Their behavior toward the clients changed once they addressed their issues to management: They now could hear the clients' issues and respond to them (Hatter, 1999, 26-28).

The unspoken knowledge of internalized oppression and of the (relative) lack of power of minority professionals may be one reason why members of a discriminated group sometimes do not seek treatment from a member of their community. Presently I am interviewing personnel and patients of mental health institutions in Berlin for a study on the significance of cultural competence. A patient in a residential psychiatric home initially stated in the presence of her counselor that she thought it was very good to have a counselor from her ethnic group and to be able to speak to someone in her mother tongue. Once he left the room, she said: "He is not good–he can't do anything for me. It would be better to have only German counselors." (I later heard that she had been making some requests which could not be fulfilled by anyone.) This is an understandable reaction in a society that allocates power to the dominant group. Generally, however, we can assume that minority clients prefer to be able to relate to someone of their own group–at least until cultural competence has become a self-understood standard for all workers in the mental health system.

Another factor is that patients may deny differences and not talk about experiences of discrimination in an effort not to place themselves in the position of the victim. This attitude may reinforce the tendency of professionals to ignore differences and racist experiences. My interviews in Berlin institutions have shown that the majority of the professionals said they will explore the effects of possible experiences of discrimination only if the patient initiates the subject.

We can, therefore, say that competence in intercultural therapeutical contexts requires professional training in combination with day-to-day learning about cultural and social differences, including differences of gender and sexual orientation and the effects of racism, sexism, homophobia and class discrimination. This implies self-reflection and a critical assessment of one's own worldview–a journey which can only add to personal and professional growth.

CULTURAL COMPETENCE AS A HUMAN RIGHTS AND AN ECONOMIC ISSUE

The cost of not providing appropriate treatment both in dollars and in human lives-is too great for the needs of ethnic minorities to be ignored. (Lu, 1999b, 22)

Cultural competence in health and mental health care

- is a human rights issue, and
- needs to be outcome oriented.

Human Rights Issue

On the basis of the UN Declaration of Human Rights and of the constitution of most Western European countries, each person has the right to equal treatment. This principle is, however, not regularly translated into practice, aside from the fact that refugees and persons without residence status often are not granted these rights.

In Germany, institutions of psychosocial and psychiatric care rarely devote themselves to patients' problems in the context of migration, racism and antisemitism. As the Black German author May Ayim writes: "While white people are faced with of choosing among a confusing range of therapy offers, Black Germans and immigrants have the difficulty of finding any appropriate therapy offers at all. Most therapists do not feel responsible for their 'special' concerns or feel incompetent and argue that the task is too much for them" (Ayim, 1997, 128).

Furthermore, as we discussed above, migration, especially involuntary migration, can cause psychic, mental and physical stress. Living in a society, where you are not welcome, as is the case for many immigrants and for Black Germans, Roma and Sinti and Jews, means chronic stress. This kind of stress can bring about or add to mental disorder. Professional help in such a situation calls for a person who speaks the language in which you feel most comfortable communicating, who has a basic knowledge of your sociocultural background, who understands the social situation you find yourself in and who has an interest in you as an individual.

For a white person of the majority culture, a mental health institution may offer a protective space, hardly however for black people, for those immigrants who belong to discriminated minorities or for Jews. In a situation in which they can no longer rely upon themselves and feel extremely helpless and dependent, all fears can rise which are based upon a variety of racist experiences. Mechanisms of resistance and survival strategies, which they had used in dealing with a (potentially) hostile and/or ignorant environment, no longer are at their disposal. Not to be understood induces fear and/or calls forth aggressions, especially with immigrants who speak little or no German. To be closed off from public life can cause feelings of panic. Jews, black persons and Roma and Sinti may distrust doctors on account of their knowledge of racism and antisemitism acted out by the medical profession during National Socialism, psychiatrists having practiced the extermination of patients before concentration camps were set up (Schultz, 1999, 156).

Cultural competence is necessary to ensure a situation where the patient can feel safe, understood and can trust people who have the power to influence her/his health and make decisions upon her/his life, a situation which guarantees the human rights of the patient.

Outcome Orientation

Certainly, economic aspects will play a decisive role in the development of culturally competent services. Professionals need to convince management of the fact that patients as well as health insurances and society at large will benefit from qualified and culture-sensitive treatment of minority persons.

The above examples demonstrated clearly the human and the financial costs of cultural incompetencies. From a systemic perspective the development of cultural competence, therefore, is necessary

- to ensure quality standards in diagnosis and treatment, and
- to contribute to cost-effective work results.

Who will then benefit from cultural competence?

- Patients and clients of minority groups.
- Patients and clients of the majority group, since greater sensitivity of professionals will have an effect on their overall performance.
- Professionals.
- Cultural competence will be of benefit not only to patients and clients of minority groups and to families and friends of clients, but also to professionals and for patients and clients of the majority group, since greater sensitivity of professionals will have an effect on their overall performance.
- Health insurances and all financing agents of the medical and social system will profit from practices of cultural competence. In the long run, cultural competence in professional contexts will have a favorable effect on society at large and the next generations.

IMPLEMENTATION OF CONCEPTS OF CULTURAL COMPETENCE

Several different levels and agents of implementation can be identified.

- the government:

Experiences in the US have shown that intervention from governmental agencies is important for implementation. This does not mean that commitment on the part of the community, of consumers and of providers is not important. But it is difficult to ensure structural reforms without governmental support.

In California, the Department of Health is exerting pressure upon institutions receiving public funds. They will have to demonstrate the fulfillment of standards of cultural competence set by the State so as to receive new funds or be refunded. Such standards need to address access and receipt of benefits, treatment of clients, family and community involvement, prevention and after-care, hiring of minority personnel, etc.

Together with educational institutions, the government needs to set up pools of qualified interpreters with basic knowledge in sociopsychology.

- the community:

If the government does not move by itself, it will be the communities which will have to demand changes in the structure and content of psychosocial care. In California, political movements of minority groups put sufficient pressure on the government to start acting.

- consumers/clients:

Certainly, this group is at the lowest level of the power scale. Still, it is important for them to make their voices heard. If they are able to take a strong position, they will put the professionals on the spot. The consumer movement in the United States has been able to impact new developments. In California, for instance, Self Help Agencies (SHAs) have been funded as adjuncts of or referral sources for Community Mental Health Agencies (CMHAs). Cooperation of the SHAs with researchers resulted in studies showing that the CMHAs "primarily deliver treatment-focused services, while the SHAs provide services aimed at fostering socialization, mutual support, empowerment and autonomy" (Segal, Hardiman, & Hodges, 2001).

- professionals:

Professionals can use their position, and academics can bring their research to bear so as to push for change. Professionals benefit in more than one way: they increase their qualifications by important aspects which will be useful in their work with all patients; they avoid making mistakes which are costly on a human and a financial level; they gain the reassurance of providing their patients with a safe setting and a culturally and medically competent treatment.

- mental health institutions including contract and private agencies:

Mental health institutions need to offer continued education in language training and in cultural competence for their personnel. Perhaps most important, they need to hire minority personnel. In the process of dehospitalization, the integration of immigrant and minority patients in resident programs is crucial.

Institutions need to set up effective community boards made up of members of the community they serve. Evaluating these processes and developing control mechanism and incentives for the fulfillment of standards is an important aspect which takes time, but is in the interest of quality management and cost effective work.

• educational institutions:

Educational institutions need to integrate cultural competence into the curriculum. In the U.S., for instance, between 1989 and 1995, the percentage of doctoral programs in counseling psychology requiring a course on multiculturalism rose from 59% to 89% (Kiselica, 1998, 5). They also need to recruit minority students for studies in medicine, psychology, psychiatry, and clinical social work.

In conclusion we can say that everyone involved will benefit from cultural competence. A comprehensive, holistic approach will include the awareness of diversity as well as the consciousness of the need to treat each person as a individual and to seek the empowerment of the individual. This kind of approach will potentially avoid longterm illness, incarceration of patients, frustration on the part of patients and their communities and high costs for the mental health system.

REFERENCES

American Psychiatric Association guidelines (1995) In: F.G. Lu (1999a) Cultural competence in mental health services and training: A 20-year perspective. The Journal of the California Alliance for the Mentally Ill. 10 (1) 12-14.

Ayim, M. (1997) Weisser Stress und schwarze Nerven. In: Ika Hügel et al. Grenzenlos und Unverschämt. (pp. 111-132). Berlin: Orlanda Frauenverlag.

Center for Mental Health Services, U.S. Department of Health (1998) Cultural Competence Standards in Managed Care. *www.mentalhealth.org*, search under "cultural competence."

Cheung, Freda K. (1999) Culture and mental health care for Asian Americans. The Journal of the California Alliance for the Mentally Ill. 10 (1), 43-45.

Gray, G.E. (1999) Providing mental health services to the African American community. The Journal of the California Alliance for the Mentally Ill. 10 (1), 24-26.

Hatter, R.A. (1999) Transference of power: Through the process of empowerment. The Journal of the California Alliance for the Mentally Ill. 10 (1), 26-28.

Hinz-Rommel, W. (1996) Interkulturelle Kompetenz und Qualität. IZA (3 + 4), 20-24.

Kiselica, Mark S. (1998) Preparing Anglos for the challenges and joys of Multiculturalism. The Counseling Psychologist. 26 (1), 155-223.

Koch, D.F. & Schulze, S. (1998) Diagnostik in der interkulturellen Therapie und Beratung. In: M. del Mar Castro Varela et al. (eds.), Suchbewegungen. Interkulturelle Beratung und Therapie (149-156), Tübingen: dgvt Verlag.

Koray, S. (2000) Interkulturelle Kompetenz-Annäherung an einen Begriff. In: Bundesweiter Arbeitskreis Migration öffentliche Gesundheit, Handbuch zum interkulturellen Arbeiten im Gesundheitsamt, Berlin/Bonn: Die Beauftragte der Bundesregierung für Ausländerfragen, 23-26.

Lawson, W.B. (1999) Diagnosis and treatment of African Americans.The Journal of the California Alliance for the Mentally Ill. 10 (1), 29-30.

Lin, K.-M. (1999) Einstein's nemesis: A journey out of the abyss. The Journal of the California Alliance for the Mentally Ill. 10 (1), 58-60.

Lu, F.G. (1999a) Cultural Competence in Mental Health Services and Training: A 20-Year Perspective. The Journal of the California Alliance for the Mentally Ill. 10 (1), 12-14.

Lu, F.G. (1999b) Exemplary practices in mental health cultural competency development. San Francisco, CA: Department of Psychiatry, San Francisco General Hospital, 16-26.

Owyang, W. (1999) Asian American perspectives on mental health. The Journal of the California Alliance for the Mentally Ill. 10 (1), 45-47.

Rodriguez, E. (1999) The heart of the matter: Worldview as a central concept in effective cross-cultural work. The Journal of the California Alliance for the Mentally Ill. 10 (1), 5-7.

Schultz, D. (1999) Ein Leben, das wir weitertragen werden. May Ayim (1960-1996) In: C. Brügge/Wildwasser Bielefeld e.V. (eds.) Frauen in ver-rückten Lebenswelten. (pp. 139.164). Bern: efef Verlag.

Schultz, D. (2002) Kulturelle Kompetenz in der psychiatrischen Versorgung von Migrant/innen und Minderheiten: Herausforderung und Chance. In: R. Geene/Chr. Hans (eds.) Armut und Gesundheit. Gesundheitsziele gegen Armut. Netzwerke für Menschen in schwierigen Lebenslagen. (pp. 240-251). Berlin: Verlag b_books.

Schultz, D. (2003) Kulturelle Kompetenz in der psychosozialen und psychiatrischen Versorgung ethnischer Minderheiten: Das Beispiel San Francisco, Kalifornien. In: T. Borde/M. David (eds.) Gut versorgt? Migrantinnen und Migranten im Gesundheits-und Sozialwesen. (pp. 167-190) Berlin: Mabuse-Verlag.

Segal, S.P., Hardiman, E.R. & Hodges, J.Q. (2001) New user characteristics in self-help and co-located community mental health agencies. Abstracts of the 3rd International Conference on Social Work in Health and Mental Health, July 1-5, 2001, Tampere, Finland, 136-137.

Smith, Michael W. (1999) Why sometimes too little is too much and too much is never enough of goldilocks and the three doses. The Journal of the California Alliance for the Mentally Ill. 10 (1), 14-16.

Thompson, C.E. & Neville, H.A. (1999) Racism, mental health, and mental health practice. The Counseling Psychologist. 27 (2), 155-223.

Valencia, M. & Yaniz, M. (1999) Toward a culturally proficient system of care: Implications for mental health services to Latinos and other minority populations. The Journal of the California Alliance for the Mentally Ill. 10 (1), 5-7.

Zeiler, J. & Zarifoglu, F. (1994) Zur Relevanz ethnischer Diskriminierungen bei psychiatrischen Erkrankungen. Psychiatrische Praxis. 21, 101-105.

Cultural and Ethical Issues
in Working with Culturally Diverse Patients
and Their Families:
The Use of the *Culturagram*
to Promote Cultural Competent Practice
in Health Care Settings

Elaine P. Congress, DSW

SUMMARY. In all aspects of health and mental health care–the emergency room, the outpatient clinic, inpatient facilities, rehab centers, nursing homes, and hospices–social workers interact with patients from many different cultures. This paper will introduce an assessment tool for health care professionals to advance understanding of culturally diverse patients and their families. *[Article copies available for a fee from The Haworth Document Delivery Service: 1-800-HAWORTH. E-mail address: <docdelivery@haworthpress.com> Website: <http://www.HaworthPress.com> © 2004 by The Haworth Press, Inc. All rights reserved.]*

Elaine P. Congress is Associate Dean at Fordham University Graduate School of Social Service, 113 West 60th Street, New York, NY 10023 USA (E-mail: congress@fordham.edu).

An earlier version of this paper was presented at the International Health and Mental Health Conference in Tampere, Finland in July 2001.

[Haworth co-indexing entry note]: "Cultural and Ethical Issues in Working with Culturally Diverse Patients and Their Families: The Use of the *Culturagram* to Promote Cultural Competent Practice in Health Care Settings." Congress, Elaine P. Co-published simultaneously in *Social Work in Health Care* (The Haworth Social Work Practice Press, an imprint of The Haworth Press, Inc.) Vol. 39, No. 3/4, 2004, pp. 249-262; and: *Social Work Visions from Around the Globe: Citizens, Methods, and Approaches* (ed: Anna Metteri et al.) The Haworth Social Work Practice Press, an imprint of The Haworth Press, Inc., 2004, pp. 249-262. Single or multiple copies of this article are available for a fee from The Haworth Document Delivery Service [1-800-HAWORTH, 9:00 a.m. - 5:00 p.m. (EST). E-mail address: docdelivery@haworthpress.com].

Digital Object Identifier: 10.1300/J010v39n03_03

KEYWORDS. *Culturagram*, cultural diversity, cultural competence, cultural and ethical issues, family assessment, culture and health care, ethical issues and health care

INTRODUCTION

The increasing cultural diversity of the United States has been the subject of news articles (Cohn, 2001; Purdum, 2000; Schmitt, 2001), as well as professional publications (Devore & Schlesinger, 1996; Gelfand & Yee, 1991; Homma-True, Greene, Lopez, & Temble, 1993; Lum, 2000; U.S. Census Bureau, 2000). While immigrants in the early 1900s originated primarily from Western European countries, current immigrants come from Asia, South and Central America, and the Caribbean. It is projected that in this century over half of Americans will be from backgrounds other than Western Europe (Congress, 1994).

CULTURAL DIVERSITY
AND CULTURAL COMPETENT PRACTICE

From the beginning the social work profession has provided services to culturally diverse clients. In the early days of the 20th century, social workers worked with immigrant populations in settlement houses. Since the late 1960s the NASW Code of Ethics has had an anti-discrimination section, and in last ten years there has been much stress on cultural competent practice. In the most recent Code of Ethics social workers are advised to understand cultural differences among clients and to engage in cultural competent practice (NASW, 1999), while the Council on Social Work Education (1996) mandates that each accredited school of social work include content on diversity. Cultural sensitivity often begins with self-assessment, and Ho (1991) has developed an ethnic sensitive inventory to help social workers measure their cultural sensitivity. The need for social workers in health care institutions to be attentive to the cultural diversity of patients has been stressed (Congress & Lyons, 1994).

Health care professionals have recently given much attention to the impact of cultural diversity on health care (Beckmann & Dysart, 2000; Chin, 2000; Cook & Cullen, 2000; Davidhizar, 1999; Dootson, 2000; Erlen, 1998). There has been some concern, however, that the curriculum of medical schools does not include content on cultural issues

(Flores, 2000). A recent Diversity in Medicine project funded by the U.S. Dept of Education, however, developed a curriculum for medical students in training on cultural factors that affect diagnosis, treatment, and communication between patient and doctor (O'Connor, 1997). Although the need for health care professionals to be culturally sensitive has been repeatedly stressed, providing health care to diverse cultural groups has been seen as one of the most challenging for health care providers (Davidhizar, Bechtel, & Giger, 1998).

While developing cultural competent practice is an ongoing goal for social workers (Lum, 2000), the diversity of clients' backgrounds, especially in urban areas, makes this process most challenging. The presence of families from 125 nations in one zip code in Queens (National Geographic, 1998) attests to the challenges that face health care social workers. How can a social worker know and understand the culture of each patient? Some literature has focused on teaching social workers specific characteristics of different ethnic populations (McGoldrick, 1998; Ho, 1987; Goldenberg, 2000).

Considering a family only in terms of a generic cultural identity, however, may lead to over generalization and stereotyping (Congress, 1994, 1997). In working with culturally diverse patients, social workers soon learn that one patient and family is very different from another. For example, an undocumented Mexican family that recently immigrated to the United States may access and use health care very differently than a Puerto Rican family that has lived in the United States for thirty years. Yet both families are Hispanic.

Even two patients from the same ethnic background may be dissimilar. For example one Puerto Rican patient who is hospitalized for a heart condition may be very different from another Puerto Rican patient with a similar medical condition. Generalizations about people from similar ethnic backgrounds may be not always give the most accurate understanding. When attempting to understand culturally diverse patients and families, it is important to assess the family from a multi dimensional cultural perspective.

CULTURAGRAM

The culturagram grew out of the author's experience in working with families from different cultural backgrounds. Two social work assessment tools, the ecomap (Hartman & Laird, 1983) that looked at families in relationship to the external environment, and the genogram (McGoldrick &

Gerson, 1985) that examines internal family relationships, are useful tools in assessing families, but do not emphasize the important role of culture in understanding families.

The culturagram (Congress, 1994; Congress, 1997) a family assessment instrument discussed in this journal article was originally developed to help social workers understand culturally diverse clients and their families. During the last seven years the culturagram has been applied to work with people of color (Lum, 2000), battered women (Brownell & Congress, 1998), children (Webb, 1996, 2001), and older people (Brownell, 1998). This article applies the culturagram to work with patients and their families in health and mental health settings.

Developed in 1994 and revised in 2000, the *culturagram* (see Figure 1) examines the following 10 areas:

- Reasons for relocation
- Legal status
- Time in community
- Language spoken at home and in the community
- Health beliefs
- Crisis events
- Holidays and special events
- Contact with cultural and religious institutions
- Values about education and work
- Values about family–structure, power, myths, and rules

Reasons for Relocation. Reasons for relocating vary among families. Many families come because of economic opportunities in America, whereas others relocate because of political and religious discrimination in their country of origin. For some it is possible to return home again, and they often travel back and forth for holidays and special occasions. Others know that they can never go home again. Some families move within the United States, often from a rural to a more urban area. Some immigrants come from backgrounds with very limited formal health care and may have associated health problems.

After relocating from their native countries, immigrant families often experience differing amounts of stress that is manifested in anxiety and depressive symptoms. There may be feelings of profound loss if they have left a land to which they can never return. Health care professionals need to understand the reasons for relocation, as this information may be helpful in understanding the physical and psychological symptoms of patients and their families.

FIGURE 1. Culturagram–2000

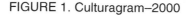

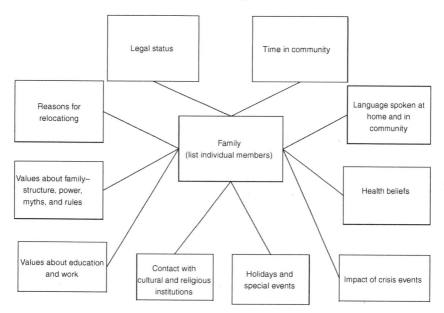

Legal Status. The legal status of a family may have an effect on patients and their families. If a family is undocumented and fears deportation, members may become secretive and socially isolated. Patients may have difficulty accessing treatment because of their undocumented status. They may also avoid seeking treatment until their health condition is very severe, less they will have to disclose their undocumented status. An important first step for the health care professional is to establish trust and to reassure the undocumented patient and family about the confidentiality of contact with health care professionals. This may not be easy especially in the patient has come from a country in which confidentiality is unknown (Congress, 1994).

Length of Time in the Community. The length of time in the community may differ for patients and their families. Often family members who have arrived earlier are more acculturated than other members. Another key factor is that family members are different ages at the time they relocate. Because of attending American schools and developing peer relationships, children are often more quickly assimilated than their parents. Children often become interpreters for parents in contacts with schools, health care providers and social service agencies.

Language. Language is the mechanism by which families communicate with each other. Often families may use their own native language at home, but may begin to use English in contacts with the outside community. Sometimes children may prefer English, as they see knowledge of this language as most helpful for survival in their newly adopted country. This may lead to conflict in families. A most literal communication problem may develop when parents speak no English, and children speak only minimally their native tongue.

Often children are used as interpreters in health care settings. Exposure of the child to sensitive health care issues and role reversals may be the unwanted results. Another concern is how can the health care provider insure that the patient has given informed consent, if it is unclear that information has been accurately understood. This points to the need for bilingual staff to facilitate the care of culturally diverse patients.

Health Beliefs. This part of the culturagram must be thoroughly explored by social workers working in health care settings. Families from different cultures have varying beliefs about health, disease, and treatment (Congress & Lyons, 1992). There are significant differences in how culturally diverse populations seek health care (Zambrana, Dorrington, Wachsman, & Hodge, 1994), view chronic illness (Anderson, Blue, & Lau, 1991; Wallace, Levy-Storms, Kinston, & Andersen, 1998), and death and dying (Parry & Ryan, 1995). Differing life expectancies have also been identified (Devore & Schlesinger, 1998).

Often health issues impact adversely on culturally diverse families, as for example when the primary wage earner with a serious illness is no longer able to work, a family member has HIV/AIDS, or a child has a chronic health condition such as asthma or diabetes. Also, mental health problems can impact negatively on families. Coping with the aftermath of losses associated with immigration, a mother may be too depressed to care for her children or a child may be acting out in school as a result of feeling an outsider in a new country. Families from different cultures especially if they are undocumented may encounter barriers in accessing medical treatment, or may prefer alternative resources for diagnosing and treating physical and mental health conditions (Devore & Schlesinger, 1996).

Many immigrants may use health care methods other than traditional Western European medical care involving diagnosis, pharmacology, x-rays, and surgery (Congress & Lyons, 1992). Some immigrants may choose to use a combination of western medicine and traditional folk beliefs.

An important issue is that of preventive care. We continually hear from early childhood about the importance of regular checkups. Managed care has reinforced the concept of regular preventive care in order to avoid future expensive medical treatment. Many new arrivals may not share American health care values about the importance of preventive care, as the following example indicates.

A mother brought her 18-month-old son to the emergency room with a very high fever. The doctor questioned if the child had been seen previously in the Well Baby Clinic. The mother responded that she had never brought the child for care previously, as he had not been sick.

When a member of a cultural diverse family is hospitalized, there may be issues in adjusting to hospital policies and procedures. For example, a family may wish to have all family members including small children come to the patient's hospital room. There may be concerns about limited visiting hours or the number of concurrent visitors. Families may want to bring the patients foods that are contrary to medically prescribed diets. The health care professional has a responsibility to explore the health beliefs of the patient and family. An important ethical dilemma arises when the health beliefs of the patient may seem contrary to those of the employing health care institution.

Crisis Events. Families can encounter developmental crises as well as "bolts from the blue" crises (Congress, 1996). Developmental crises may occur when a family moves from one life cycle stage to another. A particular stressful time for culturally diverse families may be when children become adolescents. Parents with expectations for adolescents to work or care for younger siblings may not accept that American adolescents often want to socialize with peers. Different familial attitudes about sexuality are often quite apparent for health care professionals who work in adolescent health clinics.

Families also deal with "bolts from the blue" crises in different ways. A family's reactions to crisis events are often related to their cultural values. For example, a father's accident and subsequent inability to work may be especially traumatic for an immigrant family in which the father's providing for the family is an important family value. While rape is certainly traumatic for any family, the rape of a teenage girl may be especially traumatic for a family who values virginity before marriage. Also, the serious illness and death of an elderly member may have tremendous impact on the culturally diverse family who look to the elderly family member for major support and decision-making.

Holidays and Special Events. Each family has particular holidays and special events. Some events mark transitions from one developmental stage to another; for example, a christening, a bar mitzah, a wedding, or a funeral. It is important for the social worker to learn the cultural significance of important holidays for the patient and family, as they are indicative of what families see as major transition points within their family. It may be particularly traumatic for culturally diverse patients who are too ill to participate in an important family celebration.

Contact with Cultural and Religious Institutions. Contact with cultural institutions is often very important for immigrant patients and their families. Family members may use cultural institutions differently. For example, a father may belong to a social club, the mother may attend a church where her native language is spoken, and adolescent children may refuse to participate in either because they wish to become more Americanized.

Religion may provide much support to patients and their families and the health care provider will want to explore the patient's contact with formal religious institutions, as well as informal spiritual beliefs. Knowledge of a patient and his/her family's religious beliefs are particularly important for health care professionals whose patients are struggling with serious illnesses.

Values About Education and Work. All families have differing values about work and education, and culture is an important influence on such values. Social workers in health care settings must explore what these values are in order to understand their patients and families. Economic and social differences between the country of origin and America can affect immigrant families. For example, employment in a low status position may be very denigrating to the male breadwinner. It may be especially traumatic for the immigrant family when the father can not find any work or only works on an irregular basis. Another very stressful event for immigrant families is when the breadwinner is not able to work because of serious illness, accident, or disability. For workers who are marginally employed there may not be worker's compensation or social security benefits to help the patient and families when the primary breadwinner is not able to work.

Immigrant families usually believe in the importance of education for their children. Yet children may be expected to work to maintain families in times of economic hardships. With a strong commitment to family, culturally diverse families with a parental member who is struggling with a serious illness may not want children to leave home to pursue further education.

Values About Family–Structure, Power, Myths, and Rules

Each family has its unique structure, beliefs about power relationships, myths, and rules. Some of these may be very unique to the cultural background of the family. The clinician needs to explore these family characteristics individually, but also understand in the context of the family's cultural background. Culturally diverse families may have differing beliefs about male-female relationships especially within marriage. Families from cultural backgrounds with a male dominant hierarchical family structure may encounter conflict in American society with a more egalitarian gender relationships. This may result in an increase in domestic violence among culturally diverse families. The health care professional needs to be sensitive to recognizing family violence within culturally diverse families.

If there are more rigidly proscribed household roles for women, there may much stress on the family when the woman/wife/mother is hospitalized and/or unable to carry out usually household responsibilities. Other female relatives who previously would have helped out during a health crisis may have remained behind in the country of origin and thus not be available to the immigrant family.

Finally, child-rearing practices especially in regard to discipline may differ in culturally diverse families. The social work in health care settings is always very alert to signs of child abuse or neglect, as social workers are mandated reporters of child abuse. Since health care professionals want to be culturally sensitive, however, they may face a dilemma about whether to report a mother who is disciplining a child using mild physical punishment that is acceptable in her country of origin.

The following case vignette will be used to illustrate how the culturagram can be used to understand better a family with its unique cultural background:

Thirty-five-year-old Mrs. Carmen Perez was seen in an outpatient mental health agency in her community because she was having increasing conflicts with her 14-year-old son Juan who had begun to cut school and stay out late at night. She also reported that she had a 12-year-old daughter Maria who was "an angel." Maria was very quiet, never wanted to go out with friends, and instead preferred to stay at home helping her with household chores. Maria was often kept out of school to accompany and interpret for her mother at medical appointments. Mrs. Perez did express concern that Maria had recently begun to menstruate. Every month she became ill with severe cramps and vomiting. *Mrs. Perez commented that this was women's cross that that there was nothing to be done about this.*

Mrs. Perez indicated the source of much conflict was that Juan believed he did not have to respect Pablo, as he was not his real father.

Juan complained that his mother and stepfather were "dumb" because they did not speak English. The past Christmas holidays had been especially difficult, as Juan had disappeared for the whole New Years weekend.

At 20 Mrs. Perez had moved to the United States from Puerto Rico with her first husband Juan Sr., as they were very poor in Puerto Rico and had heard there were better job opportunities here. Juan Sr. had died in an automobile accident on a visit back to Puerto Rico when Juan Jr. was 2. Shortly afterwards she met Pablo who had come to New York from Mexico to visit a terminally ill relative. After she became pregnant with Maria, they began to live together. Pablo indicated that he was very fearful of returning to Mexico as several people in his village had been killed in political conflicts.

Because Pablo was undocumented, he had only been able to find occasional day work. He was embarrassed that Carmen had been forced to apply for food stamps. Pablo was beginning to spend more time drinking and hanging out on the corner with friends.

Carmen was paid only minimum wage as a health care worker. She was very close to her mother who lived with the family. Her mother had taken her to a spiritualist to help her with her family problems, before she had come to the neighborhood agency to ask for help. Pablo has no relatives in New York, but he has several friends at the social club in his neighborhood.

After completing the culturagram (see Figure 2), the social worker was better able to understand the Perez family, assess their needs and begin to plan for treatment. For example, she noted that Juan's undocumented status was a source of continual stress in this family. She referred Juan to a free legal service that provided help for undocumented people in securing legal status. The social worker also recognized that there had been much conflict within the family because of Juan's behavior. She has also concerned that Maria might have unrecognized medical problems and referred her for a health consultation. She also helped Maria and her mother talk to an adolescent health educator who was bilingual and bicultural. Finally she was keenly aware of family conflicts between Pablo and his stepson Juan. To help the family work out their conflicts the social worker referred the family to a family therapist who was culturally sensitive and had had experience in working out intergenerational conflicts.

The culturagram has been seen as an essential tool in helping social workers work more effectively with families from many different cultures. Initial evaluation of the culturagram has been positive, and there

FIGURE 2. Culturagram–2000

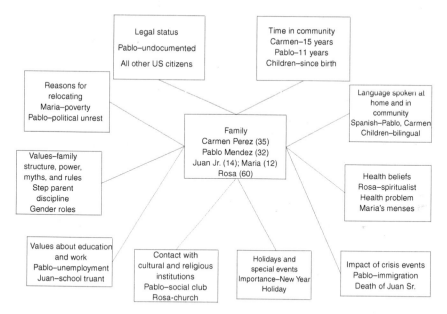

are plans to assess the effectiveness of the culturagram in promoting culturally competent practice.

Implications

Developing culturally sensitive practice, however, is only the first step. In addition, the health care social worker has an important responsibility to educate other health care providers about the beliefs of culturally diverse patients and their families. Fandetti and Goldner (1988) stress the important role of the social worker as cultural mediator. In a previous article Congress and Lyons (1994) outlined the following guidelines for social workers in health care settings:

1. increase sensitivity to culturally diverse beliefs;
2. learn more about clients' beliefs about health, disease, and treatment;
3. avoid stereotyping and emphasize individual differences in diagnostic assessments;
4. increase the ability of culturally diverse clients to make choices;
5. enlarge other health care professionals' understanding of cultural differences in the health beliefs of clients; and

6. advocate for understanding and acceptance of differing health beliefs in the health care facility and in the larger community. (pp. 90-92)

A crucial role for the social worker in a health care setting is that of advocate on a micro and macro level for the culturally diverse patients and families (Congress, 1994).

Culturally sensitive health care social workers, however, may face an ethical dilemma between advocating for a patient's right to choose alternative health care and the health care practices and policies of employing institutions. Goldberg (2000) describes a challenge for social workers between respecting the beliefs of all cultures versus supporting basic human rights. This conflict has important implications for social workers in health care settings. While social workers are respectful of different beliefs about health treatment, what if the cultural practice is potentially life threatening? For example, how does the health care provider work with a culturally diverse family who chooses visits to a faith healer and special herbs, rather than chemotherapy and radiation for a child diagnosed with leukemia?

In addition to responsibility to clients/patients, social workers also have an ethical duty to follow the policies of their employing agency (NASW, 1999). What if the behaviors of a culturally diverse patient are contrary to hospital policies and procedures? How does the social worker work with a hospitalized culturally diverse patient who wants her two-year-old child to visit, whose mother brings in special food contrary to the hospital diet? When and where should the health care social worker clearly set limits with the patient or advocate for a change in hospital policy? These questions continue to be challenges for social workers in health care settings.

REFERENCES

Anderson, J., Blue, C., and Lau, A. (1991). Women's perspectives on chronic illllness: Ethnicity, ideology and restructuring of life. *Social Science and Medicine 33*(2) 101-113.

Beckmann, C. and Dysart, D. (2000). The challenge of multicultural medical care. *Contemporary OB GYN 45*(120) 12-25.

Brownell, P. (1997). The application of the culturagram in cross cultural practice with elder abuse victims. *Journal of Elder Abuse and Neglect, 9*(2), 19-33.

Brownell, P. and Congress, E. (1998). Application of the culturagram to assess and empower culturally and ethnically diverse battered women. In A. Roberts (ed). *Battered women and their families: Intervention and treatment strategies* (pp. 387-404). New York: Springer, Press.

Chin, J.L. (2000). Culturally competent health care *Health Forum 115*(1), 25-37.

Colon, D. (2001, March 16). Immigration Fueling Big U.S. Cities *Washington Post*, Section A, p. 1.

Congress, E. (1994). The use of culturagrams to assess and empower culturally diverse families. *Families in Society*, 75, 531-540.

Congress, E. (1996). Family crisis–life cycle and bolts from the blue: Assessment and treatment. In A. Roberts (ed.), *Crisis intervention and brief treatment: Theory, techniques, and applications* (pp. 142-159). Chicago: Nelson Hall.

Congress, E. (1997). Using the culturagram to assess and empower culturally diverse families. In E. Congress, *Multicultural perspectives in working with families* (pp. 3-16). New York: Springer Press.

Congress, E. and Lyons, B. (1992). Ethnic differences in health beliefs: Implications for social workers in health care settings. *Social Work in Health Care*, *17*(3), 81-96.

Congress, E. and Lynn, M. (1994). Group work programs in public schools: Ethical dilemmas and cultural diversity. *Social Work in Education*, *16*(2), 107-114.

Cook, P. and Cullen, J. (2000). Diversity as a Value in Undergraduate Nursing Education. *Nursing and Health Care Perspectives 21*(4) 178-191.

Davidhizar, R., Bechtel, G., and Giger, J.N. (1998). A model to enhance culturally competent Care. *Hospital Topics 76*(2) 22-26.

Davidhizar, R., Havens, R., and Bechtel, G. (1999). Assessing culturally diverse pediatric clients. *Pediatric Nursing 25*(4) 371-386.

Devore, W. and Schlesinger, E. (1999). *Ethnic-sensitive social work practice*. Boston: Allyn and Bacon.

Dootson, G. Adolescent Homosexuality and Culturally Competent Nursing. *Nursing Forum 35*(3) 13-25;

Erlen, J. (1998). Culture, ethics, and respect: The bottom line is understanding. *Orthopaedic Nursing 17*(6), 79-85.

Flores, G. (2000). The teaching of cultural issues in US and Canadian medical schools *Journal of the American Medical Society 284*(3), p. 284-290..

Gelfand, D. and Yee, B. (1991). Trends and forces: Influence of immigration, migration, and acculturation of the fabric of aging in America. *Generations 15*, 7-10.

Goldberg, M. (2000). Conflicting Principles in Multicultural Social Work. *Families in Society 81*(1), 12-33.

Hartman, A. and Laird, J. (1983). *Family oriented treatment*. New York: The Free Press.

Ho, M.K. (1987). *Family therapy with ethnic minorities*. Newbury Park, CA: Sage.

Homma-True, R., Greene, B., Lopez, and Temble, J. (1993). Ethnocultural diversity in clinical psychology. *Clinical Psychologist 46*, 50-63.

Lum, D. (2000). *Social work practice and people of color: A process-stage approach* (2nd ed.). Pacific Grove, CA: Brooks Cole.

McGoldrick, M. and Gerson, R. (1985). *Genograms in family assessment*. New York: W.W. Norton.

National Association of Social Workers. (1999). *Code of ethics*. Washington DC: NASW Press.

National Geographic (September, 1998). *All the world comes to Queens*.

O'Connor, B. (1997). Applying folklore in medical education. *Southern Folklore 54*(2) 67-78.

Parry, J. and Ryan A. (1995). A cross-cultural look at death, dying, and religion. Pacific Grove, CA: Wadsworth.

Purdum, T. (2000, July 4). Shift in the mix alters face of California. *The New York Times*. Section A, p. 1

Schmidt, E. (2000, April 3). US has biggest 10-year population rise ever. *The New York Times*. Section A, p. 10.

U.S. Census Bureau. (2000). *Redistricting Public Law 94-171*, summary file, Tables PL 1 and PL2.

Wallace, S., Levy-Storms, L., Kinston, R., and Andersen, R. (1998). The persistence of race and ethnicity in the use of long term care. *Journal of Gerontology 53*(2), 104-113.

Webb, N.B. (1996). *Social work practice with children.* New York: Guilford Press

Webb, N.B. (2001). *Helping culturally diverse children and their families.* New York: Columbia University Press.

Zambrana, R., Ell, K., Dorrington, C., Wachsman, L, and Hodge, D. (1994). The relationship between psychosocial status of immigrant Latino mothers and use of emergency pediatric services *Health and Social Work 19,* 93-102.

Transforming the Legacies of Childhood Trauma in Couple and Family Therapy

Kathryn Basham, PhD, LICSW

SUMMARY. A multi-theoretical couple/family therapy clinical social work practice model synthesizes various social, family, trauma, and psychodynamic theories to inform a biopsychosocial assessment that guides clinical interventions. The client population involves adult partners who have negotiated the impact of childhood trauma, i.e., physical, sexual, and emotional abuses, including culturally sanctioned trauma. Couples may also be dealing with the aftermath of acute trauma related to interpersonal violence, political conflict, and/or the dislocations related to refugee or new immigrant status. Clinical examples demonstrate the usefulness of the model as well as contraindications when active physical violence is present. The construct of resilience remains a central focus in assessment and treatment. Specific attention to cultural and racial diversity enriches both assessment and treatment interventions with these high-risk couples and families. This practice model will be explicated in depth in an

Kathryn Basham is Associate Professor, Smith College School for Social Work, Lilly Hall, Northampton, MA 01063, USA (E-mail: kbasham@smith.edu).

Presented at the 3rd International Conference in Health and Mental Health, Tampere, Finland, July 1-5, 2001.

[Haworth co-indexing entry note]: "Transforming the Legacies of Childhood Trauma in Couple and Family Therapy." Basham, Kathryn. Co-published simultaneously in *Social Work in Health Care* (The Haworth Social Work Practice Press, an imprint of The Haworth Press, Inc.) Vol. 39, No. 3/4, 2004, pp. 263-285; and: *Social Work Visions from Around the Globe: Citizens, Methods, and Approaches* (ed: Anna Metteri et al.) The Haworth Social Work Practice Press, an imprint of The Haworth Press, Inc., 2004, pp. 263-285. Single or multiple copies of this article are available for a fee from The Haworth Document Delivery Service [1-800-HAWORTH, 9:00 a.m. - 5:00 p.m. (EST). E-mail address: docdelivery@haworthpress.com].

upcoming publication from Columbia University Press titled *Transforming the Legacies of Trauma in Couple Therapy*. *[Article copies available for a fee from The Haworth Document Delivery Service: 1-800-HAWORTH. E-mail address: <docdelivery@haworthpress.com> Website: <http://www.Haworth Press.com> © 2004 by The Haworth Press, Inc. All rights reserved.]*

KEYWORDS. Childhood trauma, traumatology, couple therapy, clinical social work practice, complex post-traumatic syndrome

INTRODUCTION

This paper introduces a clinical social work practice model that synthesizes both social and psychological theories to assist high-risk couples and families who have negotiated the impact of childhood trauma. Attention is focused on the resilience of adult partners who have suffered childhood trauma (i.e., physical, emotional, and sexual abuses). Many clients live in multicultural urban U.S. cities, dealing with oppression due to racism, poverty, or discrimination that further compounds the legacies of childhood trauma. Clients in need may also be wrestling with the aftermath of acute trauma related to interpersonal violence, political conflict, and/or the dislocations due to refugee or new immigrant status (Mock, 1998; Walker, 1979). The disturbing political landscape of post-September 11 in the USA and the Iraq War adds even another layer of traumatizing events related to terrorist attacks and threats that have stirred major emotional upheaval for many families who are now coping with additional stressors. This range of health and mental problems affects all sectors of our society, demonstrating a vivid need for clinical social work services in a range of settings including family service agencies, mental health programs, outpatient and inpatient health facilities, and a range of community agencies.

This micro-couple/family therapy approach focuses on issues of power, control, attachment, and shame always within social context. Efforts are made to shift the "victim-victimizer-bystander" dynamic, which often permeates the relationships of trauma survivors (Herman, 1992). Faced with a daunting complexity of themes, this innovative clinical social work practice model draws from (1) social constructionist, feminist, and racial identity development theories to understand the social context; (2) intergenerational and narrative family theories to understand the family of origin influences; and (3) trauma, attachment, and object relations theories to understand the influence of trauma on an individual's adaptation and inner world. This synthesis of social and psychological theories serves to inform a thorough biopsychosocial assessment that subsequently guides practice interventions.

Without question, legacies of childhood trauma often affect adult lives in both elusive and fairly direct manners. Although some trauma survivors approach their adult lives with unique zestful resilience, other adult survivors of childhood abuses experience difficulties in their capacities for attachment and intimacy (O'Connell & Higgins, 1994; Rutter, 1993). Pain and distress may occur not only on an internal or individual level, but also in interactions with other people, on the interactional level. Since many adults strive toward maintaining satisfying and productive partnerships, the majority of adult trauma survivors find themselves in relationships that require active work. In addition to issues of intimacy and control in decision-making in these partnerships, parenting also assumes primary importance for many survivors. Although some research studies suggest a low incidence of intergenerational transmission of abusive behaviors from parents who were abused as children, there is also a population of adult survivors who actively struggle to make use of the most effective, non-abusive methods of discipline with their children (Kaufman & Zigler, 1987; O'Connell & Higgins, 1994).

RATIONALE

In the midst of a current political climate in the United States that denigrates relationally based practice while overvaluing clinician productivity and rapid behaviorally defined progress, it is imperative that we continue to advocate for culturally sensitive, relationship based, theoretically grounded clinical social work practice. A question inevitably arises as to why a couple and family therapy approach with trauma survivors is important or even needed. In the field of traumatic stress, treatment has usually focussed on individual and group psychotherapy as well as psychopharmacology (Courtois, 1988; Krystal et al., 1996; Shapiro & Applegate, 2000; van der Kolk, 1996). Within the past two decades, feminist oriented clinicians have also facilitated empowerment models with psychoeducational support to partners and families (Bass & Davis, 1988; Gil, 1992). More recently, the use of cognitive-behavioral interventions such as eye movement desensensitization reprocessing (EMDR) and dialectical behavior therapy have been popular and useful models for some clients (Compton & Follette, 1998). Yet, once again, the primary therapy goals involve the remediation of individual aftereffects of trauma.

Another central question emerges: What effects do traumatic experiences of childhood have on adult partnerships and family interactions? Aftereffects of childhood trauma do not restrict themselves solely to the individual. In fact, family members are not only affected by the legacies of childhood trauma; they also influence, both positively and negatively, the survivor's experience. And so, it is important to pay attention to couple and family therapy with adult survivors of childhood trauma that relies on social, psychological, and neurobiological theories to shed clarity on the sociocultural, interactional, and individual influences within the couple (Basham & Miehls, 1998).

Although I refer to family as well as couple therapy practice, the unit of focus is actually the couple whose presenting issues may range from parenting concerns, relationship ruptures, conflict around roles and responsibilities, communication problems, sex and intimacy, financial strains, adaptation to a new culture, or spiritual ennui. If active physical violence exists, then an advocacy approach is recommended while couple/family therapy is contraindicated. With such a wide spectrum of concerns, it is useful to rely upon a range of psychological and social theories to assess a couple from different perspectives. Changes in the couple's capacities and needs may also call for continuing flexibility from the clinician in formulating assessments and treatment plans.

There are many integrative couple and family therapy models that aim to incorporate parts into a whole. However, since the process of integration involves a blending or melding of constructs, the notion of synthesis seems more useful. Synthesis involves combining discrete and, at times, contradictory constructs into a unified entity. Such an approach has usually been equated with eclecticism, an often devalued approach in social work. Negative stereotypes are often needlessly hurled at practitioners who weather accusations of randomly constructing a potpourri of unassimilated theoretical constructs. A more accurate definition of eclecticism refers to a choice of the best elements of all systems. Still, this definition differs from synthesis, which aims to build a unified plan with disparate constructs. A serendipitous benefit of a synthetic practice model is the high value placed on flexibility with different lenses to understand the uniqueness of each client. The use of metaphor is helpful in describing this synthetic stance. If you visualize staring at a crystal, the texture and color look different depending on what part of the multi-faceted crystal you are observing. Similarly, the fabric of this theoretical synthesis may shift color and shape over time during the course of different phases of the couple therapy.

In a similar fashion, a case specific practice model changes the synthesis of theoretical models depending on the unique features and needs assessed for each couple. Therefore, the assessment and therapy process sustains a continuing dynamic flow of theory models that advance to the foreground while other theoretical models remain in place, momentarily, in the background. This phase-oriented couple therapy model attends differentially to the centrality of the presenting issues. Important decision-tree processes occur at the point of initial contact with the couple, during the assessment phase, and during the phases of treatment. Although a range of social and psychological theories are available in the knowledge base of the clinician at any given moment, data forthcoming from the couple's presenting concerns determine which set of theoretical lenses advance to the foreground.

Certain theoretical models are used from the onset of therapy. For example, since a relationship base provides the foundation to the practice model, it is essential to understand relationship patterns through the lenses of object relations, attachment, and relational theories (Kudler, Blank, & Krupnick, 2000). In addition, social constructionist, racial identity and feminist theories shed clarity on the family's social context (Manson, 1997; Marsella, Friedman, Gerrity & Scurfield, 1996; Pouissant & Alexander, 2000). As a couple reveals their shared narrative, the presenting issues further signal which theoretical approaches may be especially relevant. Stated concerns about social interactions relating call for the use of an historical family perspective to explore family patterns, family rituals, and family paradigms. A narrative family perspective may also illuminate the multiple unique meanings of the trauma narrative (Sheinberg & Frankael, 2001; Trepper & Barrett, 1989; White & Epston, 1990). Symptoms of clinical depression may signal the need to employ a cognitive-behavioral lens to explore affect regulation and cognitive distortions. In general, a review of the cognitive, affective, and behavioral functioning of each partner also addresses mastery, coping, and adaptation (Compton & Follette, 1998). Finally, in the individual arena, trauma theories focus on the short- and long-term neurophysiological effects of trauma on brain function, particular memory and affect regulation (Krystal et al., 1996; Schore, 2001; van der Kolk, 1996). Although an assessment of each partner's trauma history is necessary in all cases, trauma theory may recede in centrality if there is an absence of trauma. However, in those situations where one or both partners suffered trauma in childhood or adult life, trauma theory should remain one of the central theoretical lenses situated in the foreground of couple therapy. In particular case situations, it becomes clear how all of the social and psychological theory lenses are present concurrently from the onset and throughout the course of therapy. However, one or more theoretical lenses may advance to the foreground in the therapy, when that perspective may be relevant to a particular presenting issue at hand.

In summary, the synthesis of biological, social, and psychological theory models informs the biopsychosocial assessment that subsequently guides the direction of practice. Holding the tension of multiple, often contradictory theoretical perspectives requires flexibility in perception, understanding, and action on the part of the clinician. Knowledgeability about these varied models and perceptiveness are also essential requirements to sustain this both ephemeral and solid stance.

DEFINITIONS AND DEMOGRAPHICS

Before proceeding further with a discussion of this synthetic practice model, the construct of trauma needs to be defined. Although social constructionists posit that the concept of trauma is relative, based on the sociocultural context at the time, this fluid definition points to the range of meanings offered by researchers and clinicians in their assessments of trauma.

Constructs of Trauma

Figley's (1987) definition is useful in a general way. He refers to trauma as "an emotional state of discomfort and stress resulting from memories of an extraordinary, catastrophic experience which shatters the survivor's sense of invulnerability to harm." Herman (1992) discusses how trauma overwhelms an ordinary system of care that gives people a sense of control, connection, and meaning in the world. Allen (1998) and Pinderhughes (1998) assert that the day-to-day racist assaults inflicted on people of color perpetuate the legacies of slavery and colonization. In addition, they believe strongly that such racist practices should also qualify as chronic repetitive trauma. For example, the cultural devastation resulting from the internment of Japanese Americans during WWII and disenfranchisement of indigenous peoples in the U.S. qualify as other examples of culturally sanctioned trauma (Daniel, 1994).

This couple/family therapy practice model focuses primarily on Type II trauma, generally defined as sequelae of childhood sexual, physical, and emotional abuses that includes chronic, repetitive, culturally-sanctioned trauma (Herman, 1992; Terr, 1999). In order to clarify the definitions of Type I and Type II trauma, Terr distinguishes the effects of a single traumatic blow, which she calls Type I trauma, as compared with the effects of prolonged, repeated trauma, which she calls Type II trauma. Regrettably, many survivors of childhood trauma also experience discrete Type I trauma (such as an accident, assault, or natural disaster) or repetitive Type II traumas (such as domestic violence) in adult life as well. And so, a clinician must be mindful of the effects of both Type I and Type II trauma. The severity of effects of trauma depends on five factors. They are (1) the degree of violence, (2) the degree of physical violation, (3) the duration and frequency of abuse, (4) the relationship of the victim to the offender, and (5) the age at which trauma occurs (Terr, 1999). When trauma intrudes during infancy, the emergence of basic trust, a sense of cohesive identity, and secure attachment are undermined. However, if trauma occurs after a child has developed a sense of cohesive self with object constancy, the aftereffects may or may not involve the full constellation of complex PTSD symptomatology, which involves alterations to identity.

Cultural Relativity of Posttraumatic Stress Disorder

Exploration of the effects of trauma raises the controversy surrounding the increasing popularity of the diagnosis of posttraumatic stress disorder (PTSD), as outlined in the widely used diagnostic classification system to understand emotional conditions and mental disorders, the American Psychiatric Association's *Diagnostic and Statistical Manual of Mental Disorders*. Before discussing the cultural critique, an explication of the diagnosis should first be introduced. Posttraumatic stress disorder is:

> a syndrome that occurs after a person has been exposed to a traumatic event in which the person experienced, witnessed, or was confronted with an event or events that involved actual or threatened death or serious injury, or a threat to the physical integrity of self or others. In addition, the person's response involved intense fear, helplessness or horror. The traumatic event is persistently re-experienced in one or more of the following ways: (1) recurrent and intrusive distressing recollections of the event, including im-

ages, thoughts or perceptions; (2) recurrent distressing dreams of the event; (3) acting or feeling as if the traumatic event were recurring (includes the sense of reliving the experience, illusions, hallucinations and dissociative flashback episodes, including those that occur on awakening or when intoxicated); (4) intense psychological distress at exposure to internal or external cues that symbolize or resemble an aspect of the traumatic event. There is also persistent avoidance of stimuli associated with the trauma and numbing of general responsiveness (not present before the trauma), as indicated by three (or more) of the following: (1) efforts to avoid thoughts, feelings or conversations associated with the trauma; (2) efforts to avoid activities, places, or people that arouse recollections of the trauma; (3) inability to recall an important aspect of the trauma; (4) markedly diminished interest or participation in significant activities; (5) feeling of detachment or estrangement from others; (6) restricted range of affect, e.g., unable to have loving feelings and (7) sense of a foreshortened future, e.g., does not expect to have a career, marriage, children or a normal life span. There are also persistent symptoms of arousal (not present before the trauma) as indicated by two (or more) of the following: (1) difficulty falling or staying asleep; (2) irritability or outbursts of anger; (3) difficulty concentrating; (4) hypervigilance; and (5) exaggerated startle response. The duration of the disturbance must be longer than one month; if the duration is less than three months, the situation is acute while a chronic state occurs when the symptoms persist beyond three months. (*DSM-IV*)

Although the heuristic nosology of a PTSD diagnosis provides a useful way of understanding the impact of trauma in diverse cultural groups, the culture-boundedness of the model limits a universal generalizability (Friedman & Marsella, 1996; Mock, 1998). An interesting research project revealed that the majority of African Americans interviewed are highly resilient and do not suffer PTSD (Allen, 1998). In contrast, a number of recent studies suggest that children who live in violent communities are at higher risk for developing PTSD symptomatology (McCloskey & Walker, 2000).

Another intriguing project launched by Becker (1999) and his colleagues at Yale explored the adaptation of Bosnian adolescent refugees who fled to the U.S. They found that many of the adolescents did not develop PTSD symptoms and, when they did, their recovery was more rapid as compared with their parents. Treatment recommendations focused on strengthening the entire family unit, as opposed to an exclusive focus on the individual, since the adaptation of the parents was a predictor for the effective adaptation of adolescents (Gibson, 1999). In this case, the cultural relativity of the diagnosis of PTSD bore fruitful discussion.

Judith Zur (1996) conducted a research study that explored perceptions of the Quiche, a group of indigenous Guatemalans, of their experiences during their Civil War. Since this conflict involved genocidal activity, a Western viewpoint might predict PTSD syndrome among survivors. This researcher points out the absence of social context in assessing PTSD and concentrates on two elements of social context. First is the Quiches' interpretation of agency and belief in fate as causal factors for violence. Such a stance relieves the offenders of any responsibility for their actions. Second is their understanding of emotions, which involves a valuation of emotional restraint. Since overt grief is only tolerated for nine days as a cultural proscription, families experience the ongoing loss of their loved ones as an economic, rather than a personal, loss. Finally, disturbing dreams, which could be viewed as PTSD symptomatology, can be relieving for the Quiches since such distressing dreams are considered valuable portents from the dead. Although these trauma survivors suffered from political genocide, these research data suggest the importance of evaluating the cultural meanings of trauma-related phenomena before recommending a treatment regimen for PTSD.

Demographic Data

As this paper is embedded in a sociocultural perspective, it is important to share the alarming demographics regarding childhood trauma in the U.S. In 1996, the third national incidence study of child abuse and neglect based on reporting from Child Protective Services revealed substantial increases in the incidence of child abuse and neglect as compared with the data gathered from the last national study, completed ten years earlier (Sedlak & Broadhurst, 1996). Rates of physical abuse nearly doubled; sexual abuse more than doubled; and emotional abuse and neglect rated two-and-one-half times earlier levels. There were no significant differences according to race. However, children from the lowest income families were eighteen times more likely to be sexually abused, almost fifty-six times more likely to be educationally neglected, and twenty-two times more likely to be seriously abused by child maltreatment or neglect as compared with children from higher income families. Sexual abuse of girls occurs three times more often than it does for boys.

Current data, although underreported, suggest that 35% of adult women report intrafamilial sexual childhood abuse, most frequently between the ages of seven and twelve. A smaller percentage (20%) of adult men reports childhood sexual abuse, often extrafamilial in nature, frequently, but not exclusively, from male friends, teachers, or coaches. Again, these data for male abuse survivors are dramatically underreported due to fears of disclosure in a homophobic environment. In any event, the increasing incidence of reports of child maltreatment is quite alarming. As these children grow to adulthood, a few fortunate individuals will emerge unscathed, while many others may wrestle with trauma-related aftereffects in their adult lives. If they partner, then trauma-related issues may arise in parenting, family dynamics, and their intimate relationship.

CLINICAL VIGNETTE

In order to explicate this model as more "experience-near" for the reader, the following clinical vignette is introduced. (All names and identities are disguised to protect the privacy of the clients.) Rod and Yolanda Johnson, an African American couple, each in their early forties, both working full-time in technical jobs, sought help following the recent adoption of an eighteen-month-old daughter, the offspring of an extended family member. (The identities of this family have been disguised; all names are changed to protect privacy.) I met with this couple for a total of 20 therapy sessions over a six month time period. After a sixteen-year marriage with a history of two miscarriages and one stillbirth of a baby daughter, Rod and Yolanda worried about potential divorce. Yolanda called to complain about Rod's "lack of involvement," her "floods of tears," and "constant verbal fights." Both partners completed high school and worked reliably at their respective jobs. Although both were reared in alcoholic families, neither currently drank alcohol. At the point of seeking help, they were engaged in vicious verbal battles constantly and considered divorce. Yolanda initiated the first telephone call at the urging of her friend, who had met with me and her husband to successfully work out issues in their marriage. Noteworthy strengths for this couple included a strong sense of responsibility to family and work, religious beliefs, sobriety, durability of a sixteen-year marriage, and loving connections with family and friends.

Developmental Histories

Yolanda, as the oldest of six children, was recruited early on to help out with younger siblings, developing caregiving skills which became a source of pride and accomplishment. When Yolanda was six years old, her father's drinking worsened. He yelled and beat her and her siblings with hangers and belts. Yolanda recalls trying to withhold her tears, yet winced when she saw her bloody scars afterwards. After also enduring sexual abuse between ages eleven and fourteen, perpetrated by an uncle, she learned to appease both her father and uncle by working as hard as hard as she could. No one believed her reports of abuse when she told an aunt and grandmother. Yolanda's exceptional school performance and her endearing personality won her accolades. Life in a primarily middle-class African American community shielded Yolanda from persistent racist attacks, however, she was acutely aware of covert racism in school and in her community.

Rod, as the third of four children, struggled with poverty and violence from his alcoholic father. He describes his father as embittered and destructive, often arriving home to greet the children after school with yelling and cursing. When frustrations mounted, he erupted by beating Rod and his brothers. At the age of eighteen, after finishing high school, Rod struck back and was banished from home, venturing north to establish a new life. Rod was shocked to note that the harsh racial insults that he had suffered during a segregated pre-Civil Rights era South occurred with frequency in the North as well. At the onset of couple therapy, Rod was completely estranged from his family of origin. In spite of some of the education and socioeconomic differences between Rod and Yolanda, and their respective histories of childhood trauma, the commonalties of mutual respect, work responsibility, loyalty to family, and shared dreams provided a strong foundation to their currently beleaguered sixteen-year marriage.

Biopsychosocial Assessment

Since each couple is unique and complex, it is necessary to engage a couple in a thorough biopsychosocial assessment that guides careful decision-making regarding sequencing and choices of practice interventions. Each clinician is urged to identify both strengths as well as possible vulnerabilities in each of the sections of the assessment outline, i.e., the sociocultural, interactional and individual (see Figure 1).

Sociocultural Factors

First, a review of sociocultural factors notes how the influences of extended family, community, the agency context, and the political climate may exacerbate or mediate the aftereffects of trauma. Relevant diversity themes (i.e., race, ethnicity, socioeconomic status, religion, age, gender, sexual orientation, and disability) also require a central focus as they affect both the incidence and aftereffects of childhood trauma (Kersky & Miller, 1996).

FIGURE 1. Biopsychosocial Assessment in Couple/Family Therapy with Survivors of Childhood Trauma (Physical, Sexual, and/or Emotional Abuse)

INSTITUTIONAL/SOCIOCULTURAL (grounded in social constructionist, feminist, & racial identity development theories)
- a.   Clinician biases & contextual understanding of trauma (e.g., vicarious traumatization, countertransference)
- b.   Extended family and community support
- c.   Service delivery context
- d.   Diversity (race, ethnicity, religion, socioeconomic status, disability, sexual orientation, gender)

INTERACTIONAL (grounded in intergenerational & narrative family theories)
- a.   Victim-victimizer-bystander
- b.   Power and control
- c.   Distancing & distrust
- d.   Sexuality & physical touch
- e.   Boundaries
- f.   Meaning of trauma narrative
- g.   Communication
- h.   Dearth of rituals
- i.   Intergenerational patterns

INDIVIDUAL/INTRAPSYCHIC (grounded in trauma, object relations, & attachment theories)
- a.   Complex PTSD symptomatology
  - F   Fears (nightmares, flashbacks, & intrusive thoughts)
  - E   Ego fragmentation (dissociation & identity distortion)
  - A   Affective changes / Addictions & compulsive behaviors/Antisocial behavior
  - R   Reenactment
  - S   Suicidality/Somatization (insomnia, hypervigilance, numbness vs. hyperarousal, startle response, bodily complaints)
- b.   Object relations and attachment
  - • Capacity for whole? Part-object? or Merger object relations?
  - • Internalized victim-victimizer-bystander dynamic
  - • Role of projective identification

Countertransference and Use of Self

Not only must a clinician be mindful of countertransference responses but she should also be aware of the impact of vicarious traumatization and re-traumatization (Chu, 1992; Francis, 1997; Pearlman & Saakvitne, 1995). There are a number of predictable countertransference traps in practice with trauma survivors. Since many trauma survivors possess an internalized relational template that involves the victim-victimizer-bystander pattern, this drama may be regularly externalized through projective identification (Miller, 1994; Herman, 1992). Projective identification is a psychological process where each partner represses, splits off, and projects onto the partner an aspect of the internal dispute that is disowned (Ogden, 1991). What is fought out are the conflicts that neither partner has been able to address internally. As a result, each partner may engage the other as well as the clinician in these projective identification dances. Of course, the clinician's unresolved personal issues factor into this equation as well. For example, the first potential countertransference trap involves slipping into a passive and indifferent bystander stance that mirrors the couple's numbness and detachment. Another trap leads to helpless victimization, or not knowing how to proceed. A rescuer theme may also be elicited in couple therapy, where the clinician finds herself extending the boundaries of sessions, losing clarity around professional role and financial compensation, or generally trying to become the quintessential omnipotent rescuer. An eroticized countertransference trap is common as well, where a range of sexualized feelings may be activated toward either partner. Caution is recommended to avoid eroticized reenactments that recapitulate the earlier childhood traumas. Behaving aggressively may be another countertransference enactment where the clinician disavows anger and behaves in a false, overly solicitous manner. In summary, enactments on the part of the clinician are inevitable. However, it is essential that the clinician understand the nature of these countertransference enactments in order to strengthen an empathic connection with the client and to minimize the occurrence of these missteps as best as possible in order to facilitate positive changes.

Now that certain sociocultural influences have been addressed in a general fashion, the specific sociocultural influences facing Rod and Yolanda are introduced. Various questions are posed to explore the nature of these forces. For example, what is the role of each partner's extended family? Community? Agency context? Clinician biases? Sociopolitical attitudes? How do diversity themes affect the adaptation of this couple? Since various diversity themes mediate the impact of trauma, which themes are most central?

Initially, Yolanda stated that Rod had no interest in therapy since it was "only for crazy people" and that he "disliked white people." Several questions emerged at this point. Was this assertion an expression of Yolanda's ambivalence about cross-racial therapy as well as Rod's? And, was Rod completely unreceptive to seeking therapy? In order to establish an alliance with Rod, I asked Yolanda if he might call me. When Yolanda rejected this plan, I offered to call Rod directly so that I would be able to hear his thoughts about the situation. After Yolanda reluctantly claimed that Rod would immediately resist any conversation, I proceeded to talk with Rod, who aired his concerns and decided to meet for one couple therapy session. He stated that it was "less shameful" to meet with a Caucasian clinician who was unrelated to his community. And so, is this tentativeness an expected "culturally congruent paranoia" understandable in cross-cultural therapy (Grier & Cobbs, 1968)? Do the couple's attitudes reflect internalized racism in choosing a clinician from the dominant culture? Or, are they choosing the clinician based on positive transference and expertise in the field? As the clinician, are there potential countertransference traps related to overly zealous "culturally-competent" rescuing tendencies? Perhaps all of these speculations require some consideration.

In summary, the Johnson couple presented race and gender as central themes that permeate their daily lives. Stereotypic gender roles influenced each partner's expectations about how they should behave as partners and parents. Their estrangement from church as a major historical source of support currently undermines their foundation in the family. Although allegiance to family and a work ethic fortify this couple, the sociocultural pressures and historical legacies impose negativity and failure that undermines a focus on strength in their capacities.

Interactional Factors

The interactional factors that are especially relevant to survivors of childhood trauma include the interplay of the victim-victimizer-bystander paradigm, trust, intimacy, power and control, communication, sexuality, and boundaries (Miller, 1994). Since survivors of childhood trauma have been subjected to abuses of power from adults designated as their caregivers, such violations set the stage for a sense of betrayal and distrust. Subsequently, these individuals find themselves in relationships during adulthood where the dynamics of a victim-victimizer-bystander pattern are reenacted in adult life. Not only might a survivor relate to other people with this pattern, she also internalizes a victim-victim-izer-bystander template that guides a vision of the world. Once again, it must be clear that a victim of violence should not be held responsible for activating violent treatment, even if this dynamic pattern operates.

For Rod and Yolanda Johnson, the victim-victimizer-bystander was pronounced. Rod and Yolanda continuously battled for control, with Yolanda presenting herself as emotionally responsive while Rod prided himself on emotional containment. Yolanda viewed herself as over-re-sponsible and Rod as under-responsible. He, on the other hand, viewed himself as more relaxed and spontaneous. Rod often felt persecuted by Yolanda, complaining that she failed to understand him and withheld sex. Yolanda rejected the notion that she was abusive, feeling justified in her at-tacks. Yolanda, herself, felt victimized by what she viewed as Rod's casual withdrawal as the neglectful bystander and the victimizer who abandoned her to do all childcare and housework. And so the victim-victimizer-by-stander dynamic played back and forth, with Rod and Yolanda assuming all three roles. This alternating *yearning* for connection mixed with a fear of loss and violation fuels a pattern of shifting victimization. These unre-lenting polarized fights always remained verbal, pointing out a noteworthy strength for this couple in their avoidance of physical altercations. Cross-racial therapy introduced additional layers of complexity to this dy-namic as well, where I was viewed alternately as the wished for rescuer-by-stander, the feared victimizer, or the helpless victim.

Individual Factors

Now that interactional factors have been explored, the individual factors and the inner world need to be assessed as well. Important influences in-clude the neurophysiological effects of trauma including PTSD or complex PTSD symptomatology (Dansky et al., 1996; Krystal et al., 1996; Shapiro & Applegate, 2000; van der Kolk, 1996). For example, the presence of flash-backs, arousal vs. numbness phenomena, and affective instability are in-cluded. Intrapersonal factors focus on each partner's object relational and attachment capacities as well as the role of projective identification.

A return to the clinical vignette reveals that the neurophysiological symptomatology of PTSD influences Rod and Yolanda. Although Rod does not suffer acute physiological symptoms, he does, in fact, respond abruptly to touch, demonstrating stimulus barrier issues that affect inti-macy. His periodic drinking reflects some effort to modulate his hyperarousal pendulum. Otherwise, the primary aftereffect of Rod's physical childhood trauma, compounded by racialized assaults, has been damage to his self-esteem. Yolanda takes reasonable care of her physical health, but is plagued with depression. She also suffers a startle response, dislikes surprises, and experiences touch as painful. Antidepressant medications, journal writing, meditation exercises, and cognitive-behavioral techniques to regulate affect were all useful methods to reduce these problematic symptoms of complex posttraumatic syndrome.

Persistent issues with diminished self-esteem remained for both partners. While exploring Rod and Yolanda's inner worlds, projective identification processes unfolded vividly. In this adaptive defensive process, the person who projects an internal, disavowed conflict onto the other person engages the other in an externalized drama where both partners fight overtly over the issue (Scharff & Scharff, 1987). A critical reminder here is that no matter how a partner behaves toward others with inciting projections, each person is held responsible for managing their anger appropriately. There is no excuse or sanction for violence. Typically, Rod projected his internal conflicts surrounding a wish for affirmation countered by experiences of punishing abuse, activating Yolanda's verbal persecution and victimization of him. Her acute criticalness usually followed experiences where Rod failed to follow through on promises. Yolanda disowns her own internal conflict surrounding her dependency needs. For example, she yearns for a loving connection, yet anticipates abandonment, and ultimately behaves in ways that precipitates Rod's withdrawal. With reasonably sound object relational and attachment capacities in place, Rod and Yolanda could bear the emotional intensity involved in the clarification of these projective identification processes. As they recognized the tenacious cycle of emotional victimization and oppression, they were better able to interrupt this destructive cycle. In summary, the sociocultural/institutional, interactional, and intrapersonal factors comprised a thorough biopsychosocial assessment of Yolanda and Rod's couple dynamic that guided the development of a couple therapy plan. Before the actual therapy course for Yolanda and Rod is described, some general guidelines for this phase oriented practice model will first be introduced.

PHASE ORIENTED COUPLE THERAPY PRACTICE MODEL

In spite of the creative variability that enters into each individual case assessment, there are some general guidelines that are useful for all biopsychosocial assessments and decision-making regarding the sequencing and choice of interventions. Overall, this couple therapy practice model functions as a phase model that parallels contemporary individual and group psychotherapy stage models with trauma survivors (Courtois, 1988; Figley, 1987; Gelinas, 1995; Herman, 1992; Miller, 1994; Pearlman & Saakvitne, 1995). However, there are distinct commonalties and differences between these models. In general, stages are similar to phases in terms of identifying certain uniform challenges, yet traditional stage models presume essential sequential development. On the other hand, this approach expects that diverse themes may be revisited at different periods throughout the work. The metaphoric image of a three-dimensional triple helix comes to mind here with the weaving together and interconnections of various themes.

The phases of couple therapy include Phase I: Safety, stabilization, and the establishment of context for change; Phase II: Reflection on the trauma narrative; and Phase III: Consolidation of new perspectives (see Figure 2). Phase I (Safety and stabilization) tasks are relevant for most, if not all traumatized couples in therapy. Here, it is essential to determine if the couple has secured basic safety in terms of food, shelter, and freedom from physical or external violence. As mentioned earlier, an advocacy role is assumed to ensure safety for a victim if physical violence is detected. A couple therapy modality is contraindicated at such times since it often inflames an incendiary dynamic. Assessment of self-care is strengthened by psychoeducational support about PTSD and complex PTSD symptomatology.

After reviewing the safety of the external environment along with efficacy of self-care, the clinician then needs to assess the extent of interpersonal supports among family, friends, and colleagues. The nature of community and spiritual community supports is explored here as well. In general, this phase involves a full range of psychoeducational, cognitive-behavioral, body-mind, spiritual, and ego supportive interventions that promote adaptation and coping.

Many couples are content to end their therapeutic work after completing Phase I tasks, having resolved their basic presenting issues. An important point to stress is that we, as clinicians, often overvalue the uncovering of traumatic memories. Even when couples have the object relational capacities to explore insight oriented work, they may decide to end their work after having grown from the range of Phase I ego-supportive interventions. Such cognitive-behavioral changes can positively influence a couple over a sustained period and can readily be accomplished within a brief time frame. Many couples may move along to Phase II work, which involves a reflection upon the trauma narrative. However, it is not necessary for all couples to follow such a therapy course in order to establish new more equitable ways of relating.

FIGURE 2. Phase-Oriented Couple Therapy with Survivors of Childhood Trauma: Treatment Phases

---

PHASE I: Safety, stabilization, and establishment of context for change

a. Assessment of safety
b. Self-care: Physical health; mental health (e.g., depression, anxiety, & unresolved grief); sleep, nutrition, & exercise; substance use & abuse; bio-behavioral strategies for stress reduction & self-soothing
c. Relevant diversity themes
d. Support systems (e.g., religion/spirituality, family, & community)
e. Communication skills
f. Assessment of partnership status (Continuation? Stasis? Dissolution?)

PHASE II: Reflection on trauma narratives

a. Exploration of meaning of traumatic experiences
b. Intergenerational legacy of "victim-victimizer-bystander" pattern
c. Exploration of different meanings of intimacy
d. Creation of healing rituals
e. Clarification of projective identification processes (Only in cases where each partner possesses the object relational capacities, sufficient ego strengths, and the ability to bear ambivalence will this intervention be indicated.)
f. Emergence of memories (Only in cases where each partner possesses the object relational capacities and ego strengths to bear the retrieval of traumatic memories might the uncovering of memories be indicated. Congruence with cultural beliefs must exist as well.)

PHASE III: Consolidation of new perspective, attitudes, and behaviors

a. Remediation of presenting issues
b. Increased empathy for resiliency and survivorship in partners' listening to each other's trauma narratives
c. Shifts in "victim-victimizer-bystander" dynamic leading toward equitable relating
d. Enhanced sexual relationship
e. Strengthened capacities for self-differentiation, object constancy, & self-care
f. Self-definition that moves beyond survivorship identity
g. Changes in parenting style
h. Strengthened social identities (e.g., gender, race/ethnicity, sexual orientation, age, disability, religion, class, etc.)
i. Shift in social consciousness

Phase II: Reflection on Trauma Narratives

Phase II involves sharing original perspectives on the childhood trauma experiences while restorying the narrative with a new focus on resiliency and adaptation. Since there has been so much controversy about the alleged benefit of uncovering traumatic memories, most couples benefit, instead, from a reflective sharing of their childhood trauma memories without full affective reexperiencing. Instead, an integration of affect, cognition, and memory become the therapy goals. In addition, increased capacity for empathic attunement often occurs during this sharing of experiences.

Congruence with sociocultural influences may also determine the usefulness of uncovering traumatic memories. If such a path promotes flooding or decompensation, uncovering work is contraindicated, especially when there are cultural prohibitions against such catharsis. For example, with one of my refugee couples from a war-torn Central American country, each partner had suffered torture and imprisonment from caregivers and prison guards during their respective childhoods. Cultural, religious, and political forces joined together to create a worldview that valued containment while devaluing expressiveness of intense affect. In this case, a cognitive reflection on the victim-victimizer-bystander dynamic helped this couple; retrieval of memories was clearly contraindicated. Finally, object relational capacities also determine efficacy of uncovering traumatic memories. If partners have not yet attained object constancy and lack the capacity to tolerate ambivalence in intimate relationships, then once again, uncovering of traumatic memories is not indicated.

An important point to revisit is that as clinical social workers, we continue to overvalue the uncovering of traumatic memories under the guise of an insight-oriented psychotherapy frame. Even when cultural congruence and object relational capacities exist, it remains preferable to focus on safety and stabilization work if the couple reports reasonable satisfaction with progress. If continued work is indicated, phase II tasks then focus on the reflection on and restorying of the trauma narrative.

Phase III: Consolidation of New Perspectives

Phase III involves a focus on family of origin work along with strengthening family and community relationships. Couples at this point report less shame, stigma, and isolation. They often move beyond self-definitions as survivors to overcomers or thrivers. While parenting becomes less problematic, couples may also express a greater sense of mastery, vitality, and joy. Resolution of the tasks undertaken during these phases of couple therapy does not follow a sequential developmental line. Instead, a more realistic path involves a revisiting of different phases throughout the course of the work.

EVALUATION OF COUPLE THERAPY PRACTICE
WITH YOLANDA AND ROD JOHNSON

In summary, Rod and Yolanda Johnson progressed steadily in their couple therapy. In the first six weeks, goals focused on the abatement of depression for Yolanda, resolution of the decision to work on the marriage rather than divorce, reduction in arguments, improvement in communication effectiveness, and enhanced understanding and self-care around complex PTSD symptomatology. As this couple proceeded to work on their relationship for the remaining three months, the focus shifted to exploring their different meanings of intimacy, the intergenerational origin of the victim-victimizer-bystander patterns, and the heart wrenching grieving for their lost children. Only after they grieved the losses of three children thorough miscarriage and a stillbirth were they emotionally freed to embrace their new adopted daughter. Since the Johnsons experienced reasonable stability and safety in their family environment and had the object relational capacities to tolerate conflict and ambivalence, they were able to reflect upon their histories of childhood abuse. As each partner shared their childhood memories, they were able to integrate a focus on their strengths and resilience in the face of adversity. Each partner was able to reflect upon the origin family and re-story their roles from victim to survivor to pioneer while sharing these reminiscences. Empathy was strengthened while their emotional and sexual relationship became more mutual and less hierarchical. As they recognized how their victim-victimizer-bystander dynamic mirrored not only their abusive childhood homes but also societal racist patterns, they expressed relief from internalized racial oppression as well as the oppression of their trauma histories.

In summary, this paper has attempted to provide an overview of this synthetic couple/family practice model with adult survivors of childhood trauma that is firmly grounded in a synthesis of social and psychological theories. Hopefully, this presentation has conveyed both the complexity and uniqueness of each couple in their impressive, oftentimes ambitious, endeavors to transform their historical legacies in positive ways. This clinical social work practice approach may be useful for the many couples and families who seek help in health, family service, or mental health settings in the months and years ahead.

REFERENCES

Allen, I. (1996). PTSD among African Americans. In A. Marsella, M. Friedman, E. Gerrity & R. Scurfield (Eds.), *Ethnocultural aspects of posttraumatic stress disorder: Issues, research and clinical implications.* (pp. 209-238). Washington DC: American Psychological Association.

American Psychiatric Association. (2001). *Diagnostic and statistical manual of mental disorders* (4th edition). Washington DC

Basham, K., & Miehls, D. (1998). Integration of object relations theory and trauma theory in couple therapy with survivors of childhood trauma. Part I. Theoretical formulations. Part II. Clinical illustrations. *Journal of Analytic Social Work 5*(3), 51-78.

Bass, E., & Davis, L. (1988). *The courage to heal: A guide for women survivors of child sexual abuse.* New York: Harper & Row.

Becker, D., Weine, S., Vojvoda, D., & McGlashan, T. (1999). *Journal of the American Academy of Child and Adolescent Psychiatry, 39*(6), 775-781.

Chu, J. (1992). Ten traps for therapists in the treatment of trauma survivors. *Dissociation,* 1-18.

Compton, J., & Follette, V. (1998). Couples surviving trauma: Issues and interventions. In V. Follette, J. Ruzek, & F. Abueg (Eds.), *Cognitive-behavioral therapies for trauma.* New York: Guilford Press.

Courtois, C. (1988). *Healing the incest wound: Adult survivors in therapy.* New York: Norton.

Daniel, J. (1994). Exclusion and emphasis refrained as a matter of ethics. *Ethics and Behavior, 4*(3), 229-235.

Dansky, B., Brady, K., Saladin, M., Killeen, T., Becker, S., & Roitzsch, J. (1996). Victimization and PTSD in individuals with substance use disorders: Gender and racial differences. *American Journal of Drug and Alcohol Abuse, 77*(1), 75-93.

Figley, C. (1987). A five-phase treatment of post-traumatic stress disorder in families. *Journal of Traumatic Stress,* (1), 127-141.

Francis, C. (1997). Countertransference with abusive couples. In M. Solomon & J. Siegel (Eds.), *Countertransference in couples therapy* (pp. 218-237). New York: W.W. Norton.

Friedman, M., & Marsella, A. (1996). Posttraumatic stress disorder: An overview of the concept. In A. Marsella, M. Friedman, E. Gerrity, & R. Scurfield (Eds.), *Ethnocultural aspects of posttraumatic stress disorder: Issues, research and clinical applications.* Washington DC: American Psychological Association.

Gelinas, D. (1995). Dissociative identity disorders and the trauma paradigm. In L. Cohen, J. Berzoff, & M. Elin (Eds.), *Dissociative identity disorder* (pp. 175-222). Northvale, NJ: Jason Aronson.

Gibson, E. (1999). The impact of political violence: Adaptation and identity development in Bosnian adolescent refugees. Unpublished Masters thesis submitted to Smith College School of Social Work.

Gil, E. (1992). *Outgrowing the pain together: A book for spouses and partners of adults abused as children.* New York: Bantam.

Grier, W., & Cobbs, P. (1968). *Black rage.* New York: Basic Books.

Herman, J. (1992). *Trauma and recovery.* New York: Basic Books.

Kaufman, J., & Zigler, E. (1987). Do abused children become abusive parents? *American Journal of Orthopsychiatry, 57* (2), 186-192.

Kersky, S., & Miller, D. (1996). Lesbian couples and childhood trauma: Guidelines for therapists. In J. Laird & R. Green (Eds.), *Lesbians and gays in couples and families*. San Francisco: Jossey Bass.

Krystal, J., Kosten, T., Southwick, S., Mason, J., Perry, B., & Giller, E. (1996). Neurobiological aspects of PTSD: Review of clinical and preclinical studies. In A. Marsella, M. Friedman, E. Gerrity, & R. Scurfield (Eds.), *Ethnocultural aspects of posttraumatic stress disorder: Issues, research and clinical applications*. Washington DC: American Psychological Association.

Kudler, H., Blank, A., & Krupnick, J. (2000). Psychodynamic therapy. In E. Foa, T. Keane, & M. Friedman (Eds.), *Effective treatments for PTSD* (pp. 176-198). New York: Guilford Press.

Manson, S. (1997). Cross-cultural and multiethnic assessment of trauma. In J. Wilson & T. Keane (Eds.), *Assessing psychological trauma and PTSD* (pp. 239-266). New York: Guilford Press.

Marsella, A., Friedman, M., Gerrity, E., & Scurfield, R. (1996). *Ethnocultural aspects of posttraumatic stress disorder: Issues, research, and clinical applications*. Washington, DC: American Psychological Association Press.

McCloskey, L., & Walker, M. (2000). Posttraumatic stress in children exposed to family violence and single-event trauma. *Journal of the American Academy of Child and Adolescent Psychiatry, 39*(1), 108-115.

Miller, D. (1994). *Women who hurt themselves: A book about hope and understanding*. New York: Basic Books.

Mock, M. (1998). Clinical reflections on refugee families. In M. McGoldrick (Ed.), *Re-visioning family therapy: Race, culture and gender in clinical practice* (pp. 347-359). New York: Guilford Press.

O'Connell, M., & Higgins, G. (1994). *Resilient adults*. San Francisco: Jossey Bass Publishers.

Ogden, T. (1991). *Projective identification and psychotherapeutic technique*. Northvale, NJ: Jason Aronson.

Pearlman, L., & Saakvitne, K. (1995). *Trauma and the therapist: Countertransference and vicarious traumatization in psychotherapy with incest survivors*. New York: W.W. Norton.

Pinderhughes, E. (1998). Black genealogy revisited: Re-storying an African-American family. In M. McGoldrik (Ed.), *Re-visioning family therapy: Race, culture and gender in clinical practice* (pp. 179-199). New York: Guilford Press.

Pouissant, A., & Alexander, A. (2000). *Laying my burden down: Unraveling suicide and the mental health issues among African-Americans*. Boston: Beacon Press.

Rutter, M. (1993). Resilience: Some conceptual considerations. *Journal of Adolescent Health, 14*, 626-631.

Scharff, D., & Scharff, J. (1987). *Object relations couple therapy*. New York: Jason Aronson.

Schore, A. (2001) The effects of early relational trauma on right brain development, affect regulation and infant mental health. *Infant Mental Health Journal, 22*(1-2), 201-269.

Sedlak, A., & Broadhurst, D. (1996). *Executive summary of the third national incidence study of child abuse and neglect.* Washington, DC: U.S. Printing Office.

Shapiro, J., & Applegate, J. (2000). Cognitive neuroscience, neurobiology and affect regulation: Implications for clinical social work. *Clinical Social Work Journal 28*(1), 9-21.

Sheinberg, M., & Frankael, P. (2001). *The relational trauma of incest: A family based approach to treatment.* New York: Guilford Press.

Terr, L. (1999). Childhood traumas: An outline and overview. In M. Horowitz (Ed.), *Essential papers on posttraumatic stress disorder* (pp. 61-81). New York: New York University Press.

Trepper, T., & Barrett, M. (1989). *Systemic treatment of incest: A therapeutic handbook.* New York: Brunner/Mazel.

van der Kolk, B. (1996). The body keeps score: Approaches to psychobiology of posttraumatic stress disorder. In B. van der Kolk, A. McFarlane, & L. Weisaeth (Eds.), *Traumatic stress: The effects of overwhelming experience on mind, body and society.* New York: Guilford Press.

Walker, L. (1979). *The battered woman.* New York: Harper & Row.

White M., & Epston, D. (1990). *Narrative means to therapeutic ends.* New York: W.W. Norton.

Zur, J. (1996 Winter). From PTSD to voices in context: From an "experience-far" to an "experience near" understanding of responses to war and atrocity across cultures. *International Journal of Social Psychiatry 42*, 305-317.

EVOLVEMENT OF VOICE OF SOCIAL WORKERS AND USERS IN INTERPROFESSIONAL AND INTERAGENCY COLLABORATION

Social Group Work: Building a Professional Collective of Hospital Social Workers

Joanne Sulman, MSW, RSW
Diane Savage, MSW, RSW
Paul Vrooman, MSW, RSW
Maureen McGillivray, MSW, RSW

SUMMARY. Deconstruction of traditional social work departments can isolate social workers from their primary source of professional affiliation,

Joanne Sulman is Research Coordinator, Diane Savage is Director, and Paul Vrooman and Maureen McGillivray are Senior Social Workers, Department of Social Work, Mount Sinai Hospital, 600 University Avenue, Toronto, Canada M5G1X5.

The authors wish to thank Lieve Verhaeghe, MSW, RSW, for her insightful comments on the manuscript, Barbara Beveridge for her technical expertise, and the members of the Department of Social Work for their ongoing evolution of the social group work collective.

This paper was adapted from a presentation given at the Third International Conference on Social Work in Health and Mental Health, Tampere, Finland, July, 2001.

[Haworth co-indexing entry note]: "Social Group Work: Building a Professional Collective of Hospital Social Workers." Sulman, Joanne et al. Co-published simultaneously in *Social Work in Health Care* (The Haworth Social Work Practice Press, an imprint of The Haworth Press, Inc.) Vol. 39, No. 3/4, 2004, pp. 287-307; and: *Social Work Visions from Around the Globe: Citizens, Methods, and Approaches* (ed: Anna Metteri et al.) The Haworth Social Work Practice Press, an imprint of The Haworth Press, Inc., 2004, pp. 287-307. Single or multiple copies of this article are available for a fee from The Haworth Document Delivery Service [1-800-HAWORTH, 9:00 a.m. - 5:00 p.m. (EST). E-mail address: docdelivery@haworthpress.com].

287

leaving them without the support to take stands on controversial patient care issues. This paper describes an alternative: the building of a powerful social work collective based on social group work theory that potentiates professional practice while transcending management forms. The model includes group supervision, but moves beyond it to utilize the social work group as a central organizing principle. At the heart of the collective are the elements of professional accountability, support, autonomy, and collaborative decision-making within democratic peer group structures. The authors highlight current management theory, distinctions that create an authentic social work value-based practice, and outcomes for social workers, their clients, and colleagues. *[Article copies available for a fee from The Haworth Document Delivery Service: 1-800-HAWORTH. E-mail address: <docdelivery@haworthpress.com> Website: <http://www.HaworthPress.com> © 2004 by The Haworth Press, Inc. All rights reserved.]*

KEYWORDS. Group supervision, hospital social work, social group work, collective, management

Social work's professional mandate in acute care is extremely ambitious. At an emergency room pace, workers respond to the crises that patients and families experience. As health care advocates, they identify patient care issues and gaps in community services. Social workers design multi-layered micro, mezzo, and macro level interventions and spearhead action plans. In teaching hospitals they anchor the constantly changing staff on patient care teams. The mediating function inherent in social group work is one of their leading interdisciplinary practice tools. In addition, social workers are the community workers for systems whose permeable boundaries flow beyond the walls of the hospital. Research and teaching are done "in their spare time."

IMPACT OF CHANGES IN HEALTH CARE
ON HOSPITAL SOCIAL WORK

Given the complexity and weight of social work tasks and roles in acute care, professional support is crucial. Regrettably, social workers have lost vital underpinnings for practice as a result of the changes in health care that have occurred over the past ten years. Around the world, health care reform is being driven by market influence on cost and quality of care (Berkman, 1996; Canadian Institute for Health Information, 2001; The Change Foundation, 1999, 2000; Cherin, 2000; Davidson, Davidson, & Keigher, 1999; Hunter, 1996; Leatt, Pink & Guerriere, 2000; Rosenberg & Weissman, 1995). Alterations in both the structure and delivery of health care have reduced institutional budgets, increased regulatory measures, and moved care from inpatient settings to the community–whether the infrastructure is ready or not.

Hunter (1996) states that the belief that health services have suffered from being over-administered and under-managed has led to attempts to increase efficiency and accountability. Typically these efforts involve close performance monitoring of staff and an abandonment of traditional hierarchical forms of organization. Mizrahi and Berger (2001) have underscored the changes in health care brought about by these market containment strategies: "Most hospitals are restructuring to achieve flatter organizational structures by moving away from professionally defined structures, such as departments of social work, nursing and medicine, to more integrative structures" (p. 170).

In Canadian hospitals the most sweeping change has been the move to *program management*. The intention of program management is to place the patient rather than the provider at the center of care. The hope is that by dissolving professional departments, and by centralizing administrative functions and decision-making in teams and programs, both efficiency and quality of care will improve (Globerman, 1999; Globerman, Davies, & Walsh, 1996).

This shift to program management has had a profound impact on social work in health care (Levin & Herbert, 1997, 1999). Because hospitals are a secondary setting for social work, the deconstruction of departments has left social workers with scant professional backing. While there are clear benefits from focusing on the needs of patients rather than providers, in three Canadian reports, staff describe serious concerns about changes to social work in hospitals that have moved to new management forms (Globerman, Davies, & Walsh, 1996; Michalski, Creighton, & Jackson, 1999, Levin & Herbert, 1999). In addition to the decrease in leadership roles in social work, staff experienced a loss of control over decisions regarding professional identity and social work functions. They felt a heightened sense of isolation from social work colleagues and voiced concerns regarding professional practice standards including diminished involvement in hiring and performance appraisals. Staff cited a loss of control over professional development funds and over decisions regarding the supervision of students. In many cases individual social workers have been required to assume all responsibility for upholding professional standards of practice and for advocating for their own needs within a program.

Globerman, Davies, and Walsh urge social workers to "embrace the opportunities embodied in autonomous practice" (1996, p. 187) that occur when departments disappear. However, Levin and Herbert state:

> While there is evidence that some social workers have coped successfully with these new practice realities (Globerman et al., 1996), others are floundering . . . These problems are compounded by the absence of a collective voice for the profession within the employing organization. (1999, p. 30)

Moreover, Michalski and his colleagues noted that as time passed, the majority of social workers whom they studied developed a more negative attitude toward program management. These authors conclude that the creation of professional practice roles and the establishment of shared governance models have been unsuccessful in meeting the clinical and academic needs of the profession in hospitals. "It seems clear from the present research that this type of mobilization of hospital social workers will not take place unless groups of social workers find opportunities to create a professional social work community within their work environment" (Michalski, Creighton & Jackson, 1999, p. 23).

Such struggles for social work are by no means confined to the health sector. A recent cross-Canada study identified the challenges to the social work profession in all settings (Stephenson, Rondeau, Michaud, & Fidler, 2000). One of the report's recommendations is to rebuild support in the workplace using low cost measures like the development of supportive networks of occupational groups.

CONFLICTS FOR SOCIAL WORK

There are obvious conflicts for social work in applying solutions to health care delivery that have grown out of industry (Hunter, 1996; Moore, 1998). According to Redmond, "access to health care in the United States is not a right but instead a commodity to be bought and sold. If you cannot afford it, you cannot have it" (2001, p. 55). Productivity is being monitored for cost rather than quality, and will continue to be measured by profitability or cost-containment. "Doing more with less" is praised, but budget reductions bring increased workloads at a time of decreased support. In addition, it is difficult to gauge social work's contribution in economic terms. For all these reasons we risk losing core social work values in climates driven by the bottom line (Sulman, Savage, & Way, 2001).

The lessening of the psychosocial role also represents conflict for social workers. In some cases the social work role is so pared down, there is only time to do the most urgent discharge planning. This leaves a host of unresolved issues, and compounds a sense of dissatisfaction, even failure, in the social work clinician. It also leaves the door open for professionals with a narrower skill set to "do social work."

In program-based practice there are two potential sources of conflict: money and affiliation. When the team holds the purse strings, social workers who advocate for patients can feel vulnerable when they take controversial stands. It is the difference between being unpopular and unemployed. With regard to affiliation, there can be a strong pull to go along with the team and its leaders in order to be viewed as "a good team player." These conflicts lead to a tension between advocacy and collaboration (Herbert & Levin, 1996) and jeopardize social work's ability to define its own scope of practice.

THEORETICAL BASIS FOR THE GROUP MODEL

Chaos and Complexity Theory

Having reviewed the current context of social work in health care, we looked for a conceptual rationale, besides our own experience, for using groups in an organizational model. One set of assumptions that seems compatible with a social group work approach is *chaos and complexity theory*. This wide-ranging theory was imported into postmodern management literature (Berreby, 1996; Kauffman, 1995) and group dynamics (McClure, 1998) from the natural sciences, and views organizations as complex adaptive systems that should mainly be left to run themselves. This is accomplished by fostering a flattened hierarchy where teams and solutions emerge from the people closest to the problem (Arndt & Bigelow, 2000; Polis, 1998; Santosus, 1998). In our model, the *social work group* is the key in a management system that runs itself and has the capacity to generate moment-to-moment solutions for all practice issues. This is in contrast to other models that place the individual worker in a hierarchical department or in a program management-based multi-dis ciplinary team. In those models there may be group supervision or team meetings (Abramson, 1989; Brown & Bourne, 1996; Cherin, 2000;

Richman, 1989), but the basis of the organization is not the professional social work group which has its roots in the radical democracy of settlement houses and the labour movement (Breton, 1990; Coyle, 1930/1979; Ephross & Vassil, 1988; Konopka, 1963; Lang, 1972, 1979; Lee, 1984; Middleman, 1968).

Social Group Work Theory

What makes the social work group different from other forms of group? To answer this question we need to look at some characteristics of groups. As Laski said in 1930: "we are all bundles of hyphens." Groups, including dyadic sub-groups, are the arena for most social transactions. Our profession is well aware that such interactions run the gamut of behavioural extremes–from nurturing and collaborative to violent and conflictual–and that the complete range of these behaviours can be found in groups (Coser, 1956). Nevertheless, we are social beings, and to engage with each other face-to-face implies the presence of group.

What are some of the features that make the groups in our model *social work groups*? At the heart of the model is collective decision-making within democratic peer group structures (Lang, 1969, 1972). *Democracy* is an essential value of social group work (Coyle, 1947; Middleman, 1968). The term not only describes a particular way of arriving at a decision, it also implies a culture of respect. Democratic groups are tolerant of differences of opinion and of the right to express them. Consensus decision-making is the ideal. Majority rule is the fallback position.

The group facilitator is a *member* of the group, and leadership is shared among members (Lang, 1969, 1979). Regarding the concept of membership, Hans Falck (1979, 1988) has challenged the construct of the individual as a discrete, autonomous entity that can exist separately from others. He and his colleague, Thomas Carlton (1986), replace the *individual* with *a single person who is a member*, and see social work practice in membership management terms. The concept is non-linear and holistic, like social group work process and complexity theory. The membership paradigm even supplants individualistic approaches that incorporate linkage concepts such as environment, system, or ecology (Germain, 1977). According to Falck, "when the individual is placed in the middle of an imaginary circle and all else is designated as the environment, the individual can indeed be understood as being overwhelmed, powerless, disenfranchised and, therefore, in need of social work help" (1988, p. 16). A similar understanding might apply to social workers in program management who are isolated from professional support.

Mutual aid is another core feature of social work groups (Steinberg, 1997). Social group work methodology values reciprocity, and carries an expectation that members will move towards each other in a genuine, helpful manner. An implication of mutual aid is that members will process conflict constructively rather than sidestep issues with false-positive support. Ephross and Vassil (1988), in their examination of working groups, discuss the interrelated concepts of value, membership and authenticity:

> Being valued implies that group members have responsibility for each other and deal with each other at a certain level of authenticity. Unquestioning approval is not valuing . . . To be a democratic microcosm, a group needs to value all of its members as potential contributors . . . The reciprocal obligation imposed on each member is one of commitment to the group. (pp. 47-48)

From this solid base of group membership comes the capacity for collective action and the power to tackle *social goals* collectively and effectively (Breton, 1995). Moore (1987) suggests that a group's environmental competence is the cornerstone of its ability to intervene in its own community situation. One of the mandates of the peer group in the collective model is to develop member competence in all levels of community intervention. These groups support members to intervene in their internal and external hospital communities via intergroup memberships on teams and in community networks (Shapiro, 2000).

Group Supervision

How is a *social group work collective* different from *group supervision*? In their important analysis of social work supervision, Brown and Bourne (1996) characterize group supervision as "largely uncharted territory looking for pioneers" and define it as "the use of the group setting to implement part or all of the responsibilities of supervision" (p. 144). In their view, the decision to use group as a supervisory vehicle is optional, depending upon the context. In our model, the social work group is the norm for supervision and for collective management.

WHAT THE MODEL LOOKS LIKE IN OUR SETTING

In the model we are describing, the *social work group* is the principal management vehicle where accountability, support, and collective decision-making occur between and among the members. The model addresses the need for a strong professional reference group that potentiates practice while transcending management forms. Features central to the model are professional accountability, support, autonomy, and collective decision-making within democratic peer group structures. The indelible values of social work and social group work infuse group process. Together the members of these groups create an available community of expertise, creativity, motivation, and practical help for each other.

Background and Evolution

How did the model originate? The model began as an experimental frontline initiative borne from crisis. Thirty years ago, when one of the authors first began practising social work, she was the only worker on the surgical service. She followed the directives of her supervisor until, in defense of a vulnerable family, she managed to raise the hackles of a prominent surgeon who let it be known to his colleagues that referring to social work was "asking for trouble." With a much-reduced caseload, the worker had a couple of quiet months to reflect on things. She speculated that additional ideas from other front-line staff might have helped her avoid this problem. About a year later, despite the director's misgivings, her colleagues agreed to a pilot project of group supervision. In this small department the group included all of the social workers, and this circumstance had a transforming effect on department culture. Because the supervision group was identical to the whole department, it was not only the beginning of a new supervisory process, but also the beginning of a profoundly different management structure (apparent only in hindsight). From the outset the group was infused with social work values and since the author was a group worker, she facilitated democratic process (e.g., when the director gave a strong opinion on a case, the author would simply ask, "What do other people think?"). As a result of this shift in management practice, the director was able to carry the group's consensus with her when she met weekly with a vice president of the hospital. The group's perspective added power to her recommendations and raised the profile of social work within the hospital. When the hospital moved to a new building five years later, the department tripled in size. Two more staff groups were added, along with a supervisors' group who met with the director. Individual supervision was retained for a worker's probationary period and could also be requested at any time. The group's influence, however, was now central to the management process.

Democratizing the model has occurred gradually, and at times in the face of opposition. The current director and group leaders (a position altered from that of a hierarchical supervisor to facilitator) have had extensive experience in the model and are advocates of consensus decision-making. Group process takes more time than directive leadership, but the strength of the empowered collective is ultimately more enduring (Breton, 1994a, 1994b).

Types of Management Groups in the Collective

Three types of groups are integral to the model. *Peer management* groups, a *coordinating* group, and *the total staff* group all have interconnected goals and functions.

Peer Management Groups

In our setting there are three peer management groups organized around service clusters. The groupings are (1) *perinatology*; (2) *medicine and Chinese services*; and (3) *psychiatry, surgery, and emergency*. The total staff designed the group composition to reflect major service flow patterns in the hospital, as well as to balance the number of social workers in each group. Groups meet on a weekly basis in a regular location at a specific time. Usually the members provide refreshments for themselves.

In addition, the total staff collective chooses facilitators or group leaders for the management groups based on criteria that staff members define. These include leadership skills such as expertise in clinical practice, teaching, research and group facilitation, as well as a demonstrated commitment to collective goals. Because the facilitator has a front-line clinical job, she or he is a fully participating member in the group. The facilitator takes nominal responsibility for minding group process, collecting agenda items and taking issues to and from a coordinating group that also meets weekly. In practice, all members have responsibility for keeping the group on track, and when the group leader is away, members take turns in assuming the role.

Groups provide many layers of support such as social, emotional, clinical, administrative, and strategic. They also establish peer expectations of performance. The social group work collective is strengths-based and encourages autonomy of practice within a set of standards. If a member brings a clinical issue to the group for consultation, the rule tends to be that unless there is a legal concern, it is up to the worker to decide on a plan. Similar to the narrative therapy concept that people are "experts in their own lives" (Horwitz, 2001, para. 1), staff members themselves are usually the best judge of the likely effectiveness of an intervention for their own cases and teams. To obtain support and peer consultation on clinical and systems issues, a worker will typically bring a situation to group for discussion, as in the following brief examples.

A client with a history of cocaine use has had two of her children taken into care by the child protection agency. She is pregnant again, but is doing well in this pregnancy, and the worker believes that the client can manage this baby safely with counseling and supervision. She asks her colleagues what they think are the best options for supporting the client.

Or perhaps a worker is struggling with a new member of his patient care team who pressures patients to leave hospital before a safe plan is in place. How would other group members handle the problem?

The groups also exchange information about the hospital and community resources, and address housekeeping tasks like coverage, time off, and overload. A worker may come to the group saying, "I have 50 new cases this month, my co-worker is still off sick, and I can't manage." The group might talk about different ways to triage referrals, might distribute some cases among the members, ask other groups for help, or if all else fails, ask the group leader to give formal notification to the interdisciplinary team that reduced coverage is necessary.

Another function of the peer management group is the development of member competence in all levels of community intervention, networks, and teams. Groups provide an opportunity to model these skills and make them visible. At the same time, they provide support for a collaborative practice that is highly empowering for staff. Workers, individually or collectively, design initiatives that take patient care issues to an articulated level of policy proposal or program change. In meetings with interdisciplinary colleagues and hospital executives, such proposals can lead to immediate improvements in service delivery or to longer-term projects. A short-list of examples includes: delaying a discharge until safeguards are in place, implementing pre-admission discharge planning protocols, and developing patient and family support groups.

A deeper mandate of the peer management groups is to ensure *accountability* for high-level clinical practice to clients, colleagues, and ourselves. To ignore the fact that a co-worker is functioning inadequately represents a breach of trust with patients, families, and the hospital community. For this reason performance appraisals are done collectively in the group as part of an ongoing process: There should be no "surprises."

When conflict occurs, one particular group norm is essential: Members expect their colleagues to take responsibility for identifying problems and for dealing directly with each other. The groups foster an atmosphere that is tolerant of differences of opinion. Members do not have to like each other, but they do have to be able to work together.

The Coordinating Group

The second type of group is the *coordinating group*, which includes each group leader and the director. The purpose of this group is to be a tracking system for issues raised in the peer groups. Staff's ideas are clarified and amplified with plans for action or are returned to the peer groups for new direction.

Our setting combines program management and departments within a matrix model and has retained the position of *social work director*. For the hospital, the role carries a traditional, hierarchical meaning, along with full-time administrative responsibilities that in program management are redeployed to teams. In the social group work model, however, the primary role of the director is threefold:

1. to act as the facilitator for the social work collective,
2. to act as its agent who takes patient care and systems issues outward to the hospital and the wider community, and
3. to bring back, through interaction with senior administration, universities, community agencies and the profession, a reciprocal understanding of hospital and community-wide issues that have impact on social workers and their clients.

Why is the coordinating group useful? Unless the total number of social workers is small enough to meet as a whole (e.g., 7-10 members), peer management groups are likely to fall along program lines. When this happens, groups end up competing for scarce resources in much the same way that specific programs in the hospital fight for priority. The coordinating group ensures that the inclusive values of patient care and the profession take priority over the exclusive, parochial demands of any given program or service.

Total Staff Groups

With a staff size of 27 social workers, major decisions can be made in the third type of group: *the total staff group*. (In our setting this term generally refers to all social workers, clerical/administrative staff, and students in the department.) For example, after a call from the vice-president, the director arranges an emergency staff meeting: "We have to cut two positions out of our budget; how are we going to do it?" For several years during the 1980s, all MSW staff decided to take a day off a month without pay rather than cut jobs. Last year after a decade of cutbacks, they felt that not enough was being done to highlight their own concerns about salaries. They did comparative research and discovered that their wages were indeed low. Staff then invited the head of human resources and the vice-president to a staff meeting where they presented compelling data in a powerful way, and won a significant increase.

The total staff group also meets for staff development programs, for research seminars, to undertake social action initiatives and, in the time-honoured tradition of social work groups, to have great parties.

Social Group Work Collective Creates Safety Net for Staff

Figure 1 is a visual description of how the collective works. The large outer circle represents the *Total Staff Group*. The three circles labeled *Perinatology*; *Medicine & Chinese Outreach Program*; and *Surgery, Emergency, & Psychiatry* are the peer management groups that meet weekly and are organized by service clusters. The circle labeled *Coordinating Group* is made up of the group leaders, selected by staff, who meet weekly with the director. The circle entitled *Staff Development Seminar* is one example of the many other types of periodic groups that make up the interactional life of the social work milieu. Other examples include social workers involved in advocacy, presentations, research projects, and committees. Because there are many opportunities for workers to exchange perspectives, these ongoing contacts help to create a safety net for staff within the wider hospital culture.

Is There Evidence That the Model Is Effective?

Ongoing peer evaluation is an important part of group process, and staff members give regular feedback about the utility of the group model. However, in order to assess the effectiveness of the model more fully, we looked at outcomes such as staff retention, quality assurance

FIGURE 1. Model of Social Group Work Collective

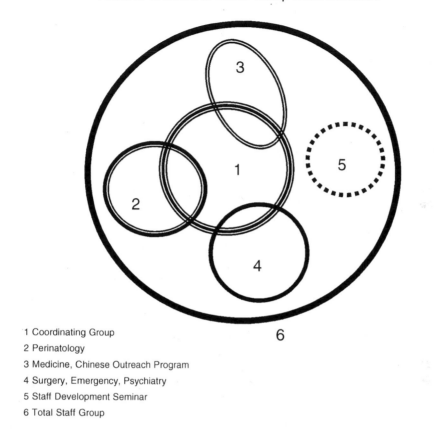

1 Coordinating Group
2 Perinatology
3 Medicine, Chinese Outreach Program
4 Surgery, Emergency, Psychiatry
5 Staff Development Seminar
6 Total Staff Group

data, and feedback from other disciplines. We also looked at client satisfaction and speculate about features of the model that promote it.

Staff Retention

Tsui and Ho (1997), in their comprehensive review of supervision, state that it "has been identified as one of the most important factors in determining job satisfaction levels of social workers" (p. 181). Moreover, when turnover is consistently low, satisfaction tends to be high (Poulin, 1994). Until three years ago, when new hiring occurred with the expansion of our "restructured" perinatology service, the average length of employment in a staff of 20 was 16 years. Currently, 16 staff have worked in the model for >15 years. Because of the move to program management and the dismantling of social work departments, Canada-wide social work retention data are currently unavailable, but it is likely that these figures compare favourably to other settings.

Qualitative Analysis of Quality Assurance Sample

In order to compare the model with other settings, a sample of four recently-hired (< 3 years) social workers with varying lengths of prior social work experience, plus one long-term staff member, were asked the following question: "Does this model differ from what you have experienced in relation to professional practice, support, and satisfaction?" Their responses clustered into five qualitative themes. The theme "professional practice" broke into three sub-themes: "patient care benefits," "comparison with program management," and "perceptions of social work." For purposes of clarity, "support and satisfaction" were merged into one theme and the theme, "drawbacks of the model" was created.

Patient Care Benefits of the Model. Staff indicated that the model supports social work values and advocacy on behalf of patients: "You can hold up the patient perspective more when you have the support," and "It gives you strength to fight battles you might not take on." In a related comment, a worker stated:

> I value the group time to discuss issues and check out my perceptions of events and cases. I want to be careful to stick to social work ethics and values. The team can tell you that you have done a bad job on a case but from a social work perspective, you may have done exactly the right thing and you need support to see it clearly and to stick with it.

Comparison with Program Management. Staff noted the isolation from social work colleagues that program management reinforces: "In program management you are an island." They also observed the negative impact that this can have on professional practice: "If you only let the team define your role, you are in trouble." Other comments included concern about the inability in program management to cover clients of workers in other programs, about having only a nurse manager as final arbiter of patient care issues, and the feeling that social work has little clout in comparison to other disciplines: "It's disheartening to work in program management where no one gives a damn about the 1 social worker compared to 80 nurses."

Perceptions of Social Work (e.g., Other Professions, Hospital Administration). In contrast, "social work is positively viewed in this hospital." Staff observed that social workers had access all the way to hospital administration if needed to deal with patient care issues; e.g., "You can get things done and have relationships with people at all levels (e.g., problem-solving with nursing unit administrators and higher to deal with a child welfare case)," and "Senior management knows our work and supports the department and the profession."

Support and Satisfaction. Perceived support is a key feature of the model: "The social work support is the most important thing here," and "social workers supporting each other doesn't exist in most places." Here social workers can "get support about practice issues, which supports the profession." Flexibility and freedom to practice were noted, as were the efficiency and effectiveness of the model in supporting practice. But primarily satisfaction related to professional collegiality: "I am here because I want to work for social workers, with social workers, to be supervised by social workers."

Drawbacks of the Model. Drawbacks reported in this small quality assurance survey related to the need to process issues amongst colleagues: "The group model can be redundant, repetitious, but is probably important for new staff," and "It can seem more restrictive–so many people you have to inform." Another worker commented: "Groups aren't easy for new staff but serve a purpose for support and consultation." Other challenges of the model are discussed later in the article.

Client Satisfaction

Another area that relates specifically to the model's effectiveness is its impact on clients. Benefits of the group model for clients include uninterrupted coverage of cases, regular clinical consultation to provide a broad rage of intervention options, and strong group support for social workers to act as advocates on clients' behalf, both within the hospital system and in the community. Clients are not only viewed as being assigned to an individual worker; they are also clients of the collective. Group members provide reciprocal coverage for each other during times of social worker overload or when workers are away. In this way, social work coverage for clients transcends the boundaries of the hospital's clinical programs.

The group model also gives strong support to the creation of programs for marginalized clients and those with special needs (e.g., parent-buddy program, sarcoma patient and family groups, Chinese community outreach program). In a quality assurance survey of 121 Chinese patients with limited English, satisfaction rates with *other hospital services* such as medicine, nursing, and nutrition were significantly higher when social workers were involved (Ng & Yau, 2002).

Feedback from Other Disciplines

Social workers are few in number in comparison to other major departments in the hospital (e.g., nursing, rehabilitation, nutrition, pharmacy) but have a strong voice in the organization. As seen above, new social work staff are quick to perceive the strength of social work in the hospital and link this strength to the model. Although the evidence is anecdotal, frequent unsolicited comments from interdisciplinary colleagues suggest social work's impact:

1. from other department heads: "Social work has such a high profile," "Social work gets a lot of recognition here," "We're fortunate to work with such exceptional colleagues";
2. from medical interns and residents who rotate through several university teaching hospitals: "I never had experience with social work before . . . didn't even know what they did till now"; "we sure could have used you at the other hospitals";
3. from physicians whose programs were transferred to other hospitals: "It's very different over there–patients don't get the same social work service," and "Social workers don't seem to be nearly as important [in the new hospital]";
4. from the hospital CEO: "This is an amazing department";
5. and from a vice president to the director: "I know. You can't give me an answer now–you have to take this back to your staff . . . "

In the context of a continually changing health care landscape, including four CEOs and five directors of social work, the social group work collective thrives. The social work department was recently named in honour of the former CEO of the hospital–at his request.

DISCUSSION

In reviewing our practice, one of the things we have discovered is the power of *social group work* as a management tool. Given the pervasiveness of restructuring in health care, as social workers we need to make our own paradigm shift back to social work. In order to position the profession in any organizational form, whether it be health maintenance organizations (HMOs), integrated delivery systems, regional health authorities, or reformed primary health care centres, we need to capitalize on our professional strengths while retaining social work's patient-focused roles and values.

The social work group is the fundamental structural and functional entity in the model. Structure includes regularly scheduled meetings of specific groups to process the broadest range of issues. Pivotal to the integrity of the model is the social work mandate to deal with conflict and to assume shared responsibility for problem resolution. There is a collective accountability, delivering continuous quality improvement, that each member owns and accepts. The fact that social group work skills are uniquely the province of social work gives us good reason to use them in our social work collectives and in our organizations. Our model provides both a theoretical and practice-based framework that promotes experiential learning as a member of a social work group and develops talent to bring to multidisciplinary teams. It also promotes the acquisition of administrative skills because leadership is carried by every member of the group.

The combination of high accountability and autonomy that is present with this model provides staff with tremendous control and influence over practice. Staff in our setting stay a long time and are continually involving themselves in new and creative activities. Despite this, not everyone is at ease with the model. Some struggle with discussing their practice in their group with colleagues, in having responsibility for difficult decisions, and with the expectation of directness in interaction. The model requires a tolerance of some personal discomfort. Identified leadership roles and the boundaries between groups must be flexible in order to diminish unnecessary conflict and negative dynamics. Ultimately, the social work collective acts as a check and balance for the integrity of the system. One of the fascinating things that we have learned in scrutinizing our model is that the exercise is long overdue. We need to use this review of practice to create a guide for new staff and to enhance the social group work skills of other members.

The ongoing evolution of a social group work collective in our setting can give clues to adapting the model to other settings. The group form gained momentum, despite reservations of directors, because from the outset, total staff group meetings were a forum for forging consensus decisions about major issues. The model is implicit in social group work, but to make it operational in the face of resistance means putting concerted energy into creating the collective. Irrespective of organizational reporting structures, any social worker in any setting can form a peer group with other social workers in order to obtain professional social work consultation and support (Levin & Herbert, 1999), although the group or network may have to meet outside formal work hours. And unless social workers in hospitals create organizational vehicles that demand attention from the policy makers and administrative power structures, they will miss vital opportunities to make lasting patient care improvements in their hospitals. This is basic small group-community development practice, and the reality of how formal organizations work.

CONCLUSION

Our search for signposts to the future required us to look again at our foundations. Embedded in the rich history of social group work theory we discovered the supportive structure that enables our practice. The portable model of radical democracy discussed in this paper keeps the critical functions of value-based social work and accountability centralized within groups. It provides a home base whether there are professional departments or unit-based programs. It will be difficult to adhere to social work values in market-driven, bottom-line climates, but it can be done. What we have described is not a band-aid solution for the new challenges in health care. It is a grass roots model that, for 30 years, has created a community of professional support for staff who put their professional values on the line for clients every day.

REFERENCES

Abramson, J. S. (1989). Making teams work. *Social Work with Groups, 12* (4), 45-63.
Arndt, M., & Bigelow, B. (2000). The potential of chaos and complexity theory for health services management. *Health Care Management Review, 25* (1), 35-39.
Berkman, B. (1996). The emerging health care world: Implications for social work practice and education. *Social Work, 41* (5), 541-551.
Berreby, D. (1996). Between chaos and order: What complexity theory can teach business. *Strategy & Business, Second Quarter* (3), 4-12.
Breton, M. (1990). Learning from social group work traditions. *Social Work with Groups, 13* (3), 21-34.
Breton, M. (1994a). On the Meaning of Empowerment and Empowerment-Oriented Social Work Practice. *Social Work with Groups, 17* (3), 23-37.

Breton, M. (1994b). Relating Competence-Promotion and Empowerment. *Journal of Progressive Human Services, 5* (1), 27-44.

Breton, M. (1995). The potential for social action in groups. *Social Work with Groups, 18* (2/3), 5-13.

Brown, A., & Bourne, I. (1996). *The Social Work Supervisor.* Philadelphia: Open University Press.

Carlton, T. O. (1986). Group process and group work in health social work practice. *Social Work with Groups, 9* (2), 5-20.

The Change Foundation, Canadian Imperial Bank of Commerce, & Arthur Anderson. (1999, September). *Making restructuring work: The current path: Hospital restructuring at the mid-point, Part one.* Toronto, Ontario, Canada: The Change Foundation.

The Change Foundation, Canadian Imperial Bank of Commerce, & Arthur Anderson. (2000, September). *Making restructuring work: Alternative paths for Ontario hospitals, Part 2.* Toronto, Ontario, Canada: The Change Foundation.

Cherin, D. A. (2000). Organizational engagement and managing moments of maximum leverage: New roles for social workers in organizations. *Administration in Social Work, 23* (3/4), 29-46.

Coser, L. (1956). *The functions of social conflict.* The Free Press: New York.

Coyle, G. L. (1979). *Social process in organized groups.* Hebron, Connecticut: Practitioners' Press. (Original work published 1930).

Coyle, G. L. (1947). *Group experience and democratic values.* New York: Woman's Press.

Davidson, T., Davidson, J. R., & Keigher, S. M. (1999). Satisfaction guaranteed . . . Not! *Health & Social Work, 24* (3), 163.

Ephross, P. H., & Vassil, T. V. (1988). *Groups that work: Structure and process.* New York: Columbia University Press.

Falck, H. S. (1979). The management of membership: The individual and the group. In S. L. Abels & P. Abels (Eds.), *Social work with groups: Proceedings of the 1979 Symposium on Social Work with Groups* (pp. 161-172). Louisville, KY: Committee for the Advancement of Social Work with Groups.

Falck, H. S. (1988). *Social work: The membership perspective.* New York: Springer.

Germain, C.B. (1977). An ecological perspective on social work practice in health care. *Social Work in Health Care, 3* (1), 67-76.

Globerman, J. (1999). Hospital restructuring: Positioning social work to manage change. *Social Work in Health Care, 28* (4), 13-29.

Globerman, J., Davies, J. M., & Walsh, S. (1996). Social work in restructuring hospitals: Meeting the challenge. *Health & Social Work, 21* (3).

Herbert, M., & Levin, R. (1996). The advocacy role in hospital social work. *Social Work in Health Care, 22* (3), 71-83.

Horwitz, U. (2001). Commonly asked questions about narrative therapy: What is narrative therapy? *The Dulwich Centre Website* (para.1). Retrieved September 16, 2002 from http://www.dulwichcentre.com.au/questions.html.

Hunter, D. J. (1996). The changing roles of health care personnel in health and health care management. *Social Science and Medicine, 43* (5), 799-808.

Kauffman, S. (1995) *At home in the universe: The search for the laws of self-organization and complexity.* New York: Oxford University Press.

Konopka, G. (1963). *Social group work: A helping process.* Englewood Cliffs, N.J.: Prentice-Hall.

Lang, N. C. (1969). *The small professionalized organizational form: An exploration of its nature and its rationalization.* Unpublished manuscript.

Lang, N. C. (1972). A broad-range model of practice in the social work group. *Social Service Review, 46* (1), 76-89.

Lang, N. C. (1979). Some defining characteristics of the social work group: Unique social form. In S. L. Abels & P. Abels (Eds.), *Social work with groups: Proceedings of the 1979 Symposium on Social Work with Groups* (pp. 18-50). Louisville, KY: Committee for the Advancement of Social Work with Groups.

Laski, H. J. (1930). *The dangers of obedience.* New York: Harper and Brothers.

Leatt, P., Pink, G. H., & Guerriere, M. (2000). Towards a Canadian model of integrated healthcare. *Healthcare Papers, 1*(2), 13-35.

Lee, J. A. B. (1984). Social work with oppressed populations: Jane Addams won't you please come home? In J. Lassner, K. Powell, & E. Finnegan (Eds.), *Social group work: Competence and values in practice* (pp.1-16). New York: The Haworth Press, Inc.

Levin, R., & Herbert, M. (1997). The social worker's domain: Perceptions of chief executives in Canadian hospitals. *The Social Worker, 65* (3), 87-97.

Levin, R., & Herbert, M. (1999). Strengthening the alliance between academics and social workers in health care: A plea to the ivory tower. *Canadian Social Work, 1*(1), 30-38.

McClure, B. A. (1998). *Putting a new spin on groups: The science of chaos.* Mahwah, NJ: Lawrence Erlbaum.

Michalski, J. H., Creighton, E., & Jackson, L. (1999). The impact of hospital restructuring on social work services: A case study of a large, university-affiliated hospital in Canada. *Social Work in Health Care, 30* (2), 1-26.

Middleman, R. R. (1968). *The non-verbal method in working with groups.* New York: Association Press.

Mizrahi, T., & Berger, C. S. (2001). Effect of a changing health care environment on social work leaders: Obstacles and opportunities in hospital social work. *Social Work, 46* (2), 170-182.

Moore, E. E. (1987). The group-in-community as the unit of attention in conceptualizing social work with groups. In J. Lassner, K. Powell, & E. Finnegan (Eds.), *Social group work: Competence and values in practice* (pp. 67-79). New York: The Haworth Press, Inc.

Moore, S. T. (1998). Social welfare in a managerial society. *Health Marketing Quarterly, 15* (4) 75-87.

Ng, J. & Yau, M. (2002). *Quality assurance survey of Chinese in-patients.* Presentation to the Patient Care Committee of the Board of Directors, Mount Sinai Hospital, Toronto, Ontario, Canada.

Polis, G. (1998). Ecology: Stability is woven by complex webs. *Nature, 395* (6704), 744-745.

Poulin, J. E. (1994). Job task and organizational predictors of social worker job satisfaction change: A panel study. *Administration in Social Work, 18* (1), 21-38.

Redmond, H. (2001). The health care crisis in the United States: A call in action. *Health & Social Work, 26* (1), 54-57.

Richman, J. M. (1989). Group work in a hospice setting. *Social Work with Groups, 12* (4), 171-84.

Rosenberg, G., & Weissman, A. (1995). Preliminary thoughts on sustaining central social work departments. *Social Work in Health Care, 20* (4), 111-116.

Santosus, M. (1998). Simple, yet complex. *CIO Enterprise Magazine, April 15.* Retrieved September 21, 2002 from http://www.cio.com/archive/041598/index.html.

Shapiro, B. Z. (2000, October). *Social justice and social work with groups. Fragile: Handle with care!* Paper presented at the 22nd Annual International Symposium of the Association for the Advancement of Social Work with Groups, Toronto, Canada.

Steinberg, D. M. (1997). *The mutual-aid approach to working with groups: Helping people help each other.* Northvale, NJ: Jason Aronson.

Stephenson, M., Rondeau, G., Michaud, J. C., & Fidler, S. (2000). *In critical demand: Social work in Canada, Volume 1* (Final report prepared for the Social Work Sector Study Steering Committee). Ottawa, Ontario, Canada: Canadian Association of Schools of Social Work-Association canadienne des écoles de service social.

Sulman, J., Savage, D., & Way, S. (2001). Retooling social work practice for high volume, short stay. *Social Work in Health Care, 34* (3/4), 315-332.

Tsui, M., & Ho, W. (1997). In search of a comprehensive model of social work supervision. *The Clinical Supervisor, 16* (2), 181-205.

Partnership in Mental Health and Child Welfare: Social Work Responses to Children Living with Parental Mental Illness

Rosemary Sheehan, PhD, MSW

SUMMARY. Mental illness is an issue for a number of families reported to child protection agencies. Parents with mental health problems are more vulnerable, as are their children, to having parenting and child welfare concerns. A recent study undertaken in the Melbourne Children's Court (Victoria, Australia) found that the children of parents with mental health problems comprised just under thirty percent of all new child protection applications brought to the Court and referred to alternative dispute resolution, during the first half of 1998. This paper reports on the study findings, which are drawn from a descriptive survey of 228 Pre-Hearing Conferences. A data collection schedule was completed for each case, gathering information about the child welfare concerns, the parents' problems, including mental health problems, and the contribution by mental health professionals to resolving child welfare concerns.

The study found that the lack of involvement by mental health social workers in the child protection system meant the Children's Court was

Rosemary Sheehan is affiliated with the Social Work Department, Monash University, Caufield, 3145, Victoria, Australia (E-mail: Rosemary.Sheehan@med.monash.edu.au).

Presented at the 3rd International Conference on Social Work in Health and Mental Health, July 1-5, Tampere, Finland.

[Haworth co-indexing entry note]: "Partnership in Mental Health and Child Welfare: Social Work Responses to Children Living with Parental Mental Illness." Sheehan, Rosemary. Co-published simultaneously in *Social Work in Health Care* (The Haworth Social Work Practice Press, an imprint of The Haworth Press, Inc.) Vol. 39, No. 3/4, 2004, pp. 309-324; and: *Social Work Visions from Around the Globe: Citizens, Methods, and Approaches* (ed: Anna Metteri et al.) The Haworth Social Work Practice Press, an imprint of The Haworth Press, Inc., 2004, pp. 309-324. Single or multiple copies of this article are available for a fee from The Haworth Document Delivery Service [1-800-HAWORTH, 9:00 a.m. - 5:00 p.m. (EST). E-mail address: docdelivery@haworthpress.com].

given little appreciation of either a child's emotional or a parent's mental health functioning. The lack of effective cooperation between the adult mental health and child protection services also meant decisions made about these children were made without full information about the needs and the likely outcomes for these children and their parents. This lack of interagency cooperation between mental health social work and child welfare also emerged in the findings of the Icarus project, a cross-national project, led by Brunel University, in England. This project compared the views and responses of mental health and child welfare social workers to the dependent children of mentally ill parents, when there were child protection concerns.

It is proposed that adult mental health social workers involve themselves in the assessment of, and interventions in, child welfare cases when appropriate, and share essential information about their adult, parent clients. Children at risk of abuse and neglect are the responsibility of all members of the community, and relevant professional groups must accept this responsibility. *[Article copies available for a fee from The Haworth Document Delivery Service: 1-800-HAWORTH. E-mail address: <docdelivery@ haworthpress.com> Website: <http://www.HaworthPress.com> © 2004 by The Haworth Press, Inc. All rights reserved.]*

KEYWORDS. Parental mental health, child welfare, social work decision-making, child protection, mental health social work, child protection social work, children's courts

Meeting the needs of children in families with parental mental illness is a recognised and increasing problem. Developments in the mental health field have meant that more people with mental illness are being managed in the community. Moreover, contemporary social policy emphasises that people with mental illness should be maintained in the community and that those who are parents should be better supported to retain their children in their care. Parents with mental illness who have dependent children need considerable support and are therefore likely to be involved with a range of professionals and services. The precarious nature of mental illness can bring these families to the attention of child welfare services when the parent's mental illness interferes with their capacity to appropriately care for their children. However, an awareness of the strong association between parental mental illness and difficulties in the development and psychosocial adaptation of their children has yet to lead to broad support for service initiatives that address the needs of both mentally ill parents and their children (Falkov 1999:7). Clearly not all children whose parents are mentally ill will experience difficulties. What is important to identify is what constellation of social and psychological factors in combination with parental mental illness will impact on child care and parenting and contribute to child abuse (Stanley and Penhale 1999).

Mental illness is an issue for a number of families reported to the Child Protection Service in Victoria (Australia) (Buist 1998), and the difficulties such families encounter challenge not only the families themselves but also the professionals who work with them. Community studies in the UK (Iddamalagoda and Naish 1993) have shown that around 60% of women with serious chronic illness have children under the age of 16 years; the same result was found from a 1998 survey of in-patients at Maroondah Hospital Area Mental Health Service (Victoria). Parental mental health problems were encountered in two of the major research studies included in the British Department of Health's examination of the workings of the child protection system (Stanely and Penhale 1999:35). Gibbons, Conroy and Bell (1995) found that 13% of children of children on the child protection register across eight English counties were living in a family where their parent had been treated for mental illness. Lewis and Shemmings (1995) found a similar association: Nearly 20% of the 220 child protection cases they studied involved a parent with a mental health problem.

What the study reported on today sought to do was investigate to what extent adult mental health problems were present in children's court matters, what difficulties these cases presented to the court, and child protection, and at how much mental health services involved themselves in the court process. A study I undertook in 1995 at the Melbourne Children's Court (Victoria, Australia) revealed that the children of parents with a psychological disorder comprised one of the groups of cases that were regularly presented at Court (Sheehan 1997). In fact, twenty-five of the ninety-two child protection hearings observed over a three-month period at the Children's Court involved parents with very poor parenting skills who might not have a recognised psychological disorder but whose difficulties as parents clearly involved mental health issues. The study reported on today set out to investigate if this is still the pattern.

THE STUDY EXPLAINED

The study findings are drawn from the child protection cases that Magistrates in the Melbourne Children's Court, Victoria, referred to a pre-hearing conference during the first six months (January-June) of 1998. Magistrates refer child protection matters to a pre-hearing conference when a parent or parents dispute the need for the Court to make a child protection order. Pre-hearing conferences are conducted by a Convenor who generally has social work or legal training. Convenors' appointments are formally made by the parliament but in practice are managed by the Victorian Attorney-General. The conference is held prior to any formal hearing so that the family, their legal representatives, and the welfare authority can see whether or not they can negotiate an agreement about a child protection order. Pre-hearing conferences were introduced into the Victorian child welfare legislation in 1994 in the belief that the use of a mediation process, with confidential discussion between the parties, could avoid difficulties inherent in the adversarial nature of court-resolved disputes.

There were 228 Pre-Hearing Conferences held during the first six months of 1998 (January-June). A descriptive survey of the Conferences was undertaken; the Convenors completed a data collection schedule for each case at the completion of the Conference. The data sought was both qualitative and quantitative. The survey schedule asked a series of standard questions about each case: the reasons for the child protection application, the nature of the child protection concerns, who were the participants in the conference, and the conference outcome. The information was drawn from what case information was available on the day of the Conference.

THE STUDY FINDINGS: PROFILE OF CASES

Of the 228 Pre-Hearing Conferences that comprised this study, 40 of these cases (29%) involved parents with mental health problems. The 40 cases involved 59 children. A case was determined to involve mental health issues when parental mental health problems were the basis of, or a significant factor in, the child protection concerns supporting the child protection application. This information was drawn from the child protection court report. Convenors noted on the data collection schedule whether parent mental illness was listed in the child protection service's Court report as a fact contributing to the child protection application. Whilst the child protection service's Court report might state that a parent's mental health status was part of the basis of their concern for a child-or the entire basis of their concern-very often there was no clear diagnostic information presented in the report. Certainly there was no checklist of mental health problems that accompanied the child protection report. Child protection workers often struggled to find out accurate information about a parent's mental health status, or a parent might conceal a history of mental health problems. Moreover, mental health problems associated with, for example, borderline personality disorder, did not readily fit the criteria for assessment and treatment in the public health mental health service. Child protection workers therefore found it difficult to get confirmation of their concerns or obtain advice about appropriate interventions from adult mental health professionals.

The child protection matters referred to a Pre-Hearing Conference included new child protection applications (n = 137); in 64 cases extensions of orders were sought; in 27 cases a breach of an existing child protection order was brought to court. Cases would either settle at the pre-hearing conference, be adjourned, or be referred to a magistrate for a contested hearing.

Of the 137 new child protection applications that came to a pre-hearing conference, 31 involved parents with mental health problems (43%). Twenty-four of the new child protection applications involved allegations of actual physical harm, or likelihood of physical harm to a child (S 63 (c)); twenty-five applications involved concerns about emotional abuse or the likelihood of emotional harm to a child (S 63 (e)). One case involved abandonment of the child (S 63 (a)); nine cases were based on a parent's or parents' inability to care for the child, eight cases involved significant harm, or likelihood of harm, to a child's physical development or health (S 63 (f)); one case involved allegations of sexual abuse to a child (see Table 1).

The children who were the subject of the 137 new child protection applications were predominantly very young, generally aged between birth and three years of age (n = 96), and at the pre-school age level (see Table 2).

The Child Protection Concerns

Cases involving parental mental health issues and child protection concerns were characterised by child neglect, domestic violence, financial and accommodation difficulties, family disorganisation, and relationship difficulties. What also emerged was significant substance abuse by the parent who had care of the child, and this appeared to exacerbate mental health difficulties. In the 31 cases that involved parents with mental health problems, from the 137 new child protection applications that

TABLE 1. Grounds for new child protection applications referred to a pre-hearing conference January- June 1998, Melbourne Children's Court. The *Children and Young Person's Act (Victoria)1989* Section 63 sets out the six grounds on which a child protection application can be made. Very often two or three grounds may be made out to support the application.

Grounds: statutory reference	Total	Percent of total
Abandoned (s.63.a)	0	0
Parents dead or incapacitated (s.63.b)	0	0
Significant harm–physical injury (s.63.c)	2	6%
Significant harm–sexual abuse (s.63.d)	0	0
Emotional, psychological harm (s.63.e)	1	3%
Physical development or health harmed (s.63.f)	0	0
Parents incapacitated (s.63.b) and emotional harm (s.63.e)	3	9%
Significant physical harm (s.63.c) and emotional harm (s.63.e)	11	37%
Significant physical harm (s.63.c) and child health harmed (s.63.f)	4	13%
Significant emotional harm (s.63.e) and child health harmed (s.63.f)	1	3%
Parent incapacitated (s.63.b), physical harm (s.63.c), emotional harm (s.63.e)	5	17%
Parent incapacitated (s.63.b), emotional harm (s.63. e), child health harmed (s.63.f)	1	3%
Abandoned (s.63.a), emotional harm (s.63.e), child health harmed (s.63.f)	1	3%
Significant harm (s.63.c), sexual abuse (s.63.d), emotional harm (s.63.e)	1	3%
Significant harm (s.63.c), emotional harm (s.63.e), child health harmed (s.63.f)	1	3%
Total	31	100%

came to a pre-hearing conference, concerns were presented to support the child protection application (see Table 3).

Sheppard's (1997) UK study found that mothers with depression were living in households pervaded by abuse and violence. Falkov (1996) found also, in his study fatal deaths in children, that domestic violence was a significant feature in the context of maternal mental health problems. The child protection concerns, in the majority of cases, in this study were grounded in similar concerns about adult functioning and focussed on the physical and psychological aspects of parenting. The problems included a parent's incapacity to provide physical care for the

TABLE 2. Ages of children who were the subject of the new child protection applications referred to a pre-hearing conference at the Melbourne Children's Court, January-June 1998.

Ages of children	No. of children	%
0-3 yrs	96	43%
4-8 yrs	66	29.5%
9-12 yrs	47	20%
13-14 yrs	10	4.5%
15-17 yrs	7	3%
Total	226	100%

TABLE 3. Child protection concerns listed (number of cases involving parents with mental illness n = 31). Typically there are a number of concerns attached to each case, which are presented in the child protection service court report as the basis for the child protection concerns.

Grounds for child protection application	N	%
Domestic violence	10	34%
Inability to provide basic care for child	7	23%
Child out of control	1	3%
Attachment difficulties	5	17%
Excessive punishment	11	37%
Hospitalisation of parent	3	9%
Transience	6	20%
Imprisonment	2	14%
Substance abuse (including use of marijuana, over-use of prescription drugs)	6	20%
Other children in care	5	17%
Social isolation	11	37%
Sexual abuse of child	3	9%
Developmental delay in child	1	3%

child; financial and accommodation difficulties included the inability to maintain accommodation and transience, and consequent social isolation and lack of supports; and poor impulse control leading to unsafe consequences for the child. Family disorganisation and relationship difficulties included issues such as:

- the chaotic lifestyle of a parent,
- parent's inability to get the child to school or to child care and to then collect the child, or to keep to access arrangements if a child was in foster care,
- parent's physical harm to a child,
- parent leaving the child in the care of multiple others,
- exposing the child to physical and sexual harm by others,
- exposing the child to domestic violence,
- exposing the child to inappropriate relationships with others,
- the parent's poor impulse control leading to unsafe consequences for the child,
- the parent's overly harsh discipline of the child,
- the poor ability of a parent to understand the consequences of their actions,
- the child having the care of the parent, siblings, meals and other household responsibilities,
- social isolation/lack of stimulation,
- developmental delay in a child.

Other concerns raised by child protection workers, in these cases, included issues such as: a parent's inability to acknowledge their mental health problems, the inability to negotiate with others about important issues (e.g., child care arrangements) and the lack of insight into their own or their children's difficulties. Another issue was the unrealistic expectations a parent may have of a child, such as around child behaviour, responsibility, and independence. Older children involved in the cases also identified these issues as concerns and a number did not want to return to their parent's care until the concerns were resolved. A smaller number of children (over 11 years) were themselves engaging in risk-taking behaviours.

Parental Mental Illness and Child Protection

The mental health concerns that brought the child to the attention of child protection overwhelmingly related to the child's mother, who tended to have sole care of the child or children. In two cases both parents had a mental illness; in two cases it was the father who had a mental illness. The particular mental health problems present in the cases were variously described as a diagnosed mental illness such as schizophrenia (n = 11) or a psychotic disorder for which the parent (predominantly the mother) was receiving treatment, a personality disorder, in particular borderline personality disorder (n = 7)–which was variously described as depression, attachment difficulties or presented as problems with domestic violence, transience and/or anger management. One mother (of two children aged 4 and 5) with a history of psychiatric disorder was in jail. Three mothers had attempted suicide and had been hospitalised. Other individual cases included the attempted strangulation of a baby; shaken baby; factitious disorder by proxy (n = 2); one case in which the mother held the fixed belief that the father had sexually abused the child (this had been disproved on a number of occasions in the three-year-old girl's life). The nature of the parental mental illness or psychological disorder was often not specified, unless a psychiatric assessment was attached to the court report or the parent was identified as a client of the adult mental health services.

Other concerns raised by child protection workers, in these cases, included issues such as: a parent's inability to acknowledge their mental health problems, the inability to negotiate with others about important issues (e.g., child care arrangements), and the lack of insight into their own or their children's difficulties. Another issue was the unrealistic expectations a parent may have of a child, such as around child behaviour, responsibility, and independence. Older children involved in the cases also identified these issues as concerns, and a number did not want to return to their parent's care, until the concerns were resolved. A smaller number of children (over 11 years) were themselves engaging in risk-taking behaviours.

The concerns expressed by the child protection service most often related to the nature and consequences of the particular parental mental illness. Issues such as how poor concentration, lack of motivation, medication side-effects, and impulsivity affect a parent's ability to participate in intervention and therapeutic programmes for their child and to carry through with agreements. Agreements made about, for example, engaging in treatment programmes, counselling services; agreements about the physical aspects of child care such as getting a child to school, etc. Adult mental illness brings with it other psychosocial problems, already noted; problems, perhaps, with financial management, maintaining accommodation, social isolation, maintaining employment. What was often clear in discussions about child protection concerns was that parents with significant psychiatric problems may struggle to understand their child's developmental needs and struggle to understand how their disorder influences their parenting capacity. What was clear was also that there was a general lack of knowledge, by professionals including legal practitioners, of the long term nature of serious mental illness, its impact on the individual's day to day functioning, and how that affects parenting. Previous findings by Sheehan (1997), that generally very little expert information was provided to the Court process by mental health practitioners; nor, did the child protection service refer to mental health knowledge and practice to explain their concerns about a child, are again confirmed.

In this study, in two cases, mental health professionals did attend Court, in their role as the case managers for parents. In so doing, they provided important information about a parent's capacity to care for the child. In general, however, neither professionals nor extended family attended court in these cases, highlighting the lack of support networks and the social isolation that is commented on by professionals and in the literature. Apart from the child protection service and lawyers, only in two cases did grandparents attend. In six other cases, support workers from community agencies attended, and the Salvation Army chaplain attached to the Children's Court attended as a support for a parent in one case.

The difficulties that bring children of parents with a psychiatric disorder to the attention of the Children's Court are particularly challenging. The lack of involvement by mental health professionals in the child protection system meant the court was given little appreciation of either a child's emotional or a parent's mental health functioning. The lack of effective co-operation between the adult mental health and child protection services also meant decisions made about these children were made without full information about the needs and the likely outcomes for these children and their parents. When mental health professionals did attend court, generally as the case managers for parents, their focus was solely on the adult client, and they appeared to minimise parental responsibilities. There was a lack of expert information for the court about a parent's capacity for rehabilitation, about the temporary or permanent nature of the disorder, what responds to treatment, what programmes work, and what do not.

How dependent child protection work is on cooperation from other professionals has been well-covered in the literature (Holt, Grundon, and Paxton 1998). Stanley and Penhale (1999), in their study of mental health assessments and child protection, found that social workers were often uncertain about how a mother's mental health problems were impacting on their child, and that there was no consistency on professional input into assessments even if it was established that there was some impact. This might in part be explained by a sensitivity to maternal mental health problems and how they are characterised.

The different frames of reference and agency functions of adult mental health and child protection services appear to impede communication, and ultimately decision-making, about child protection cases (Holt, Grundon, and Paxton 1998:266). Moreover, how child welfare/child protection is conceptualised by services and their providers has a significant influence on service responses to families with a mentally ill parent. The Australian child protection system looks for single incidents of child abuse, or for actions that have precipitated a crisis in a family, to confirm the need for intervention. However, parents with mental illness, and their dependent children, will often have problems that are ongoing in nature, problems that are poorly accommodated by both child protection and adult mental health services, problems that may very well be exacerbated by bringing such problems to the Children's Court.

System Responses

This inter-agency cooperation is difficult to obtain and, the literature suggests, bedevils attempts to assess adult mental health implications for dependent children (Holt, Grundon, and Paxton 1998; Reder and Duncan 1997; Buist 1998). However, Byrne et al. (2000) in their recent Australian study found that service providers did acknowledge difficulties and problems specific to parents with a serious mental illness and their offspring. It was the lack of liaison between agencies, and the lack of coordinated service provision, that was the barrier to effective service delivery. They found that, despite an awareness of the overall problem in working with parents with mental illness, very few agencies had written policy guidelines for the management of these clients. In fact details about whether adult clients had parental responsibilities or whether children were present in the home were not recorded on client files (Byrne et al. 2000).

The reasons why effective collaboration between the child welfare and adult mental health services might be difficult were canvassed by the *Icarus Project* (1998-2000), a cross-national study developed by Brunel University (England), to investigate the nature and level of support in the community for children and parents in families where there is parental mental illness. What was found was that the structural separation between mental health and child welfare services, each with separate governing authorities in Australia, is markedly different from other countries, in particular the Scandinavian and continental European countries. The lack of a shared discourse across the Australian system, and authority to cross service boundaries between child welfare and adult mental health services, means there are differing views about when parental mental illness constitutes a risk to a child. This hinders the development of practices that provide information about the whole family, and a more complete understanding of a family's functioning, which will assist the legal system in its responses to vulnerable families.

Countries in which the two services were co-located, or where multi-disciplinary teams responded to child and family welfare problems, increased the potential for good communication between professionals (Hetherington et al. 1999). Where the professionals in the team could obtain information about the whole family, then a more complete understanding of a family's functioning was possible. The more specialised the organisation of child welfare and mental health services became, the more likely it was to have barriers between services, over information, access to resources and to programmes. In Australia, the right of a parent to maintain that information about a mental illness is confidential is a source of conflict for both mental health and child protection services. Child welfare professionals commented that they found it difficult to discuss, and seek information about, the impact of significant mental illness on a parent and other family members. In Australia, many primary health carers would be reluctant to involve child protection services unless it was absolutely necessary, as social workers are regarded with some suspicion and closely identified with child removal.

Statutory intervention in families in Australia has to be legally justified rather than based on social work discretion. There is considerable emphasis on the importance of due process, attention to individual rights and legislative obligation. What this means in practice is a need to establish fault with parents, to permit the involvement of welfare services, rather than propose that need is the basis for the involvement of the child protection service in a family's life.

How child welfare/child protection is conceptualised appeared also to have a significant influence on service responses to families with a mentally ill parent. The Australian child protection system looks for single incidents of child abuse, or for actions that have precipitated a crisis in a family, to confirm the need for intervention. Parents with mental illness, and their dependent children, will often have problems that are ongoing in nature, problems poorly accommodated by both child protection and adult mental health services.

Meeting Needs

The significance of developing services that will work together, and share knowledge frameworks and responsibility for children at risk, is pivotal to the effective functioning of child protection. Where the child protection system intersects with the legal system in order to protect a child from harm, it needs to provide the courts with reasons for its actions. To do this effectively and appropriately it needs to draw on the expertise of other professionals who work with families, and this will include mental health professionals, when parenting and family difficulties are the result of parental mental illness. Where there is little inter-agency collaboration, problems such as those evident in the study described herein, impede decision-making.

Falkov (1999:19) identified a number of important principles in working with families in which there is parental mental illness. Principles, which when combined with services that recognise and support parent competencies, and emphasise resilience factors for children, may reduce the need for statutory, and legal, responses:

- Mental illness should be seen as one of a number of adversities that influence the quality of life of many families.
- The health and social care needs of children and parents should be considered jointly.
- A life span perspective that emphasises children's changing developmental needs over time and recognises the lifelong implications of severe mental illness for all family members. This points to the need for preventative and pro-active interventions that may need to extend beyond crises.

These principles that re-frame how a parent's, and child's, needs might be understood and when cases are referred to the Children's Court, and they involve parental illness, the legal decision-makers have a context in which to decide present an future outcomes for children. Campbell (1999) emphasised that the best place for solving problems is the community where they occur, and where services will work together there is a better chance that problems can be solved this way, leaving only those problems that cannot be resolved for statutory attention.

The Victorian service system has recognised the importance of community-based and multi-disciplinary services and put in place a range of services (for example, the Parent Project, Maroondah Adult Mental Health Service, the Mothers Support Programme, Prahan Mission, *Keeping Kidz in Mind, Hidden Children Hard Words* MHRI, 1997), that focus on prevention and early intervention to help parents cope with mental illness and its impact upon them and other family members. Child and adolescent and adult mental health services, the child protection service, maternal and child health nurses would also see many of this client group, So too do drug and alcohol services, youth and family services, schools, medical practitioners, and the juvenile justice system. Other initiatives also provide a range of approaches for service cooperation: outposting mental health workers in child protection teams, introducing case review processes to review clients who may require multiple service responses; providing mental health consultation to child protection staff. All provide professionals with the opportunity to develop informal networks that encourage consultation and the exchange of information between mental health and child welfare workers.

CONCLUDING COMMENT

These issues will not receive priority unless attention is paid to the following pivotal issues. First, knowledge of the risks for emotionally abused or stressed children must be shared between all services and providers. Second, adult mental health services must put more emphasis on the parenting responsibilities of their clients with dependent children and have stronger links with family support and child welfare services. Third, mental health must be accepted as everybody's business although there must also be a realistic acknowledgement of the opportunity and restraints on all. A shared systems interactional "mental model" will see the whole complex picture where multiple needs need to be addressed through "joined up" services. These changes must be driven by social polices that are not just welfare and health based, but include attention to child welfare legislation (Sheehan, Birleson, and Bawden 2001). The development of inter-agency cooperation and inter-professional confidence is essential if families are to receive the support they need, and if the legal system is to have confidence that the best interests of children and vulnerable families are properly met.

REFERENCES

Ayre P (1998) "Significant Harm: Making Professional Judgements" *Child Abuse Review*, Vol. 7, pp. 330-342.

Buist A "Mentally Ill Families: When are Children Safe" *Australian Family Physician* Vol. 27, No. 4 pp. 261-265.

Campbell L (1999) "Collaboration: Building inter-agency Networks for Practice Partnerships" in Cowling V. (ed.) (1999) *Children of Parents with Mental Illness*, Australian Council for Educational Research, Melbourne, Victoria.

Commonwealth Department of Health and Aged Care (2000) *National Action Plan for Promotion, Prevention and Early Intervention for Mental Health 2000*, Canberra ACT.

Department of Justice, Victoria *Statistics of the Children's Court of Victoria*, 1998/9, 55 St Andrews Place, Victoria.

Dingwall R, Eckelaar JM and Murray T (1983) *The Protection of Children: State Intervention and Family Life*, Basil Blackwell, Oxford, 1983.

Falkov A (1997) "Adult Psychiatry–A Missing Link in the Child Protection Network: A Response to Reder and Duncan," *Child Abuse Review*, Vol. 6, pp. 40-45.

Falkov A (ed) (1999) *Crossing Bridges: Training resources for working with mentally ill parents and their children*, Department of Health, HMSO, London.

Glaser D and Prior V (1997) "Is the Term Child Protection Applicable to Emotional Abuse" *Child Abuse Review*, Vol. 6, pp. 315-329.

Glaser D "Defining and Identifying Emotional Harm, Assessment and Notification" Keynote Paper, *Working Together for Children at Risk Conference*, Monash University, Melbourne, 18-19 November, 1999.

Glaser D and Prior V (1997) "Is the Term Child Protection Applicable to Emotional Abuse" *Child Abuse Review*, Vol. 6, pp. 315-329.

Hallett C (1993) *Inter-agency Work on Child Protection and Parental and Child Involvement in Decision Making* in NSW Child Protection Council Seminar Series No. 1, NSW Government Printer.

Hallett C (1995) *Interagency Coordination in Child Protection*, Studies in Child Protection, HMSO, London.

Hetherington R, Cooper A, Smith P and Welford G (1997) *Protecting Children: Message from Europe*, Russell House Publishing, Lyme Regis, UK.

Hetherington R, Baistow K and Johanson P (1999) *Executive Summary of the Interim Report to the European Commission, May 1999, The Icarus Project*, Centre for Comparative Social work Studies, Brunel University, Middlesex.

Hetherington R, Baistow K, Johanson P and Mesie J (2000) *Professional Interventions with Mentally Ill Parents and their Children: Building a European Model*, Centre for Comparative Social Work Studies, Brunel University, Middlesex.

Holt R, Grundon J, and Paxton R (1998) "Specialist Assessment in Child Protection Proceedings: Problems and Possible Solutions" *Child Abuse Review*, Vol. 7, pp. 266-279.

Human Services Victoria, Victoria's Mental Health and Protective Services *Working Together: A Guide for Protective Services and Mental Health Staff*, February, 1998.

Hunt J and McLeod A (1997) *The Last Resort: Child Protection The Courts and the 1989 Children Act 1989*, Centre for Socio-legal Studies University of Bristol.

Iddamalogda K and Naish J "Nobody cares about me: Unmet needs among children in West Lambeth whose parents are mentally ill" cited in *The needs of children of parents with a mental health problem*, (1999) Lanarkshire Health Board, England.

Offord DR, Kraemer AE, Kazdin AE, Jenson PS, and Harrington R (1998) Lowering the Burden of Suffering from Child Psychiatric Disorder: Trade-offs among Clinical, Targeted and Universal Interventions. *Journal of the American Academy of Child and Adolescent Psychiatry* 37: 686-694.

Pietsch J and Cuff R (1995) *Hidden Children: Families Caught Between Two Systems. CHAMP Report: Developing Programs for Dependent Children who have a Parent with a Serious Mental Illness.* Melbourne: Mental Health Research Institute of Victoria.

Reder P and Duncan S (1997) "Adult Psychiatry–A Missing Link in the Child Protection Network" *Child Abuse Review* Vol. 6, pp. 35-40.

Rutter M and Quinton D (1984) Parental Psychiatric Disorder: Effects on Children. *Psychological Medicine* 40: 1257-1265.

Sheehan R (1997) "Mental health issues in child protection cases" *Children Australia* Vol. 22 No. 4, pp. 13-21.

Sheehan R (2001) *Magistrates' Decision-Making in Matters of Child Protection*, Ashgate, Aldershot, Hants., U.K.

Sheehan R (2000) "Family preservation and child protection: The reality of Children's Court decision-making" *Australian Social Work*, Vol. 53, No. 4, pp. 41-46.

Sheehan R, Pead-Erbrederis C. and McLoughlin A (2000) *The Icarus Project: A Study of Professional Interventions with Mentally Ill Parents and their Children; The Australian Contribution*, Dept. of Social Work, Monash University, Melbourne, January 2000.

Sheehan R, Birleson P and Bawden G (2001) " Working Together for Children at Risk" Report on the Conference held at Monash University, Victoria, Australia, 18-19 November, 1999, *Children Australia*, Vol. 26, No. 3, pp. 33-37.

Stanley N and Penhale B (1999) " The Mental Health Problems of Mothers Experiencing the Child Protection System: Identifying Needs and Appropriate Responses" *Child Abuse Review*, Vol. 8, pp. 34-45.

Stevenson O (1996) "Emotional Abuse and Neglect" *in Child and Family Social Work*, No. 1, pp. 13-18.

Changing Practice:
Involving Mental Health Service Users in Planning Service Provision

David M. Rea, PhD

SUMMARY. Changes to professional work now ensure that social care and health care workers should be accountable to service users, and not only to their professional colleagues. This paper seeks to explore how this may eventually be realised in new working relationships that will profoundly affect mental health social work.

These changes are driven by factors that are external to the social work profession–in policy initiatives that introduce measures of performance that incorporate the service user in both evaluating and planning services, in efforts to build new relationships, and in a breakdown of barriers between social work practitioners and service managers. While these changes are sometimes likely to be resisted by practitioners and

David M. Rea is affiliated with the Centre for Health Economics and Policy Studies, School of Health Science, University of Swansea, Singleton Park, Swansea, SA2 8PP, UK (Website: http://www.healthscience.swan.ac.uk/) (E-mail: d.m.rea@ swansea.ac.uk).

The author would like to acknowledge the service users and staff whose support was invaluable to this research.

This paper is a revision of a paper presented for the Social Factors, Prevention and Empowerment stream of the 3rd International Conference on Social Work in Health and Mental Health, July 1-5, 2001, Tampere, Finland.

[Haworth co-indexing entry note]: "Changing Practice: Involving Mental Health Service Users in Planning Service Provision." Rea, David M. Co-published simultaneously in *Social Work in Health Care* (The Haworth Social Work Practice Press, an imprint of The Haworth Press, Inc.) Vol. 39, No. 3/4, 2004, pp. 325-342; and: *Social Work Visions from Around the Globe: Citizens, Methods, and Approaches* (ed: Anna Metteri et al.) The Haworth Social Work Practice Press, an imprint of The Haworth Press, Inc., 2004, pp. 325-342. Single or multiple copies of this article are available for a fee from The Haworth Document Delivery Service [1-800-HAWORTH, 9:00 a.m. - 5:00 p.m. (EST). E-mail address: docdelivery@haworthpress.com].

service users alike, the demands of policy makers for a new professional accountability to service users can be used to pave the way for effective dialogue. The paper outlines the steps necessary to build confidence among both service users and service providers. This requires sensitive management and leadership. It also requires that action demonstrably follows from such dialogue. The paper uses evidence from Community Mental Health Teams in Swansea, over a three-year period, to demonstrate how the policy and management imperatives faced by service providers can be reconciled with the expressed desires of mental health service users. *[Article copies available for a fee from The Haworth Document Delivery Service: 1-800-HAWORTH. E-mail address: <docdelivery@haworthpress.com> Website: <http://www.HaworthPress.com> © 2004 by The Haworth Press, Inc. All rights reserved.]*

KEYWORDS. Leadership, teamwork, service user involvement, mental health, empowerment, change management

INTRODUCTION

The days when social work could practice independently as a profession–if they ever existed–have passed. Social work practice cannot be isolated from management and policy making. Accountability can no longer be restricted to professional accountability, but must also incorporate accountability to service users and a wider population.

This paper is intended to identify some of the more important management challenges arising from involving service users in planning mental health services. It focuses on user involvement which is often limited to consultation or to participation in decisions initiated by service providers. The focus here, however, will be on strengthening user involvement to the point where users actively take part in leading services towards change.

In the UK, as elsewhere, the challenges faced by management arise from national and local government policies which include user involvement in measures of performance, the desire of service users to have greater say in how the service delivers, and the willingness of managers and service providers to improve the quality of the services they provide. The will to involve service users is considerable and it is not new, although some might impatiently question why relatively little has occurred.

In some countries, where the state has taken less responsibility for provision and has encouraged private provision, service user involvement has sometimes progressed significantly beyond expectations. The virtue (and the vice) of private provision is that services can be developed *ad hoc*. However, the UK shares with many states a tradition of state responsibility and (at best) paternalism in service provision. While present policy developments incorporate notions of service, consumer, and responsiveness, mental health services are provided within a statutory framework that includes a high degree of compulsion. Within the contradictions of this framework, there are severe obstacles to user involvement and these can be presented–by service users as much as by social work practitioners–as reasons to do little or nothing.

This paper uses evidence from community-based mental health services (in Swansea, UK) to demonstrate some of the steps necessary to meet these challenges. Swansea is probably not typical. Judged by the evidence of recent social service inspectorate reports, Swansea is probably ahead of most in the UK (NAW-Social Services Inspectorate for Wales, 2001; NAW and the Audit Commission, 2000).

Elsewhere, a perceived lack of leadership, or the wrong kind of leadership, has increasingly concerned policy makers and service providers in health and social care. In Swansea, the Social Services Inspectorate also noted that user involvement developments were not widespread and occurred only where individuals took the initiative. This implies a similar diagnosis as elsewhere–that leadership is necessary before policy initiatives are taken up and incorporated into professional practice and managerial routines.

This paper seeks to contribute to this debate by identifying strategies that place service users at the centre of change affecting their services. Specifically, the paper argues that leadership needs to be conceptualised flexibly and needs to include team building, team-working, and networking where teams and networks *include* mental health service users who are empowered to drive forward change.

The needs of service users would lead the service and come to the fore through these networks. This concept of leadership is clearly distinguishable from concepts of transactional leadership or transformational leadership which focus on the leader as hero (Bryman, 1996). The importance of the concept of leadership is in the recognition that achieving (beneficial) change is what is not possible in conventional public sector bureaucratic structures, although their continued existence is probably necessary. User representation in these bureaucratic structures is unlikely to affect change. In the very recent past, public sector management has been in thrall to a singular model of management where a manager is defined as someone who imposes his will on others (Geenen, 1985; Pollitt, Harrison, Hunter, & Marnoch, 1991).

That this is an unlikely model for change has been recognised more recently by politicians and policy makers, as well as educationalists and trainers. They have re-discovered leadership. 'Re-discovered' because it is far from a new idea and has been around long enough for everyone concerned to know of its conceptual and empirical limitations (Bryman, 1996). But governments have recognised that issuing policy, providing financial incentives and penalties, and restructuring formal 'authority' in health and social care organisations is not sufficient. In the UK, the importance of leadership in health care has led to more policy documents (NHS Executive, 1999), expensive training schemes for executives, and the NHS Plan has promised a national Leadership Centre (DoH, 2000). Nevertheless, it remains difficult to detect what concept of leadership is being promoted by these initiatives.

Leadership, in this paper, is conceived of as dispersed among teams, 'leading others to lead themselves' (Sims & Lorenzi, 1992, p. 295), and more concerned with processes and skills than with who is formally designated as a leader.

So, the paper takes issue with much of the general management literature which is frequently concerned with role specificity (Carignani, 2000; IBM Corporation, 1993; Katzenbach & Smith, 1993; Margerison & McCann, 1985; Obeng, 1994; Ramcharan, Grant, Parry-Jones, & Robinson, 1999), while the presence of clearly defined professional boundaries and current legal requirements act to prevent the flexibility required for multi-disciplinary teamwork (Payne, 2000). Networking in a manner that allowed for service users to take a leading role would therefore pose enormous problems for public service accountability and for measuring the performance of those charged with providing services.

The aim of involvement where users are involved with leading the service is therefore likely to remain a distant prospect. The necessity for it, however, will be illustrated by the research discussed in this paper. Payne's model of open teams and networking arrangements is the most promising model of leadership from which to proceed, and it will be used as a framework in the analysis that follows later. However, at this point, it may help to stress that open teamwork does not require new structural arrangements, but affects ways of working across existing structures.

Rather than outline this and other models of leadership separately from any empirical evidence, the paper seeks to examine teambuilding, networking and user-involvement, citing empirical evidence integrated within the discussion. It must be stressed that the benefits of this model cannot be demonstrated by this empirical work which only serves to indicate that further development is required. This can be understood if we first address the problems faced by further user involvement. In particular, there is an apparent dichotomy to be faced between an increased stress on leadership within the public sector, on one hand, and greater user involvement, on the other.

Before discussing this in more detail, however, the context of present policies towards measuring performance, involving users, and improving public sector management (leadership) can usefully be reviewed.

PERFORMANCE MANAGEMENT AND POLICIES TO INVOLVE USERS

User involvement–from involvement in deciding their own care through to involvement in policies and planning–has emerged in a distinctly modern form. Once associated with the radical movements of the 1960s, user involvement is now incorporated within what some writers have identified as the new public management (Barberis, 1998; Ferlie, Ashburner, Fitzgerald, & Pettigrew, 1996; Hood, 1991). Managers are made accountable for providing quality services with the money they spend (OECD, 1992). While policy directives insist that quality–as defined by service users–must be incorporated into measures of quality performance, definitions and measurements of quality still tend to be determined by providers, not service users.

Definitions of quality and the degree of user involvement remain contentious–this is an inevitable consequence of change. Practitioner, managerial, and user definitions of quality differ, as does its measurement. Involvement can vary from the minimum of consultation through to regular case reviews (for individuals) and routine structured representation.

Routine structured involvement has developed in the UK through joint commissioning of services involving service uses and voluntary bodies. A recent policy document, the *NHS Plan* (DoH, 2000), cites an example of joint commissioning from Somerset (p. 71). Other examples of 'partnership' trusts involving health and social care providers, with service users included in the decision making structures, are developing. At the time of writing, Norwich and West Sussex are two examples in England, while in Wales plans for partnership arrangements are out for consultation (NAW-Health Service Strategy Team, 2001).

The requirement to involve mental health service users in Wales is also evident in a raft of policy papers (NAW, 2001; Welsh Office, 1998a; Welsh Office, 1998b; Welsh Office, 1998c; Welsh Office, 1998d). The NAW's mental health strategy said:

> User and carer empowerment and their full participation in all aspects of mental health services is a fundamental principle of this Strategy. This involves partnership at three distinct but related levels. The first is in the assessment of individual need and agreeing the response to that need; the second is in joint planning, development and monitoring of services and thirdly in the running and management of services themselves. (NAW, 2001, 21)

Current policies are enacted through the establishment of targets and standards against which performance is measured. The results or performance measures are publicized. Performance is also enforced through audit and inspection. This is a common approach within public sector management, whatever sector. The standards for mental health services are expressed through the *Mental Health National Service Framework* (DoH, 1999), which states as its first guiding principle that 'People with mental health problems can expect that services will involve service users and their carers in planning and delivery of care' (p. 4). Further, on p. 17, it states 'All mental health services must be planned and implemented in partnership with local communities, and involve service users and carers.' However, all the standards relate to individuals and their care, and no standard for user involvement is specified. So user involvement may be limited to the provision of evidence from surveys (graded as Type V evidence, p. 6).[1]

In Wales, a *National Service Framework for Mental Health* has set December 2003 as a target by which all providers will have 'introduced arrangements to ensure constructive user and carer participation in the planning, design, delivery and, monitoring and evaluation of mental health services' (Welsh Assembly Government, 2002, p. 10).

However, it is not clear that user involvement for statutory agencies and service providers means the same as it does for service users (Barnes, 1999). Involvement can range from, at a minimum, the incorporation of a select number of views into policy and practice to, at a maximum, provider accountability to service users. There are difficulties in ensuring user representatives can adequately represent a diverse range of service user views (Bowl, 1996; Croft & Beresford, 1990). Any degree of representation may seem inadequate for service users who will argue that it may mean very little unless users are also involved in appointing staff (Brandon, 1992).

While the majority of staff welcome user input, some may take the view that service providers are unable to represent themselves adequately because their judgment is affected by their condition or by its treatment (Barnes & Wistow, 1994). Others may resist user involvement because they sense they are already over-burdened with work and that it has lesser priority than service provision (Dewa, Horgan, Russell, & Keates, 2001). It is also apparent that service providers have little of the skills necessary for systematic or meaningful research designed to establish what users want or what they think of the service (Rea, 1999). Under pressure for evidence, a 'plethora' of satisfaction surveys lacking theoretical foundation is of mounting concern (Edwards & Staniszewska, 2000).

Few providers budget to routinely measure service user views. Measurement of service quality poses a challenge to some mental health professionals who deny their work can be 'reduced' to quantifiable data. Others may accept the idea but see measurement too narrowly, in terms of clinical effectiveness (reduction of symptoms, of risk, or in the need for medication) (Rea & Rea, 2000).

These obstacles ensure that, because government policy requires user involvement, what little is done tends to be sporadic and the result of a few committed individuals. When social workers and other providers perceive links between finance and their performance, or when providers see that career opportunities depend on the public's perception, bias is likely. Surveys may merely establish whether users were satisfied with services and whether the service was achieving the goals set by the professionals (Godfrey & Wistow, 1997, p. 326).

One alternative that seeks to avoid this bias is where service users themselves evaluate the service (Rose, Ford, Lindley, Gawith, & Group, 1998). While this should be empowering for the service users involved, there may too be questions about the commitment of the service providers to change as a result of this sort of involvement. This sharing of commitment is central if involvement is to be turned into action. The emphasis now placed on leadership development may address these issues provided leadership is defined as dispersed leadership. The next section illustrates what is meant by this.

LEADERSHIP AND EFFECTIVE USER INVOLVEMENT

These obstacles to user involvement are apparent in several local initiatives in Swansea's mental health services. However, some progress is evident.

Mental health services in the Swansea are provided jointly by health and social services through four community mental health teams (CMHTs). In-patient beds are available, as well as a variety of day services, a resource centre, and specialist services. While the pattern of responsibility is changing radically, social services are an arm of local government while health services are provided through a national service, the National Health Service (NHS).

In Wales, this is complicated by the recent devolution of government to the National Assembly for Wales (NAW) responsible for health care policy. Local government and health authorities have both been reconfigured over the past five years–a process that is continuing with the abolition of health authorities. At present, social care staff are employed by the City and County of Swansea, and health care staff employed by the Swansea NHS Trust.

The lack of clear direction from the top–which may be viewed as an opportunity–accounts for local variations in service development and initiative. The CMHTs have devised multi-disciplinary working, some more so than others. The range of user involvement initiatives have been previously reported elsewhere (NAW-Social Services Inspectorate for Wales, 2001; Rea & Rea, 2000).

As elsewhere, the main focus has been on assessing service user views of the service, responding with information and policy changes, and followed by further user involvement in assessing user views.

These processes are highly reliant on the will of the individuals concerned and are not easily mapped onto the bureaucratic structures of health and social services. The process of policy change–in response to service user views–is not easily formalised. It relies on changes to professional practice, the willing adoption of changes to clinical practice and care management. It principally relies on communications and dialogue between service users and providers. Usually, however, user involvement is perceived as a structural mechanism.

Structures for User Involvement

An example of how user involvement is easily demonstrated in Swansea. The comment of a recent Social Services Inspectorate (SSI) report is worth examining:

> While some productive mechanisms for involving users in service planning were in place, . . . further efforts needed to be made to encourage wider representation of users, carers and the voluntary sector. (NAW-Social Services Inspectorate for Wales, 2001, p. 2)

To view involvement as occurring and existing though 'mechanisms' and structures of 'wider representation' is a product of a quasi-legal Inspectorate examining what is expected to be bureaucratic. Obviously, community mental health services *are* delivered through bureaucratic organisations, with a separate legal status, separate funding, and clearly demarked patterns of responsibility and accountability.

However, multi-disciplinary work, using a variety of agencies, can also be viewed as organised in ways that cannot be adequately represented as a hierarchical bureaucracy. It avoids the nature of the work CMHTs need to do to be an effective community-based team.

Payne's idea of 'open teams,' for example, cannot be represented well as a bureaucracy (Payne, 2000). He represents open teams pictorially as:

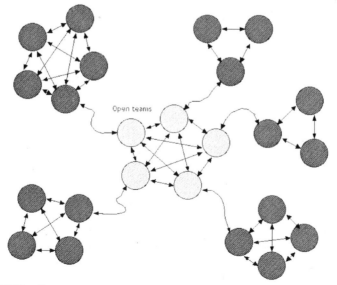

(Payne, 2000, p4)

This is a diagram intended to show how teams exist in relation to other teams. There are many definitions of teamwork, but some characteristics are common to all definitions. A team is not a group. Nor is a team a group of people working to a common person in charge over them (McGregor, 1960). Teams have common goals. Its members share information, decision making, and responsibility. Its decisions are made to work. There is open criticism matched by trust. Everyone must lead, at some time or another. Drawing largely on Harrington-Mackin (1993), Payne argues that leadership roles must be shared, nobody can opt out, and they need to focus on administration, quality, production, processes, training, supplies, work environment, and service user relationships (pp. 205-210).

In community mental health work, teams must work with and relate to teams in other agencies. And there is every reason why these relations should be extended to include service users–whether as isolated individuals or as members of representative bodies.

Open team working and networks should allow people to work together, whether they are paid employees or service users. Of course, bureaucratic relationships co-exist, and it would be foolish to ignore them. However, user involvement is unlikely to be organised neatly in a way that dovetails with bureaucratic hierarchies. This is likely to concern some, because services and the extent of user involvement will vary. The SSI report on Swansea, for example, is concerned about the structural mechanisms which were said 'to be inadequate and all planning partners recognised the need to develop a more innovative approach to achieving a wider representation of views' (NAW-Social Services Inspectorate for Wales, 2001, p. 20). But, equally, service users are unlikely to be entirely comfortable with the hierarchies and bureaucratic arrangements that some service providers feel more comfortable with. However, as the examples provided below illustrate, service users can be involved as part of a network, taking the lead sometimes in service developments, provided the key elements of open team working outlined below are fostered.

User Involvement and Building Dialogue

In Swansea, one of the CMHTs has attempted to build a dialogue between itself and its users over the past three years using a process of surveying what users think of the service and feeding this into professional practice and information provision. This strategy has increasingly been recognised as enhancing dialogue and, in 2001, the process was extended across the whole area. Moreover, in 2001, the draft questionnaire was reviewed with service users and questions added or altered. The questionnaire was therefore the result of work by health and social service staff, service users, and this author.

It is important to appreciate that this survey should not only be assessed by its ability to represent user views accurately by means of an objective scientifically validated instrument. It does not offer comparison over time or with other services. Its importance is as a means of opening dialogue.

The results of the survey are made public knowledge throughout the service, including principally the service users. It is intended to be a document for them when they want to argue for change. Over subsequent years, they will be able to measure progress. It is also intended to guide policy and management decisions, and to ensure service providers know what service users want of them. It provides service providers with the information they need to act, but it will also make them accountable to service users.

Building a dialogue that both service users and service providers value takes time and leadership skills. It takes time because service users have to test that it is genuine and because service providers have to see that it is valuable to users, and not a threat to themselves.

When service providers are being compelled to listen to user views, then professionals and services users are likely to view a survey as merely a requirement of the system. It is extra work for service providers and service users, and they may think the only likely benefit is to the people at the top. Service users have to see the results. They have to be able to comment on the results. They have to be able to look back and see that beneficial change occurred and that it can be attributable to the information provided earlier.

While survey evidence requires some sensitivity in its interpretation, the CMHT survey does provide some evidence of the necessary dialogue. It is apparent in a number of key indicators. One straightforward indication that service users value the survey as a means of communicating their wishes is whether they take part–and continue to take part, although we might also expect people to weary of filling on forms. The first survey, in 1998, was limited to one of the four CMHTs, and the response rate was 63%. By 2001, this had dropped to 54%. But in 2001, the survey was conducted in all four CMHT areas for the first time and the average was 37.7%. These are ambiguous data; respondent fatigue may have caused the reduction in the first area. Workload pressures may have prevented the survey being administered fully in the other areas. However, the fact that 54% of service users were willing to take part in 2001 does indicate some measure of its perceived value to them.

In planning the first survey (1998) it was decided to ask whether service users had enough information about their condition and their diagnosis. Informally, some CMHT staff indicated reservations about this question and doubted it would be of value to ask about it. The survey revealed, however, that 68% felt fully informed of their diagnosis and that 78% of these respondents found this information helpful. More seriously, 31% said they had not been told their diagnosis, and of these 68% said they would find it helpful. Decisions to change practice were made, but in 2001 the survey reported that only 58% had information and 33% said they did not. There were more respondents in the later survey from this CMHT area, and people may have different expectations, but otherwise this has to be interpreted as a failure to amend practice sufficiently.

Similarly depressing figures emerged when users were asked about whether they had enough information about their treatment or the services available to them. In 1998, 82% said they had enough information about their treatment, and 83% said they had enough information about local services. By 2001, for the same area, 74% said they had enough information about their treatment, and 77% said they had enough information about local services. Again, these figures need interpretation–especially with the word 'enough' in the question–as expectations may have altered. In response to the first survey in 1998, leaflets have been issued about treatments and services. This may have affected service user expectations, but otherwise these figures are disappointing.

Direct comparison between surveys is otherwise impossible because the later survey has incorporated many more questions than its earlier counterpart. However, the comparisons above offer a salutary lesson that gathering information about what service users want from their service can only be regarded as a first step in the process of change. Need for further action has been clearly identified and one response by the providers is to devise an information strategy. Since the latest survey, service users have been active in improving the care management process, taking part in improving review procedures. They have also worked on user-focused monitoring: devising, administering, and analysing their own surveys. These initiatives illustrate that some progress has been made in confidence and trust building.

The paper now outlines what is necessary to ensure action follows.

Team Building for User Involvement

Confidence building and establishing a dialogue are necessary first steps, but others are needed. Following Payne's discussion (on pp. 205-210), these steps are set out below. However, we should note that current job descriptions and performance management measures that stress the needs of the seriously mentally ill cannot assist in this kind of support. If it happens at all, it takes place outside of work hours.

> *Support:* Effective team leadership recognises that staff need support from their peers–sympathy, understanding, and encouragement, as well as practical help, such as information. The same is equally true of mental health service users if they are to be effectively involved in planning services. In Swansea, CMHT staff have begun working on this aspect of networking only during the past year. Service users have become involved in projects, and equally, some staff are beginning to offer support for service user projects. While staff may get praise for this, it is not a requirement of their role as defined in job contracts. As with all these efforts, the work frequently is an addition to their recognised workload and frequently involves out-of-hours work.

> *Conflict Resolution:* the literature on teambuilding generally recommends starting with a small project around a problem that needs solving. It also requires a sense of urgency. Clear rules of behaviour need to be established (confidentiality, 'no sacred cows,' and above all 'everyone does real work'), people need to be kept informed, and people need to spend time together. The potential for conflict while mental health service users are involved has to be recognised and worked on. Again, current job definitions do not encourage staff to work with service users on team building and involvement in planning service delivery. It is a role which is taken more seriously when there is a complaint or an investigation.

> *Training and Support for Team Members' Development:* The organisation of service users so they can contribute requires they

know how to communicate with each other. That takes money (for postage and room hire for meetings). It also takes skills, typically how to work together in meetings and how to carry ideas into action. At a less basic level, service users need to be able to speak publicly and confidently about their needs. They also need to be able to contribute workable ideas for improvement. These abilities are frequently lacking in full-time work organisations, so the difficulties for mental health service users cannot be underestimated. Their involvement in service planning requires training that they are infrequently made available to them. In Swansea, in recent months, money for training and support has been made available to service user organisations. This is fortunate and has occurred quite independently of service providers. But in the long-term, this is something service providers must take seriously if they wish to encourage service user involvement and their ability to lead the service. The support will also need to encompass other service users.

Less optimistically, we can note that users were involved with staff appointments under previous organisational arrangements. The new unitary authority (City & County of Swansea) has adopted a fair selection policy, however, that requires training. Service users have not had any access to this training and so can no longer take part. Organisational boundaries and policies do not always allow for the sort of collaboration needed for open teams and networks, or respect the rights of service users to be involved in planning their service. So training needs also to cross those organisational boundaries and, in this example, would empower users significantly.

Social Climate: Payne stresses the need for politeness, warmth and consideration. People need to take an interest in people's non-work lives. 'Humour is a useful part of team life, provided it is not sarcastic or destructive' (Payne, 2000, p. 208). A structure of representation, and the development of procedures and protocols for service user involvement can be put in place. Service providers will then have met the performance management targets set by government. When they occur, these are welcome developments. But they are not sufficient. This point is a reminder that it is the informal aspects of work that provide meaning to people's work life. Service users can too easily be seen as outsiders by provider organisations, especially where teambuilding has worked narrowly to include only those within the formal organisation. Open networking and user involvement require, above all else, that staff and professionals involved in service provision are open and respectful of others. Teambuilding has to be inclusive of service users, and that also means being warm, considerate, and even building a shared sense of humour.

Leadership and Supervision: Payne, this time drawing on Chandler (1996), argues that supervision has to provide opportunities for testing out ideas, not just checking on what has been done, and that leadership is required to ensure the team is developing. This has to be extended out into the community so that mental health service users benefit.

These are probably the bare minimum of what is required for service users to be involved and to participate fully in open networks. In Swansea, there is some evidence that some of these things are happening, but not all. Much more needs to be done. Moreover, Swansea probably provides one of the more advanced services in Wales. So, it is likely that further work is needed elsewhere.

CONCLUSION–
RECONCILING POLICY AND MANAGEMENT IMPERATIVES WITH USERS' EXPRESSED DESIRES

This paper has highlighted some of the difficulties inherent in involving mental health service users in service planning. Policy directives and modern forms of management are increasingly demanding they have a say. However, for service users to find their voice and ensure it is heard, further empowerment is required. Foremost among the steps that can be taken to empower them is the idea that they be involved through open networks. An opportunity exists in the UK for management of services to move in this direction, through the government's recent stress on leadership skills. These have yet to be defined adequately by central government.

However, the definition of leadership does not have to come from central government. Managers, educationalists, service provider professionals, and service users can work together within this framework to encourage team leadership that involves service users in affecting change. A structure of representation can assist in this process, but it is not always required, and it is not all that is required. Far more important is that service users be empowered and encouraged. Their views have to be sought and acted upon, and be seen to be acted upon.

The kind of leadership necessary for these developments to occur is unlikely to be top-down leadership in the 'hero' mould. This requires that the accountability of those with formal leadership positions should specify what they have done to lead others to lead themselves, rather than what they themselves have achieved. Dispersed leadership makes accountability and responsibility difficult. But, leadership has to develop within teams of people working together across–or in spite of–formal organisational boundaries and financial systems. This development requires policy and organisational boundaries to be re-thought.

There are useful, even obvious, lessons to be learned from the concepts of leadership within teams, and Payne's model of open teams provides a way in which user involvement can be developed in the future so that the service is user-led at appropriate times. Considerable problems have to be overcome, however, and the benefits of this model cannot be demonstrated empirically. However, it may provide a vision for future user involvement.

NOTE

1. *http://www.jr2.ox.ac.uk/bandolier/band12/b12-1.html*

REFERENCES

Barberis, P. (1998). The new public management and a new accountability. *Public Administration, 76*, 451-470.

Barnes, M. (1999). Users as citizens: Collective action and the local governance of welfare. *Social Policy & Administration, 33*(1), 73-90.

Barnes, M., & Wistow, G. (1994). Learning to hear voices: Listening to users of mental health services. *Journal of Mental Health, 3*, 525-540.

Bodwell, D. J. (1996). *High Performance Teams.*

Bowl, R. (1996). Legislating for user involvement in the United Kingdom: mental health services and the NHS and Community Care Act 1990. *International Journal of Social Psychiatry, 42*(3), 165-180.

Brandon, D. (1992). *Skills for people: Annual report and national conference report.* Newcastle-upon-Tyne: Skills for People.

Bryman, A. (1996). Leadership in organizations. In S. R. Clegg, C. Hardy, & R. Nord (Eds.), *Handbook of organization studies.* London: Sage.

Carignani, V. (2000). Management of change in health care organisations and human resource role. *European Journal of Radiology, 33*, 8-13.

Chandler, J. (1996). Support for community psychiatric nurses in multi-disciplinary teams: An example. In M. Watkins (Ed.), *Collaborative Community Mental Health Care* (pp. 292-306). London: Edward Arnold.

Croft, S., & Beresford, P. (1990). *From paternalism to participation: Involving people in social services.* London: Open services Project/Joseph Rowntree.

Dewa, C. S., Horgan, S., Russell, M., & Keates, J. (2001). What? Another form? The process of measuring and comparing service utilization in a community mental health program model. *Evaluation and Program Planning, 24*, 239-247.

DoH. (1999). *A National Service Framework for mental health: Modern standards & service models.* London: DoH.

DoH. (2000). *The NHS Plan: A plan for investment, a plan for reform.* (Vol. Cm 4818-I). London: HMSO.

Edwards, C., & Staniszewska, S. (2000). Accessing the user's perspective. *Health and Social Care in the Community, 8*(6), 417-424.

Ferlie, E., Ashburner, L., Fitzgerald, L., & Pettigrew, A. (1996). *The new public management in action.* Oxford: Oxford University Press.

Geenen, H. (1985). *Managing.* London: Granada.

Godfrey, M., & Wistow, G. (1997). The user perspective on managing for health outcomes: The case of mental health. *Health and Social Care in the Community, 5*(5), 325-332.

Harrington-Mackin, D. (1993). *Keeping the team going: A tool kit to renew and refuel your workplace teams.* New York: American Management Association.

Hood, C. (1991). *Public management reform in the 1980s: Reflections on national variations.* Paper presented at the Calculating health in the new public sector? Workshop on changing notions of accountability in the UK public sector, London School of Economics and Political Science, Department of Accounting and Finance.

IBM Corporation. (1993). *Ideas on Teams and Teamwork*: IBM Corporation.

Katzenbach, J. R., & Smith, D. K. (1993). *The wisdom of teams: Creating the high-performance organization.* Boston, MA: Harvard Business School.

Margerison, C., & McCann, D. (1985). *How to Lead a Winning Team.* Bradford: MCB University Press.

McGregor, D. (1960). *The human side of enterprise.* New York: McGraw-Hill.

NAW. (2001). *Adult mental health services for Wales: Equity, empowerment, effectiveness, efficiency: Strategy document.* (September 2001 ed.). Cardiff: NAW.

NAW-Health Service Strategy Team. (2001). *Improving health in Wales: Structural change in the NHS in Wales.* Cardiff: National Assembly for Wales.

NAW-Social Services Inspectorate for Wales. (2001). *Inspection of adult mental illness services in the City and County of Swansea.* Cardiff: National Assembly for Wales.

NAW and the Audit Commission. (2000). *Learning the lessons from Joint Reviews of Social Services in Wales, 1999/2000.* Oxford: Audit Commission.

NHS Executive. (1999). *Leadership for health: The health authority role.*

Obeng, E. (1994). *All change!* London: Financial Times/Pitman.

OECD. (1992). *The reform of health care systems: A comparative analysis of seven OECD countries.* (Vol. 2). Paris: OECD.

Payne, M. (2000). *Teamwork in multi-professional care.* London: Macmillan.

Pollitt, C., Harrison, S., Hunter, D. J., & Marnoch, G. (1991). General management in the NHS: The initial impact 1983-88. *Public Administration, 69,* 63-83.

Ramcharan, P., Grant, G., Parry-Jones, B., & Robinson, C. (1999). Roles and tasks of care management practitioners in Wales–revisited. *Managing Community Care, 7*(3), 29-37.

Rea, C., & Rea, D. (2000). Responding to user views of service performance. *Journal of Mental Health, 9*(4), 351-363.

Rea, D. M. (1999). Towards routine user assessment of mental health service quality performance. *International Journal of Health Care Quality Assurance, 12*(4), 169-176.

Rose, D., Ford, R., Lindley, P., Gawith, L., & Group, a. t. K. C. a. W. H. A. M. H. M. U. (1998). *In our experience: User-focused monitoring of mental health services.* London: Sainsbury Centre for Mental Health.

Sims, H. P., & Lorenzi, P. (1992). *The new leadership paradigm.* Newbury Park: Sage.

Welsh Assembly Government. (2002). *Adult mental health services: A National Service Framework for Wales.* Cardiff: Welsh Assembly Government.

Welsh Office. (1998a). *Better health: Better Wales: A consultation paper.* (Vol. CM3922). Cardiff: Welsh Office.

Welsh Office. (1998b). *Improving local services through best value.* Cardiff: Welsh Office.

Welsh Office. (1998c). *NHS Wales: Putting patients first.* (Vol. Cm3841). Cardiff: Welsh Office.

Welsh Office. (1998d). *NHS Wales: Putting patients first: Local Health Groups preliminary guidance.* Cardiff: Welsh Office.

ADVANCING INCLUSIVE AND EMPOWERING PRACTICE

Postmodern Social Work in Interdisciplinary Contexts: Making Space on Both Sides of the Table

Marty Dewees, PhD, LICSW

SUMMARY. This paper describes a university-based, maternal child health, interdisciplinary training project designed to assist health professionals in working with neurodevelopmentally at-risk children and their families. It discusses a role for social work educators and practitioners that brings to the table varied, conceptual questions that are intertwined with more traditional social work intervention in a postmodern approach to interdisciplinary teaming. A case example illustrates the integration of these two approaches and the inquiries that social work can initiate to

Marty Dewees is Associate Professor, Department of Social Work, 443 Waterman Building, University of Vermont, Burlington, VT 05405 (E-mail: mdewees@zoo.uvm.edu).

Based on a paper presented at 3rd International Conference on Social Work in Health and Mental Health, Tampere, Finland, July 4, 2001.

[Haworth co-indexing entry note]: "Postmodern Social Work in Interdisciplinary Contexts: Making Space on Both Sides of the Table." Dewees, Marty. Co-published simultaneously in *Social Work in Health Care* (The Haworth Social Work Practice Press, an imprint of The Haworth Press, Inc.) Vol. 39, No. 3/4, 2004, pp. 343-360; and: *Social Work Visions from Around the Globe: Citizens, Methods, and Approaches* (ed: Anna Metteri et al.) The Haworth Social Work Practice Press, an imprint of The Haworth Press, Inc., 2004, pp. 343-360. Single or multiple copies of this article are available for a fee from The Haworth Document Delivery Service [1-800-HAWORTH, 9:00 a.m. - 5:00 p.m. (EST). E-mail address: docdelivery@haworthpress.com].

facilitate "making space" both between the team and family and between members of the team in a dynamic, postmodern, interdisciplinary context. *[Article copies available for a fee from The Haworth Document Delivery Service: 1-800-HAWORTH. E-mail address: <docdelivery@haworthpress.com> Website: <http://www.HaworthPress.com> © 2004 by The Haworth Press, Inc. All rights reserved.]*

KEYWORDS. Interdisciplinary teams, postmodern approaches, social work roles

I brought food to the hungry,
and people called me a saint;
I asked why people were hungry,
and people called me a communist.

Dom Helder Camara, Archbishop of Recife, Brazil
Cited in Gil, (1998) *Confronting Injustice and Oppression,* p. 127

The Vermont Interdisciplinary Leadership Education for Health Professionals (VT-ILEHP) program is a training project funded by the U.S. Department of Health and Human Services Maternal and Child Health Bureau. It is designed to make a positive impact on children and adolescents with special health needs and their families. The twelve participating disciplines, including social work, are committed to culturally competent, strengths-based, family-centered intervention in neurodevelopmental disabilities. While the work is frequently focused on a combination of medical, educational, and speech-language interventions, the emphasis on family-centered, culturally competent practice represents commitment to the framework of family empowerment, family goals, and liberation from domination by experts.

This paper discusses a role for social work educators and practitioners that brings to the table varied, conceptual questions that are intertwined with social work intervention in a postmodern approach to interdisciplinary teaming. It will be useful to situate this project in its professional/historical context before describing the specific content of the social work role.

INTERPROFESSIONAL PRACTICE

Interdisciplinary teaming, particularly for children's health concerns, is not a new structure for social work. Because of social work's traditional, person-in-environment focus, abiding interest in the family, and long-term role in health care, interdisciplinary practice is a natural method for it.

Children are complex creatures with multiple developmental concerns along many biopsychosocial dimensions. While there is support for the agency of both infants and children as active social participants (see Satka, 2001; Stern, 2000), young children are largely dependent on the macro environments into which they are born. This in turn implicates such aspects as poverty or cultural identity, which intersect with the experience of childhood. Children with special health needs present particularly complex scenarios, and most of their families require the direct-service intervention of a variety of professionals, as well as financial and social supports (Prelock, Beatson, Contompasis, & Bishop, 1999). In this context, successful interdisciplinary teaming integrates numerous biopsychosocial facets into ecological services (Guralnick, 2000; Johnson & Johnson, 1987; Nagi, 1991; Roberts-DeGennerao, 1996; Sameroff, 1993). The overall goal is an improved quality of life for individual children and families (Dennis, Williams, Giangreco, & Cloninger, 1993).

Interdisciplinary teaming can also create some stressors. Beyond "the myth of good intentions" (Compton & Galaway, 1999, p. 440) the interdisciplinary context requires the ability to suspend the tendency to evaluate difference as right or wrong. Tolerance for conflict, negotiation of boundaries, and willingness to confront competitiveness are all indicated in effective, relational, interdisciplinary work. Abramson (1984) stresses the importance of agreement on key ethical issues as well as a regular time to process their meaning.

The arena of difference in interdisciplinary work can become murky. While individual variations in style, adherence to agreed-upon norms, and capacity for conflict may represent strengths, professional training and socialization can, on some occasions, present a strong set of obstacles. Social workers may become caught, for example, in a conflict between client advocacy, one of its core values, and team consensus about a recommended discharge plan. In another situation, the culture of social work, which tends to preclude "dual relationships," may clash with another profession that does not address them in that way. For example, the U.S. National Association of Social Workers Code of Ethics (NASW, 1996) is explicit about avoiding dual relationships with people who are clients, particularly during the period of their clienthood. But members of other disciplines may assume additional roles, as private citizens, which they feel *obliged* to take up in the name of family-centered care. Profession-bound lenses do not abdicate easily for the sake of unity, but need rather to be raised as open and normative concerns for exploration.

Family-Centered Approach as Postmodern

While incorporating interdisciplinary approaches, service delivery methods have undergone a paradigm shift from reliance upon professional expertise(s) to a collaborative, family-centered approach (Prelock et al., 1999). This represents a significant change in focus that is consistent with postmodern approaches to working with people. Postmodern thinking tends to question assumptions and indeed, " . . . does not accept claims of knowledge and understanding at face value" (Payne, 1997, p. 30). Professional child experts, then, are not seen as inscrutable interventionists who necessarily know best. Families are more likely to be recognized as the single most influential force in the life of a child (see Delaney & Kunstal, 1993). Family-centeredness values the family as the constant, cultural, and experiential expert on the child's life. It respects the family as decision makers for their children and respects their rights as consumers (McBride, 1999). In addition, it is committed to:

- working with families as partners
- facilitating multilevel collaboration, ranging from individual care to policy development
- exchanging complete, unbiased communication
- honoring cultural diversity
- recognizing diverse coping strategies
- recognizing strengths
- encouraging parent-to-parent connection and support
- facilitating flexible, accessible services (see Shelton & Stepanek, 1994).

While the family as the "unit of work" (Hartman, 1981) has ben a long standing tenet of social work practice, the focus has not always been salutary, particularly in the arena of culturally different customs and expectations. The more current emphasis on family as participant in the work has yielded several "choicepoints" (Briar-Lawson, 1998, p. 544) that distinguish among varying aspects and degrees of family as center of the work. The contemporary shift to family-as-expert can be seen as an example of the postmodern perspective regarding the nature of epistemology, privilege, and political hegemony (Alcoff, 1997). A benchmark of postmodern thinking is reflected in its critical stance regarding the nature of truth and reality as they are traditionally formulated. In the context of family work, this suggests that practitioners of all the professions reexamine the political and social arrangements of their clients' lives with an eye to their interests and benefits.

Family-centeredness, like interdisciplinary teaming, is less sanguine than first glance might suggest. As an ideal, its currency is sometimes more rhetorical than real. Both professional literature and consumer folklore uncover families charging they have not been honored as the approach would warrant. Many professionals have struggled to release their expertise without abandoning their wisdom and surrendering their values. Nursing, nutrition, and medicine, among others of the medical model tradition, may face an even greater challenge as they attempt to relinquish their particular hold on an objective and scientific truth.

Social Work as Critical Construction

Within the context of interdisciplinary, family-centered, culturally competent practice, the department of social work brings its own focus to the work. Committed to a strengths perspective, social justice, human rights, and social construction, its participation on an interprofessional team is highly shaped by its worldview. Social construction offers another standpoint within postmodern thinking and a useful method for understanding social work (Lum, 1999; Witkin, 1999). Constructionists believe that people, within their social contexts, are active in the shaping of their own realities through an intersubjectivity of knowledge and experience (Weick, 1993). Critical, dialogic inquiry into practice/theory assumptions is an important expression of the constructionist position (Gergen, 2000). It considers that the realities of the social world are not objective, scientific facts, but agreed-upon understandings generated through social and linguistic processes. For example, the assertion that anyone who cooperates can access good health care, and the corollary that if one is not getting good health care, one is not cooperating enough (see Fadiman, 1997, for a striking demonstration of this assumption), reflects more about beliefs resulting from collective sense-making in a particular context than it does about neutral objectivity. Challenging the absolute quality of such equations, critical social constructionist thinkers are likely to ask who benefits from such arrangements as inaccessibility, limited health care, and poverty; who is silenced, and whose influence is most valued as the dominant or popular opinion (Laird, 1995). The differences uncovered in this examination are seen as instrumental to the process of inquiry.

Further, in the social work context, as in special education and many others, this view has raised questions about the language of dominance (Dewees, 1999; Freedman & Combs, 1996; Weedon, 1987) and the phenomenon of subjugated voices (Hartman, 1994). Dietz (2000) suggests that the manner in which an issue is described in language tells us a great deal about how it will be addressed (p. 370). Kalyanpur and Harry (1999a) discuss language as a critical component in the construction of the meaning of the term disability and the establishment of objective, hierarchal boundaries that medicalize and give birth to expertise (Kalyanpur & Harry, 1999b) among professionals. The social world of families and its forms are made concrete through everyday talk and interaction (Gubruim & Holstein, 1993). On a more direct level, with metaphoric inference, Blatt describes the power of language and giving voice:

> language is such a miracle! . . . language stirs people to make love, to initiate wars, to lay their lives down for their country, or their God, or their youth, or their excesses . . . nothing is more certain than that there are inescapable consequences of language . . . not to have it is to be in such serious trouble . . . (p. 116)

In this context, family-centered practice seeks to make space for the language and voices of families. At the same time, the constructionist practitioner will recognize the potential for the language of dominance to appear within the team. In some cases this is reflected in the jargon of a particular profession. In others it may reflect subtle (or less so) status levels among the professions. This may present an exceedingly difficult phenomenon to confront while maintaining good will and a cooperative spirit.

Social Work Roles

Cook (2000) proposes three roles for social workers in family-centered interdisciplinary teams: (a) ethnographic assessment, (b) support, and (c) empowerment. Many social workers recognize these as solid professional functions in almost any context, quasi-traditional to postmodern. Multiple meanings lie within them, however, that will influence the work depending on how they are experienced by providers. If, for example, family-centeredness is taken up as the perspective of beleaguered parents, a disenfranchised mother with developmental disabilities, or a ferociously proud father, it will look quite different from family-centeredness from the perspective of the recalcitrant teen, the confused ten year old, or the near adult child tied to his bed for "safety." These perspectives in turn influence the work of assessment, support, and empowerment.

Ethnographic Assessment. There is a growing body of literature on ethnographic interviewing theory and techniques applicable to social work practice (Dewees, 2001; Laird, 1996; Leigh, 1998; Lum, 1999). In general, the postmodern social worker works within the theme that there are "many ways of knowing" (Hartman, 1994) and social workers assume a position of "not knowing" (Anderson-Goolishian, 1992). Leigh (1998) advises that it is the worker's responsibility to gain knowledge of the client's culture as she or he places the client in the role of teacher. In this project, the notion of "culture" may refer to ethnic differences, class, or age and also to the culture generated by those experiencing disabilities in their families.

Among several useful techniques in this process is the examination of cover terms and global questions (Greene, 1997; Leigh, 1998). Cover terms are those words or groups of words that signify the particular experience or meaning to the person interviewed. For example, an examination of the phrase "disabled child" as it is used in common parlance may suggest a specific meaning to the parent of a child with, for example, autism. As such terms are made explicit, the practitioner can become more attuned to the meanings they hold for clients. Global questions may arise from the considerations that occur to the worker prior to or during the interview when a cover term is explored. For example, if one senses that labeling is a highly sensitized issue for the family, one might ask "What does it mean to your family when your child is identified as disabled?" This kind of exploration can reveal how the family understands its circumstance and the beliefs it has about the child. It can facilitate a responsive relationship as it conveys genuine respect for the family's expertise and experience and also opens the way for the family's description of other variables that characterize their child, such as "sweet natured," or "loving," or "funny," which may add balance and fullness.

More direct inquiry, utilizing ethnographic methods, might address the areas of stresses, resources, and family home environment (Krauss & Jacobs, 1990). Because high levels of stress are frequently associated with how well the family can meet its needs, it is important to explore the meanings attributed to it. Here it is particularly important for social workers to attend to the environmental issues that may serve as "background" material for other team members. Cultural isolation, loss of a parent, lack of transportation, and lack of decent housing are among the influences that carry very different implications within U.S. culture.

Identification of resources, coping strategies, methods for relaxation, and maintenance of optimism are all integral components of this aspect of the work. Here the significance for the family is elicited and explored through their narratives. In this sense, then, assessment is a misnomer as it implies an expertise (Laird, 1995) that is avoided in the ethnographer's situating of her or himself. Laird suggests that the process is characterized by collaboration (a dialogue to generate new possibilities), reflexivity (recognizing that one's stories are in flux and are influenced by each telling), and multiplicity (a recognition of many possible understandings of one situation) (1995, p. 159).

Support. Most workers agree that supporting the family includes a focus on its strengths and the facilitation of its access to helpful resources. Within the last twenty years, strengths-based intervention has been introduced to many different social work fields of practice, including families (Kaplan & Girard, 1994). Saleebey (1992, 1997) identified several overall principles guiding a strengths perspective: (a) every individual, group, family, and community has strengths; (b) trauma and abuse may be deleterious, but may also provide the forum for challenge and opportunity; (c) the upper limits of the capacity for growth are not known; (d) clients are best served through collaboration; and (e) every environment is full of resources. All of these points speak to the needs of parents who find themselves in a role they never envisioned. Conceiving support as an effort to emphasize the strengths of parents as caregivers, social workers can adapt any of the solution-focused therapy question types that Saleebey has adopted (1997). These include (a) survival questions; (b) support questions; (c) the exception question; (d) possibility questions; and (e) esteem questions. These are important tools for building relationship; they impart the workers' assumptions of strengths and capacities, at the same time, recognizing and validating hardship. The implementation of a strengths-based practice, however, is not always easy. U.S. culture tends to support a problem focus and has a resilient respect for models that highlight pathology. More recently, Saleebey (2000, 2001) calls for the same degree of detailed, refined description of strengths as is found in the diagnostic categories of the *DSM-IV-TR* (2000). This calls on team members to think another way, combating old, internalized ideologies (Gil, 1998).

Referral to other supportive networks is likewise an important part of working with families. Organizations like Parent-to-Parent provide significant sources of support in a manner that is consistent with family-centered practice. Parents can choose how the agency can be helpful to them (if at all) and connect with other parents of children with disabilities. The roles of advocacy, information sharing (e.g., assistance with a Medicaid application), and camaraderie are for some families a lifeline to the rest of the world. Many highly esoteric concerns that families with children with disabilities face are immediately recognized and honored without lengthy explanations. The language of resilience and strengths is the norm, and the dreams and hopes of families are taken seriously. Connecting families with other families experiencing similar stresses may open the way for their own sense of empowerment, both personally, and with regard to a growing capacity to intervene in the many systems they encounter (Boyd-Franklin, 1993).

Empowerment. The concept of empowerment is embedded in the core of social work practice. For well over 100 years ago, social workers have sought to facilitate the empowerment of clients. In some of the interdisciplinary literature, empowerment refers to the family's ability to obtain resources and advocacy (Cook, 2000), the prominence of family-driven services (Cooley & Olson, 1996), and the quality of helpgivers' relational interactions (Dunst & Trivette, 1996). Social work, too, emphasizes empowerment as "reflexive activity" (Simon, 1994) that can be facilitated (not accomplished) by the professional, as it "resides in the person, not the helper" (Lee, 1996, p. 224). Its interpersonal dimension is nurtured through effectiveness in influencing others (Gutierrez, 1991). A more sociopolitical dimension points to the intersection of personal effectiveness with the environment and its resources (Rappaport, Reischl, & Zimmerman, 1992). Lee combines these aspects in identifying three dimensions of empowerment "(a) the development of a more positive and potent sense of self; (b) the construction of knowledge and capacity for more critical comprehension of social and political realities of one's environment; and (c) the cultivation of resources and strategies, or more functional competence, for attainment of personal and collective social goals, or liberation" (p. 224).

Because social work has traditionally (although not consistently) been concerned with oppression and social reform (Abramowitz, 1998; Haynes, 1998; Specht & Courtney, 1995), it often makes a more explicit connection between the personal and the political than is made in more medically-based professions. Injustice and discrimination constitute the very "stuff" of social work intervention (Gitterman, 1991). While social workers are by no means unified on the degree to which they believe, for example, that poverty is responsible for people's private troubles, they are probably more likely to look earlier to structural aspects of the family's context than are many other professions. This is made more complex by the fact that disabilities in children can and do appear in all sociocultural groups; the focus is often on the individual family's functioning. These distinctions may highlight team differences when the emphasis on empowering the family is bounded in what seems like narrowly focused internal mechanisms to social workers, who are especially sensitized to the role of more institutional arrangements, such as poverty, oppression, and lack of access. At this intersection, social workers can create space among their colleagues by facilitating their understanding of the social conditions that shape their clients' lives. This understanding will require that "our messages . . . touch people's hearts as well as their minds" (Witkin, 1998).

All of these practice roles–assessment, support, and empowerment–and their many subsets in a family-centered interdisciplinary practice, are designed to open the practice context, to amplify the voices of families, honor the meanings they hold, and strengthen their capacities even as they differ from the notions of professional expertise. In a parallel process, team members also make meanings of these concepts, also have voices, and are different one from another. Constructionist social workers can facilitate the making of space on both sides of the conference table; that is, they can assist in raising the differences among team members as well as between the team and the family.

CASE ILLUSTRATION: PLAYING IT OUT AND ASKING THE QUESTIONS

Early in the academic year, a social work graduate student had completed the required training with her colleagues (four other trainees and fellows). Bringing a strongly constructionist stance to her work, and being something of a respectful iconoclast, she began to develop her place in the program by asking what the team meant by family-centered care. Since this is one of the most emphasized tenets of the program, this seemed to her to be a critical inquiry, particularly because it was arising out of the practice context of her first assignment, which follows.

Wayne's Story

Wayne is a man in his mid-thirties with significant developmental delays. He has experienced a difficult childhood, adolescence, and young adulthood, as a person in need of resources and a great deal of support. He has become a multiple service recipient, with a fair amount of reluctance. He has not always seen the purpose of recommended services and generally perceives himself at odds with authorities who seem to try to control him. He is pleasant and friendly but is reticent about involvement in services whose purposes he sees as interfering with the course of how he wants to live his life.

Wayne fathered a child with Ellen, whom he met in a brief stay at the state institution serving developmentally delayed youths, after he had had a behavioral episode in his own home. When their daughter was born, Ellen developed a post-partum response which complicated her already-questioned capacity to care for a child adequately and safely. Choosing not to take up the nurturing role, she relinquished her parental rights very soon after the child's birth. Wayne, on the other hand, attached quickly to the child, Ellie, named after her mother, and was determined to make a home for her. By this time, Wayne had had a series of part-time jobs and received a supplemental disability allowance. He was able to keep an apartment, with Section 8 assistance, obtain subsidized child care, and was, for the first few years, Ellie's single, custodial parent.

Wayne also had, along with his motivation to parent, a pervasive need for affiliation. One of his friends had a history of sexual aggression against children and was well known to the community. Receiving limited services from the state child protection team, Wayne was warned that he must keep his friend away from his apartment in order to keep Ellie safe. Because he rarely could afford to go out, and because he wanted to spend more time with Ellie, most of his social life occurred at his apartment. He did not comply with the condition that his friend be restricted from visiting when Ellie was around, and several friends (including the sexual offender) visited frequently. Ellie slept in a bedroom immediately off the living room in which Wayne's friends slept when they spent the night. Wayne was repeatedly warned that Ellie's safety was at risk as was his continuing custody of her. Wayne was offered services that would assist him in maintaining the standards required by child protection authorities (help in locating a larger apartment, respite, etc.). He refused them. When Ellie began to exhibit sexualized behaviors at school, child protection initiated a custody hearing. There were no grounds to support sexual abuse nor did Ellie demonstrate overt symptoms consistent with abuse. Rather Ellie was thought to have witnessed consensual adult sexual activity, probably on numerous occasions. The grounds for removing Ellie from Wayne's home rested in his inability to keep her separated from his friend with a record of predatory behavior. When Ellie was placed in foster care, Wayne tried hard to maintain the schedule for visiting her. He was disheartened and angry about the removal of Ellie from his custody and continued to be determined to get her back.

Ellie was referred for interdisciplinary consultation by members of the school team. She demonstrated various difficulties in learning, speaking, and socializing appropriately with peers. She performed significantly below grade level on standardized tests of ability and progress. Ellie's new foster parents, Dave and Liz, also supported the referral to the interdisciplinary team and were reportedly interested in adopting her if she became available. Personnel at the new school (in the county in which Dave and Liz resided) were very supportive of them, but found Wayne's inclusion in any of the intake, planning, or community clinic assessments to be problematic. During the course of the evaluation period, child protective services made it clear that they would support termination of Wayne's parental rights. This position created further tension in the ambiguity of the assessment process. The termination procedure, however, was described as likely to take nearly two years before a final determination could be made and likely appeals could be settled.

Student Intervention. In the beginning, to strategize her practice role as the coordinator of the assessment process, the intern wondered where to start. Family-centered work seemed to be particularly complex in this constellation with its disrupted lives and multiple caretakers acting as parents. The first team meeting in which the genogram and ecomap were drawn set the stage for what would become a familiar process. The mapping activity raised several questions as to the meaning that members made of this family's background. How should Wayne be placed vis a vis the foster parents? Was his place "legitimate"? What does being a parent mean to team members who have ideas, very different from Wayne's, around safety issues for children? What level of protection is required to be a "real" parent? What bias did members have around exposure to sexual expression that is different from their own views? What sociocultural issues were raised when a parent refused services that child protection authorities recommend to assist him in retaining custody? What role did gender play in consideration of an adequate parent? Is a man with developmental disabilities inherently less preferred to raise a girl-child? Any child?

In drawing the ecomap, further questions arose regarding the placement of the project. What was the team's role here? Should the project take a position with family court on who should be parent in the child's best interest? Was it the role of the team to enter that dialogue? How could the team continue its advocacy for Wayne whether he loses parental rights or not? How would such advocacy be perceived by other agencies? How did poverty and disability influence the ability to parent? How did they influence the team's view of its work? (For a discussion of the effect of poverty on family-centered services in occupational therapy, see Humphrey, 1995.) Did family-centeredness imply the child's best interests? The parent's best interests, or did it imply that the interests are one in the same? How did we construct family-centered practice on this team?

An early visit at the school in which Ellie was then a student revealed that the foster parents were considered the "family" by those working with her. Because the school personnel had no knowledge of or contact with Wayne, they saw the state's custodial arrangement as the dominant one even though Wayne retained legal parental rights at the time. More questions arose: Whose perspective prescribed the membership of this family? Was the team's role to harmonize differing perspectives within families? What were the biases that team members brought to the interdisciplinary table, regarding poverty, custom, parental incompetence, compliance, and cultural variations in perceptions of optimal childcare? How did a family-centered stance meet a child-centered one?

Intervention Related to Roles. Returning briefly to Cook's conception of social work's roles, we can focus on similar questions. Who should be included in an ethnographic family *assessment*? Whose story was preferred over others? Whose was discounted? Whose understanding was taken as "accurate" or "reasonable"? Whose was not? Whose motives were suspect? Whose were honored? Who was to be *supported*? The parent about to lose parental rights? The child in foster care? the foster parents? The school personnel? How were these mutually exclusive (or not)? What strengths did Wayne have? How could the team facilitate his resilience without misleading him? What was support and what collusion? Who on the team saw this the same way? How did differences impede the work to be done with Ellie? The *empowerment* of whom? The child? What might it mean to empower the developmentally delayed father in this situation? Were the "best interests of the family" one thing?

Differences. Each one of these questions raised issues of values, professional orientation, biases, cultural expectations, and in some cases idiosyncratic experiences. Each presented a break in the usual routines in consultation and service delivery. Each also provoked a sometimes reluctant recognition in team members at the least and a modified epiphany at best. These questions and others like them disrupted an otherwise smooth interprofessional process because they raised differences among team members about the nature of its work and about the nature of individual and collective worldviews.

These questions are not the stuff of easy resolution. Collectively team members, each a strong participant in her or his profession, and each a committed individual, were not poised to abandon their positions for the sake of diminishing the disruption. They were, however, inclined to come to some kind of understanding about how their stances would impact the family and its members. They were also ready to examine which areas required an agreed upon interaction and which did not.

Much of the literature on teaming emphasizes the phenomenon of learning new ways to work and be together, respecting each profession and its potential contribution to the family (Guralnick, 2000; Garner, 1994). Professional differences in defining good practice and appropriate relational contexts arise in the process. The importance of listening to these differences and establishing common ground is seen as critical (Stoneman, 1995). A postmodern approach to social work can play a useful role by helping to uncover, bring to light, and work through the differences on the professionals' side of the table while it maintains its content roles of assessing, supporting, and empowering families. This has the potential to strengthen not only particular social work values, but also the human values of most workers committed to the welfare of children. It also can enlighten team members about the family's experience in trying to give voice.

In this scenario, the role of the social worker was played by a second year graduate student intern. Through this practicum experience this student was able to experience her mentors and colleagues at a depth that is uncommon in most social work agencies. While the student still carried out the more traditional roles involved in an interdisciplinary project concerned with assessment and service delivery, she was routinely welcomed into a space that students rarely even visit–that of the soul searching and thought confrontation of her current and future colleagues. In return, her colleagues recognized the contributions she made through her questioning as well as more standard social work roles.

CONCLUSIONS

Interdisciplinary teams with a family-centered approach hold great potential in the provision of consultation and services in complex cultures in which children with disabilities and their families are frequently isolated and disempowered. Social work designed from the standpoint of critical construction can offer a postmodern component to the work that helps to clarify and make transparent professional expertise through raising differences and assumptions, honoring the multiplicity of ideas and possibilities, and reflexively working through them. It can make space at the table for differing professional views as well as differences between the team and the family. The sacrifice is a tranquil, if stifled, sense of unity, which is sometimes difficult to release. Yet even as we encourage our clients to differ from us, so as to make their voices heard, we need to encourage *us* to differ from us as well. The integrity of our work with families depends on it.

REFERENCES

Abramowitz, N. (1998). Social work and social reform: An arena of struggle. *Social work, 43* (6), 512-526.

Abramson, M. (1984). Collective responsibility in interdisciplinary collaboration: An ethical perspective for social workers. *Social work in health care, 10* (1), 35-43.

Alcolff, L. (1997). Cultural feminism versus post-structuralism: The identity crisis in feminist theory. In L. Nicholson (Ed.). *The second wave: A reader in feminist theory* (pp. 330-355). New York: Routledge.

American Psychiatric Association (2000). *Diagnostic and Statistical Manual IV-Text revision.* Washington, DC: The American Psychiatric Association Press.

Anderson, H. & Goolishian, H. (1992). The client is the expert: A not-knowing approach to therapy. In S. McNamee & K.J. Gergen (Eds.) *Therapy as social construction.* Newbury Park, CA: Sage.

Blatt, B. (1981). How to destroy lives by telling stories. *In and out of mental retardation: Essays on educability, disability, and human policy* (pp. 115-135). Baltimore, MD: University Park Press.

Boyd-Franklin, N. (1993). Race, class, and poverty. In F. Walsh (Ed.). *Normal Family Processes.* 2nd Ed. (pp. 361-376). New York: Guilford Press.

Briar-Lawson, K. (1998). Capacity building for integrated family-centered practice. *Social work, 43* (6), 539-551.

Compton, B.R. & Galaway, B. (1999). *Social Work Processes* (6th edition). Pacific Grove, CA: Brooks/Cole.

Cook, D.S. (2000). The role of social work with families that have young children with developmental disabilities. In M. Guralnick, *Interdisciplinary Assessment of Young Children with Developmental Disabilities,* (pp. 201-218).Baltimore, MD: Paul H. Brookes.

Cooley, C. & Olson, A. (1996). Developing family-centered care for families of children with special health care needs. In G.H. Singer, L.E. Powers & A. Olson (Eds.), *Redefining family support* (pp. 239-257). Baltimore: Paul H. Brookes Publishing.

Delaney, R.T. & Kunstal, F.R. (1993). *Troubled transplants.* Wooden Barnes Publishing Co.

Dennis, R.E., Williams, W., Giangreco, M.F., & Cloninger, C.J. (1993). Quality of life as a context for planning and evaluation of services for people with disabilities. *Exceptional children, 59,* 499-512.

Dewees, M.P. (1999). The application of social constructionist principles to teaching social work practice in mental health. *Journal of teaching in social work,* 19 (1/2), 31-47.

Dewees, M.P. (2001). Building cultural competence for work with diverse families: Strategies from the privileged side. *Journal of cultural and ethnic diversity,* 9 (3/4), *33-51.*

Dietz, C. (2000). Responding to oppression and abuse: A feminist challenge to clinical social work. *Affilia,* 15 (3), 369-389.

Dunst, C.J. & Trivette, C.M. (1996). Empowerment, Effective helpgiving practices and family-centered care. *Journal of Pediatric Nursing, 22* (4), 334-344.

Fadiman, A. (1997). *The spirit catches you and you fall down: A Hmong child, her American doctors & the collision of two cultures.* New York: Farrar, Strauss, & Giroux.

Freedman, J. & Combs, E. (1996). *Narrative therapy: The social construction of preferred realities.* New York: WW. Norton.

Garner, H.G. (1994). Critical issues in teamwork. In H.G. Garner & F.P. Orelove (Eds.). *Teamwork in human services* (pp. 1-18). Woburn, M: Butterworth-Heinnemann.

Gergen, K. (2000). *An Invitation to Social Constructionism.* Thousand Oaks, CA: Sage Publications.

Gil, D. (1998). *Confronting injustice and oppression: Concepts for social workers.* New York: Columbia University Press.

Gitterman, A. (1991). Introduction: Social work practice with vulnerable populations. In A. Gitterman (Ed.). *Handbook of social work practice with vulnerable populations.* New York: Columbia University Press.

Greene, J.W. (1997). *Cultural awareness in the human services: A multi-ethnic approach.* Boston: Allyn & Bacon.

Gubrium J.F. & Holsstein, J.A. (1993). Family disclosure, organization embeddedness, and local enactment. *Journal of family issues, 14* (1), 66-81.

Guralnick, M. (2000). *Interdisciplinary clinical assessment of young children with developmental disabilities.* Baltimore: Paul H. Brookes Publishing Co., Inc.

Gutierrez, L.M. (1991). Empowering women of color: A feminist model. In M. Bricker-Jenkins, N.R. Hooyman, & N. Gottlieb (Eds.). *Feminist social work practice in clinical settings* (pp. 199-214). Newbury Park, CA: Sage Publications.

Hartman, A. (1981). The family: A central focus for practice. *Social work, 26,* 7-13.

Hartman, A. (1994). In search of subjugated knowledge, In A. Hartman (1994). *Reflection & Controversy: Essays on social work* (pp. 23-28). Washington, DC, NASW Press.

Haynes, K. (1998). The one-hundred year debate: Social reform versus individual treatment. *Social work, 43,* 501-511.

Humphrey, R. (1995). Families who live in chronic poverty: Meeting the challenges of family-centered services. *The American Journal of Occupational Therapy,* 49 (7), 687-694.

Johnson, D., & Johnson, F. (1987). *Joining together: Group theories and group skills.* Englewood Cliffs, NJ Prentice Hall.

Kalyanpur, M. & Harry, B. (1999a). Legal and epistemological underpinnings of the construction of disability, *Culture in Special Education*, (pp. 15-45). Baltimore: Paul H. Brookes Publishing Co.

Kalyanpur, M. & Harry, B. (1999b). The role of professional expertise and language in the treatment of disability, *Culture in Special Education* (pp. 47-75). Baltimore: Paul H. Brookes Publishing Co.

Kaplan, L. & Girard, J. (1994). *Strengthening high risk families: A handbook for practitioners*. New York: Lexington Books.

Krauss, M.W. & Jacobs, F. (1990). Family assessment: Purposes and techniques. In S.J. Meisels & J.P. Shonkoff (Eds.). *Handbook for early childhood intervention* (pp. 303-325). Cambridge, United Kingdom: Cambridge University Press.

Laird, J. (1995). Family-centered practice in the postmodern era. *Families in society*, *76*, 150-162.

Laird, J. (1996). Family-centered practice with gay and lesbian families. *Families in society*, *77*, 559-572.

Lee, J.A.B. (1996). The empowerment approach to social work practice. In F. Turner (Ed.). *Social work treatment*. (4th Ed.), pp. 218-249. New York: Free Press.

Leigh, J.W. (1998). *Communicating for cultural competence*. Boston: Allyn & Bacon.

Lum, D. (1999). *Culturally competent practice: A framework for growth and action*. Pacific Grove, CA: Brooks/Cole.

McBride, S.L. (1999). Family-centered practice. *Young children*. May, 1999, 62-68.

Nagi, S.Z. (1991). Disability concepts revisited: Implications for *prevention*. *Disability in America: Toward a National Agenda for Prevention* (pp. 309-327). Institute of Medicine: Committee on a National Agenda for the Prevention of Disabilities.

National Association of Social Workers (1996). *Code of Ethics*. Washington, DC: Author.

Payne, M. (1997). *Modern Social Work Theory*. 2nd Ed. Chicago: Lyceum Books.

Prelock, P., Beatson, J., Contompasis, S. & Bishop, K.K. (1999). A model for family-centered interdisciplinary practice in the community. *Topics in Language Disorders*. May 1999.

Rappaport, J., Reischl, T.M. & Zimmerman, M.A. (1992).Mutual help mechanisms in the empowerment of former mental patients. In D. Saleebey (Ed.). *The strengths perspective in social work practice* (pp. 84-97). New York: Longman Press.

Roberts-DeGennarao, N. (1996). An interdisciplinary training model in the field of early intervention. *Social Work in Education*, *18*, 20-29.

Saleebey, D. (Ed.). (1992). The strengths perspective in social work practice. New York: Longman.

Saleebey, D. (1997). The strengths approach to practice. In D. Saleebey, *The strengths perspective in social work practice*. (2d. Ed.), New York: Longman.

Saleebey, D. (2000). Power in the People: Strengths and hopes. *Advances in social work*, *1* (2), 127-136.

Sameroff, A.J. (1993). Models of development and developmental risk. In C.H. Zenah, Jr. (Ed.), *Handbook of infant mental health* (pp. 3-13). New York: Guilford Press.

Satka, M., & Mason, J. (2001). Questioning the implications of a post World-War II conceptualisation of childhood for child welfare. Paper presented at the International Conference on social Work in Health and Mental Health. Tampere, Finland.

Shelton, T.L., & Jeppson, E.S. (1994). *Family-centered care for children need specialized health and developmental services* (3d Ed.). Bethesda, MD: Association for the Care of Children's Health.

Simon, B. (1994). *The empowerment tradition in American social work.* New York: Columbia University Press.

Specht, H., & Courtney, N. (1995). *Unfaithful angels: How social work has abandoned its mission.* New York: Free Press.

Stern, D. (2000). The *interpersonal world of the infant: A view from psychoanalysis and developmental psychology.* New York: Basic Books.

Stoneman, Z., & Malone, D.M. (1995). The changing nature of interdisciplinary practice. In B.A. Thyer, & N.P. Kropf (Eds.). *Developmental disabilities: A handbook for Interdisciplinary practice* (pp. 234-247). Cambridge, MA: Brookline Books.

Weedon, C., (1987). *Feminist practice and postructuralist theory.* Oxford, UK: Basil Blackwell Ltd.

Weick, A. (1993). Reconstructing social work education. In J. Laird (Ed.). *Revisioning social work education: A social constructionist approach* (pp. 11-30).

Witkin, S. (1998). Is social work an adjective: [Editorial]. *Social work, 43,* 483-486.

Witkin, S. (1999). Constructing our future [Editorial]. *Social work, 44* (1) 5-9.

Using Music as a Therapy Tool
to Motivate Troubled Adolescents

Alexander W. Keen, MSocSc (SW) (Natal)

SUMMARY. Children and adolescents with emotional disorders may often be characterized by having problems in peer and adult relations and in display of inappropriate behaviours. These include suicide attempts, anger, withdrawal from family, social isolation from peers, aggression, school failure, running away, and alcohol and/or drug abuse. A lack of self-concept and self-esteem is often central to these difficulties.

Traditional treatment methods with young people usually includes cognitive-behavioural approaches with psychotherapy. Unfortunately these children often lack a solid communication base, creating a block to successful treatment. In my private clinical practice, I have endeavoured to break through these communication barriers by using music as a therapy tool.

This paper describes and discusses my use of music as a therapy tool with troubled adolescents. Pre- and post-testing of the effectiveness of this intervention technique by using the *Psychosocial Functioning Inventory for Primary School Children* (PFI-PSC) has yielded positive initial results, lending support to its continued use.

Music has often been successful in helping these adolescents engage in the therapeutic process with minimised resistance as they relate to the music and the therapist becomes a safe and trusted adult. Various techniques such as song discussion, listening, writing lyrics, composing music, and performing music

---

Alexander W. Keen is a Clinical Social Worker in Private Practice, South Africa.

[Haworth co-indexing entry note]: "Using Music as a Therapy Tool to Motivate Troubled Adolescents." Keen, Alexander W. Co-published simultaneously in *Social Work in Health Care* (The Haworth Social Work Practice Press, an imprint of The Haworth Press, Inc.) Vol. 39, No. 3/4, 2004, pp. 361-373; and: *Social Work Visions from Around the Globe: Citizens, Methods, and Approaches* (ed: Anna Metteri et al.) The Haworth Social Work Practice Press, an imprint of The Haworth Press, Inc., 2004, pp. 361-373. Single or multiple copies of this article are available for a fee from The Haworth Document Delivery Service [1-800-HAWORTH, 9:00 a.m. - 5:00 p.m. (EST). E-mail address: docdelivery@haworthpress.com].

362 *Social Work Visions from Around the Globe: Citizens, Methods, and Approaches*

have proven to be useful in reaching the child, facilitating self-expression, projecting personal thoughts and feelings into a discussion, enhancing self-awareness, stimulating verbalization, providing a pleasurable, non-threatening environment, facilitating relaxation, and reducing tension and anxiety. I have found that by using music in this way, the distrustful adolescent has come to regard me as a positive adult. Music has thus provided a safe, non-confrontative means of expression. This has helped in creating more socially acceptable ways of venting anger and fears, increasing self-awareness, self-confidence, and self-esteem. *[Article copies available for a fee from The Haworth Document Delivery Service: 1-800-HAWORTH. E-mail address: <docdelivery@haworthpress.com> Website: <http://www.HaworthPress.com> © 2004 by The Haworth Press, Inc. All rights reserved.]*

KEYWORDS. Music, adolescents, post trauma stress, therapy

THE DIFFICULTIES OF INTERACTING WITH ADOLESCENTS IN THE THERAPY SITUATION

In South Africa today most if not all children are at risk. They are regularly confronted by news of tragedies–the TV and media are packed with images of murder, hijacking, hold-ups, assaults, break-ins, senseless shootings, school violence, tragic taxi, bus and other motor accidents, as well as other community disasters–flooding, fires, and so on. Many children are more directly impacted by crime and violence as they become the targeted victims or are the innocent bystanders (Lewis, 1999).

Children are unprepared for and have a limited capacity to understand and deal with these traumatic situations. They are forever changed. Often the only way that they can express the effects of such intense stress and anxiety in their lives is in their outward behaviour. It is therefore not uncommon to see adolescents presenting with deterioration in academic performance, aggressiveness or withdrawal from peers, a decreased enjoyment in and motivation towards activities and hobbies, tobacco, alcohol and drug abuse, promiscuous sexual and risk taking behaviour, irritability and excessive rebelliousness at home, insomnia and other somatic symptoms such as weight loss, headaches, and general aches and pains. Although emotional turbulence with negative behaviour often accompanies the emerging adolescent as he or she grapples with the difficulties of assuming adulthood, the behaviours I have described are often so uncharacteristically intense and forceful in nature that further exploration is necessary. It is at this point that the emotional scarring as a result of being the victim or witness to a traumatic event surfaces (Alexander, 1999).

Adolescents often find it difficult to communicate their feelings to an adult, and by the very nature of their "anti-social" behaviours are then confronted with a battlefield of demanding and critical parents, teachers, and other significant adult figures. It is therefore not unusual to find the teenager sitting beside you in therapy, having been forced there by his or her parents, suspicious and antagonistic towards yet another "authority" figure. They are as yet unskilled in expressing their real feelings, they do not trust the counsellor, and they perceive themselves to be in another situation where demands for which they are unprepared, are going to made on them. It is no wonder that this teenager may remain unresponsive and cannot wait to be "released" from the therapy session!

Being exposed to trauma has emotionally wounded these adolescents. Their lives will never be the same. Untreated, the effects may last a lifetime and leave them hopeless and vulnerable to chronic depression and even suicide.

USING MUSIC AS A THERAPY TOOL WITH ADOLESCENTS

In my practice situation, music has shown itself to be useful as one journeys through the heart, mind, body, and soul of teenagers suffering from the trauma of having been raped, having been involved in horrific accidents, and having to come to terms with losing a loved one, losing a limb, or receiving a spinal cord injury resulting in permanent paralysis, having been violently hijacked, experiencing the trauma of confronting a burglar in their homes, or being physically assaulted (Keen, 1989; Gaston, 1968). This paper presents the use of music as a means to interact with adolescents in order to gain their trust and confidence, so that the healing process may be facilitated to regain their appreciation for life and themselves. To illustrate more effectively, one case example is presented.

Assessment

The Problems Presented

Tracey, aged 13 years, was brought to me by her mother who indicated that she was at her wits' end with her daughter. Tracey is the youngest of four siblings. She attends an exclusive private girls' school. Her father is a prominent medical doctor, and her mother has raised all four children at home. What follows is part of what Tracey's mother told me in my initial consultation with her alone:

Last weekend, Tracey had two of her close friends visiting her . . . They went to play badminton on the lawn . . . things went wrong . . . Tracey stormed upstairs . . . when I went to talk with her, she burst into tears and a tirade followed: "You don't love me . . . You don't want me for a daughter . . . You should have dumped me when I was born . . . I'm going to live in Brazil, far away from you and leave you in an old age home . . . " She wouldn't let me hug or touch her. The next afternoon (after another seemingly small situation going wrong), Tracey snapped at me again: "Why don't you put me in a black refuse bag and dump me on the street? You can all have a big grin then." Tracey went and hid in the garden. She later grazed her knee from a fall. That night, she wouldn't let me kiss her goodnight. She turned and faced the wall and started to shout at me again: "You don't know how sore this knee is . . . You don't care at all about it . . ." She performed about how she would have to keep her leg out of the blankets, how cold it would be, but it was too sore, and nobody cared how cold she would be. I've noticed that this year Tracey is not so responsible with her schoolwork. She loses work that she has completed, then there is a panic, and abuse hurled at me because she can't find it and I'm not helping. She forgets to take the necessary work to school, forgets to bring home the right books for home-work, and is generally not coping as well with school as she has in the past. She doubts herself, lacks self-confidence and won't try anything. She is causing immense tension in the home. She is sulky, rude, slams doors, complains about pains and when I ask her what is wrong she retorts: "You don't care . . . You don't help . . . You don't listen to me, one day I won't speak anymore . . ." She is jealous if our dogs lie by me or sit on my lap. She says the dogs are doing it to show her they prefer me. She recently pulled out a chair making a big noise. I rushed in because I thought she had fallen. Tracey: " Well, would it have mattered if I'd fallen?" She has stopped play-ing tennis or swimming at school, saying that people laugh at her . . . that they don't want her in the team. She says: "Funny I was a good swimmer. Now I'm not. I can't do anything right." When she is sick she complains that nobody is interested in her: "I wish there was someone who cared about me. I've got diarrhoea. I never told you this morning because I know you wouldn't care or do anything about it." When her granny has phoned and asked to speak to her, she has refused to pick up the telephone. "Gran is so mean. She always says how gorgeous Sarah (Tracey's older sister) was as a baby. She's not really interested in me." After a small altercation with her father, Tracey stormed off with: "All I want is to be a wanted child. You never know one day I may end up in the streets begging. Everything's wrong with me." Other statements have included: "Why didn't you just kill me when I was born?" "Why don't you kill me and take me to an orphanage?" She is scared of sleeping alone. If she is playing games with her friends and starts to lose, she stops trying. She won't go on school excursions, complains of having a sore tummy. At home it's like living on an active volcano. We are never sure when and how she is going to erupt. As a result there is enormous tension at home. Her teachers like her but say she lacks confidence; she won't answer questions or talk in a group. I am so hurt by what Tracey says and how she treats me. I try to be very tolerant, supportive, understanding, and not to correct her too often–but I'm not winning. It's difficult to know how to correct or discipline her–whichever way I try it ends up with her saying she is "unloved." I am now finding it very difficult to enjoy being at home with her, and am finding it very hard to enjoy her company. Please help me–I'm at my wits' end!

Music in the Initial Consultations

In my first session with Tracey, as she was not forthcoming about herself, I chatted to her about myself in an attempt to help her feel more comfortable with me. As I knew that she would be attending a concert of a visiting Irish pop group, *Westlife*, we listened to some of their music that I had brought to the session. Adolescents generally relate to the music of their peer culture, and find it easier to express themselves and their feelings when familiar music is playing. In this instance the music provided a safe, non-threatening environment where the therapist-client relationship was significantly enhanced. She visibly relaxed, smiled and at the end of our time together, agreed to complete an open-ended questionnaire entitled *"Discovering Myself*!" at home and to see me again. At the subsequent session, Tracey returned the homework, which had been neatly completed and then, whilst appropriate pop music was played in the background, she willingly answered the *Child Functioning Inventory for Senior Primary School Children* (CFI-Snr Prim). When one knows that this session will be used to complete any assessments, it is often useful to ask the adolescent to bring one or two CDs of her favourite music with her. This is the music that is then played, allowing the teenager to feel "at home" and empowered and provides a further opportunity for relationship and trust building. Music is a familiar and therefore a "safe" medium to most adolescents. Using a technique such as song discussion and listening is a non-confrontative tool, which often facilitates the projection of personal thoughts and feelings into the therapy session.

Results of Assessment

The social work profession over the last two decades has made great strides in its development of high-quality measurement tools to improve its effectiveness and accountability in service delivery. Since children are less verbal and less powerful than adults in the traditional family hierarchy, the therapist working with a child has to move quickly to empower the child and to incorporate his/her perceptions of the world. The Child Functioning Inventories (CFI) have been developed and validated by the *Perspective Training College (South Africa)*.

The CFI-Snr Prim is a paper and pencil self-report measure designed to evaluate the social functioning of children between the ages of 13 and 18 years by obtaining an assessment of child problems in 24-28 different areas of functioning. The results of the CFI are graphically presented. This visual profile facilitates clinical discussions with clients.

The results of the CFI-Snr Prim completed by Tracey indicated the following:

Section A: Positive Functioning Areas

> Perseverance (72), Satisfaction (81), and Future Perspective (75): These results were all in the recommended range with an overall score of 76%.

Section B: Self-Perception

> **Anxiety (62 *)**, **Guilt feelings (44 *)**, Lack of self-worth (31), Isolation (18), **Responsible for consequences against others (75 *)**, **Lack of assertiveness (56 *)**. (see Graph 1)

Section C: Trauma Dynamics

Memory loss (75 *), **Frustration (42 *)**, **Helplessness (62 *)**, At-
titude towards adults (5), **Mistrust (45 *)**, **Stigma (75 *)**, Body
Image (38), Personal Boundaries (14), **School problems (57 *)**,
Alcohol/Drug use (Not completed/not applicable).

The overall score was 45%. Scores above 40% (*) indicated problem
areas. Graphic results of these scores may be seen at the end of the paper
(see Graph 2).

Section D: Relationship Scores

Relationship with friends (93), Relationship with mother (100), Relationship with father (68), Relationship with family (81): Overall
score was 85%. Scores of less than 60% indicate a need for improvement, and thus Tracey's scores were all within the recommended range.

The Overview Profile of all these results indicated that Tracey's
self perception and trauma dynamics sometimes impair her positive
functioning areas and relationships to the extent that she cannot always deal with them in an effective way. Her overall functioning
was therefore described as being fluctuating pointing to an adolescent who was troubled and possibly the victim of some kind of
trauma.

Using Music To Facilitate Emotional Discussion

When showing her the graphs and discussing these results with her,
Tracey broke down crying. The use of background music during this
discussion (e.g., an acoustic guitar playing *Cavatina* by Myers) will often facilitate and ease the way for an adolescent to share emotional issues. The therapeutic process is enhanced as well as resistance being
lowered because the adolescent client is "tuned-in" to the music and not
the therapist whose role as a safe and trusted adult is accepted. In this
consultation with Tracey, with limited verbal encouragement from the
therapist, just soft, soothing background music playing, the following
story emerged:

When coming home in the car with my Mom from Church on a Sunday night in 1998 (NB: 2 years, 8 months prior to my seeing Tracey) *I was talking to her about how everyone should wear seatbelts, when suddenly we saw headlights coming straight for us. My Mom didn't have time to swerve away but she slammed on brakes. I managed to put my hand on the dashboard but before we knew it, we had been hit and glass was shattering all around me. When I realised what had happened, I looked across to my Mom to see if everything was OK. Her head was on the steering wheel with her eyes closed and blood was streaming down her face. I shouted to her: "I love you Mom!" and just kept on calling "Mom! Mom! Mom!" but there was no reply. Someone opened my door, asked if I was OK and helped me out of the car. After I had given this person my home telephone number, she phoned my Dad and brother to come. She then went to my Mom. Another person came to me and asked me if anything hurt. I told her that my thumb and hand did. This person fetched a blanket and umbrella for me because it was raining. Two ambulances arrived. One took me to hospital accompanied by my brother's girlfriend who had arrived with him and my Dad. When I arrived at the hospital I had x-rays, and a doctor put a plaster of paris cast on my left arm and a neck brace. I felt really uncomfortable and actually thought I was going to die! After that, I was put in a wheelchair, and my brother's girlfriend took me to where the trauma unit staff was by now working on my Mom. I only saw her for a split second. She was lying on a stretcher, with a bandage wrapped the whole way around her head, and her eyes were closed. She was then wheeled away and I heard a nurse say: "This is a bad one!" I was then taken home. I wasn't hungry, as I knew my Mom could be dead. I went to bed very uncomfortable. I couldn't sleep. I was worrying so much.*

Final Assessment

Tracey's responses, results of the CFI-Snr Prim, her behaviours as described by her Mom, Dad, family and teachers, all pointed to an assessment of a chronic Post Traumatic Stress Disorder with delayed onset (309.81) as described by the *Diagnostic and Statistical Manual of Mental Disorders* (4th Edition) (1994)–DSM-IV.

GRAPH 1. Self-Perception Scores CFI-Snr Prim (Tracey)

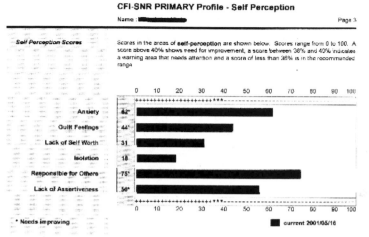

CFI-SNR PRIMARY Profile - Self Perception

Name : ▮▮▮▮▮▮▮   Page 3

Self Perception Scores

Scores in the areas of self-perception are shown below. Scores range from 0 to 100. A score above 40% shows need for improvement, a score between 36% and 40% indicates a warning area that needs attention and a score of less than 36% is in the recommended range

Area	Score
Anxiety	62*
Guilt Feelings	44*
Lack of Self Worth	31
Isolation	18
Responsible for Others	75*
Lack of Assertiveness	56*

* Needs improving   ■ current 2001/05/16

GRAPH 2. CFI-Snr Prim Trauma Dynamics Scores (Tracey)

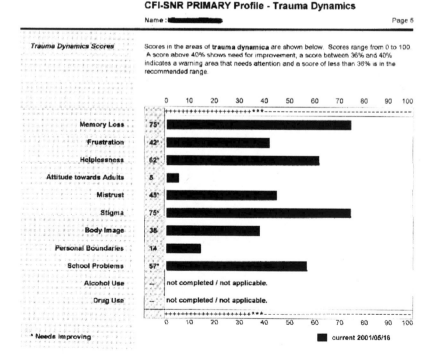

CFI-SNR PRIMARY Profile - Trauma Dynamics

Name : ▮▮▮▮▮▮▮   Page 5

Trauma Dynamics Scores

Scores in the areas of **trauma dynamics** are shown below. Scores range from 0 to 100. A score above 40% shows need for improvement, a score between 36% and 40% indicates a warning area that needs attention and a score of less than 36% is in the recommended range.

Area	Score
Memory Loss	75*
Frustration	42*
Helplessness	62*
Attitude towards Adults	8
Mistrust	45*
Stigma	75*
Body Image	38
Personal Boundaries	14
School Problems	57*
Alcohol Use	— not completed / not applicable.
Drug Use	— not completed / not applicable.

* Needs improving   ■ current 2001/05/16

Upon further investigation, it was found that Tracey's mother had been unconscious for two days, and had remained in hospital for over a month, most of the time being cared for in the Intensive Care Unit. She subsequently had to return to hospital on two further occasions for orthopaedic treatment. During this period, the family's focus was on Tracey's mother–more so with her father being a doctor. Tracey was sometimes left alone with strangers or her granny. When with groups of people or in the family, all they spoke about was her Mom. She just had to "get on with things" such as returning to school and particularly being available to help around the home because her mother was not there, or her mother was unable to move or walk when she did return home. In addition, the family had to support her Mom through a criminal court hearing whilst she gave evidence in the trial of the driver of the other vehicle who had been charged with reckless and drunk driving after the accident. Tracey has been attempting to cope with the emotional trauma of being injured in a serious motor accident, very nearly losing her mother in the accident, and overwhelming family and friend support for her mother over an extended period. It is understandable that this girl who was 10 years at the time is now reacting to her perceived reality of not being important to the family and is expressing these toxic emotions in negative attitude and behaviour towards her mother who she perceived as having received all the care and attention.

When all this emerged, it made sense to Tracey's mother, father, and family. The restoration and healing process was initiated. The initial focus has been on Tracey, with active affirmation and positive reinforcement for all achievements, however small. The expectations of her day-to-day performance and activities at school and at home have been lowered. She has been regularly reassured about her seemingly confused, and frightening fears and thoughts. Her parents and family have been encouraged to indulge Tracey's special needs for a time so that a sense of personal and family security may be reconstructed.

Intervention

Using Music To Enhance the Healing Process

During the individual sessions with Tracey, she has been encouraged to re-tell and to re-experience the "accident." Music has played a constructive part in this. Tracey has first been taught progressive relaxation techniques accompanied by soothing relaxation type music. Music has helped to prevent her mind from wandering and has reinforced her ability to focus on relaxation. Harp music and sounds of the ocean and nature have been particularly useful in this process. She has then been taught to focus her thoughts on the present moment, again accompanied by familiar music. At this point, in a state of deep muscle relaxation, a "special personal place" where she can express her thoughts and feelings in safety has been created through a visualization process. Together we have created a seaside scene, where her senses of sight, hearing, smell, taste, and touch have been acutely sensitised by vivid descriptive imagery (Bourne, 1995). For example:

> *Imagine yourself walking along a very beautiful, expansive beach . . . the sand is very fine and white in appearance . . . feel it between your toes . . . hear the roaring sound of the surf . . . watch the waves . . . the colour of the ocean is a relaxing shade of blue . . . notice a tiny sailboat skimming easily across the surface of the sea . . . take a deep breath and take in the fresh, salty smell of the sea air . . . notice a seagull flying gracefully across the waves . . . imagine yourself having the freedom to fly . . . feel the sea breeze blowing against your face . . . the warmth of the sun on your shoulders . . .*

Using the same piece of music on each occasion has assisted Tracey to "enter" this special place by herself. She is then able to use this music at home, when travelling in the car or elsewhere to enhance a sense of wholeness and well-being. Once she has visualised herself in this place, and feels emotionally safe, therapy has consisted of using slow, emotive classical music, e.g., the *Violin Concerto No 1 in G Minor, Opus 26–Adagio by Bruch, to* guide the imagery process back to the accident, encouraging desensitisation to physical reaction whilst allowing emotional expression to personal feelings. The music has facilitated a cognitive engagement whilst reinforcing relaxation during the "re-living" of the stressful event. Upon conclusion of the music, Tracey has been emotionally drained but has expressed feelings of warmth, safeness, closeness to family members, especially her mother, of being at peace within herself and a general sense of contentment.

The playing of a theme song jointly chosen has at this point concluded therapy. Generally such theme songs should be positive, engender a sense of courageousness and hope for the future. For Tracey this has been the song by Mariah Carey entitled *The Hero.*

Evaluation

Evaluation of the Therapy Process

Therapy has still to include other family members although Tracey's mother has been included as an important part of this initial process. Post therapy results using the CFI-Snr Prim as the test instrument has shown positive changes. Tracey has been encouraged to write letters to her mother and father.

Significant parts of these letters include:

> Dear Mom,
>
> . . . You are the greatest mom ever. You always care for me in such a unique way. You will always stay in my heart as the sweet, kind person who always makes me happy! Thank you for always understanding and loving me and for being there when I need you . . .
>
> Dear Dad,
>
> . . . Thank you for asking how my day was. Thank you for being willing to listen to me when I don't make sense. Please could you help me with practising tennis? . . .

Although there are still essential changes to take place, it is important to note that Tracey has made crucial strides in a short space of time. Initial assessment using the CFI-Snr Prim assisted positively in identifying areas of concern and opening up the possibility of a previous traumatic incident. The non-verbal aspect of the music used made it an excellent resource for reaching this adolescent and facilitating self-expression. The music used provided a relaxing, non-threatening environment where Tracey was able to safely risk trying new experiences that could then be transferred to other areas of her life. Within two sessions, Tracey was able to regard the adult therapist as a friend and important role model. Music afforded Tracey the opportunity to express her fears, anger, and hurts in a non-confrontative environment where levels of tension and anxiety were reduced. Her defences were lowered and she found herself more motivated to attempt life tasks again. More appropriate co-operative behaviours were noticed within the home environment.

CONCLUSION

In this paper, the deliberate but careful use of music to reach a traumatised adolescent has been described. Because of its non-verbal, creative and emotional qualities it proved to be a useful technique in the therapy process. In the case example given, music provided a constructive tool for the therapist to establish a therapeutic relationship, to facilitate interaction, self-awareness, and personal change within a relatively short period of time. The motor accident that Tracey survived did not make headlines. It was an explosion of glass and metal that happened in the midst of other day-to-day events that did make news that day. For Tracey though, it was one of the most life-altering, profound experiences she has ever known. For those of us who are privileged in our work to come alongside young people who have suffered in some traumatic situation, music may prove to be a unique tool to open up new perspectives and insights as we gently guide them through the therapy process on the path of personal healing and development.

NOTE

Names and identifying details have been changed for the purposes of confidentiality.

REFERENCES

Alexander, D W (1999) *Children changed by trauma–a healing guide. Oakland*: New Harbinger Publications

American Psychiatric Association (1994) *Diagnostic and Statistical Manual of Mental Disorders* (4th Edition), Washington, DC: American Psychiatric Association

Bourne, E J (1995) *The anxiety and phobia workbook* (2nd Edition), Oakland: New Harbinger Publications

Gaston, E T (1968) *Music in therapy.* New York: Macmillan

Keen, A W (1989) Use of music as a group activity for long-term hospital patients. *Social Work Practice.* Issue 1, 4-6

Lewis, S (1999) *An adult's guide to Childhood Trauma–Understanding traumatised children in South Africa* Claremont: David Philip Publishers

_____ (2000) *Post-traumatic Stress Disorder Treatment and Referral Guide.* Compiled by the Scientific and Advisory Board Members of the Depression & Anxiety Support Group (SA), Johannesburg

_____ (2000) *Technical Manual: Child Functioning Inventories for Pre-, Primary and High School Children.* Noordbrug: Perspective Training College Publications (E-mail: perspekt@lantic.net)

Mental Health, Social Inclusion and the Green Agenda: An Evaluation of a Land Based Rehabilitation Project Designed to Promote Occupational Access and Inclusion of Service Users in North Somerset, UK

Paul Stepney, MA
Paul Davis, MA

SUMMARY. The current debate about social inclusion in the field of mental health reveals a tension between the political and economic objectives of social policy. The former utilises the language of citizen empowerment and rights, whilst the latter is concerned with reducing welfare dependency through labour market activation. A central question here is whether a suitable programme of therapeutic work, training

Paul Stepney is Lecturer in Social Work, University of Wolverhampton, West Midlands, UK (E-mail P.M.Stepney@wlv.ac.uk). Paul Davis is Senior Practitioner, Community Mental Health Team, North Somerset Social Services, Somerset, UK.

An earlier version of this paper was presented to the 3rd International Conference on Social Work in Health and Mental Health, 'Visions from around the Globe,' University of Tampere, Finland 1-5 July, 2001.

[Haworth co-indexing entry note]: "Mental Health, Social Inclusion and the Green Agenda: An Evaluation of a Land Based Rehabilitation Project Designed to Promote Occupational Access and Inclusion of Service Users in North Somerset, UK." Stepney, Paul, and Paul Davis. Co-published simultaneously in *Social Work in Health Care* (The Haworth Social Work Practice Press, an imprint of The Haworth Press, Inc.) Vol. 39, No. 3/4, 2004, pp. 375-397; and: *Social Work Visions from Around the Globe: Citizens, Methods, and Approaches* (ed: Anna Metteri et al.) The Haworth Social Work Practice Press, an imprint of The Haworth Press, Inc., 2004, pp. 375-397. Single or multiple copies of this article are available for a fee from The Haworth Document Delivery Service [1-800-HAWORTH, 9:00 a.m. - 5:00 p.m. (EST). E-mail address: docdelivery@haworthpress.com].

Digital Object Identifier: 10.1300/J010v39n03_10

and support will produce better outcomes than those predicted by either a clinical diagnostic assessment or indeed open employment in the labour market.

This article evaluates a research project with mental health users designed to develop pathways towards inclusion. The principal means for achieving this was a programme of 'green' land-based activities, training and social support. The researchers employed a mixed method approach, utilising a quasi-experimental design with a hypothetical control and standardised testing. This was followed by interviews with users, staff and focus group discussion.

The evaluation produced some unexpected findings; for example, it was found that no strong correlation existed between diagnosis and performance. Many users performed better than had been predicted by their diagnostic assessment. However, the reasons for this remained unclear until the qualitative interviews enabled users to give accounts of the problems they faced, explain what inclusion meant for them, and outline how the project had brought gains in confidence, motivation and self belief.

The data gathered during the research derived from different epistemological positions. This can be seen as representing two ways of 'slicing the reality cake' rather than producing one complete view of mental health users reality. One construction related to how 'the system' diagnosed, processed, and 'objectively' managed them. The other was about how users' responded to their situation, utilised the opportunities available, and made 'subjective' sense of their experience. *[Article copies available for a fee from The Haworth Document Delivery Service: 1-800-HAWORTH. E-mail address: <docdelivery@haworthpress.com> Website: <http://www.HaworthPress.com>*

KEYWORDS. Mental health, inclusion, project evaluation, mixed method research, horticulture, rehabilitation, empowerment

SOCIAL ISOLATION, MENTAL HEALTH AND THE SOCIAL POLICY OF INCLUSION

Living in a community is more than cashing a benefit cheque . . . social isolation damages health and the quality of life. (Bates, 1996)

Mental health services in Britain, as elsewhere, are frequently characterised by inadequate resources, bureaucratic processes, and medical terminology. Many users refer to these services as 'the system,' which confirms their subordinate status in a restricted world that denies them access to work, training, and social support. It follows that any project concerned with enhancing occupational access and inclusion must start by listening to what mental health users have to say about the problems they face in the community, the labour market and the wider society. This implies recognising the centrality of social isolation as a problem that shapes their lives.

Bates drew a bleak picture from research conducted amongst mental health service users in Nottingham, as the quote above indicates. Sociologists have consistently attributed a range of social problems to isolation and alienation. House et al. (1988) reviewed twenty years research in a meta-analysis and concluded that socially isolated people are twice as likely to die at any given age compared with those who enjoy strong social ties. However, relationships within households are not necessarily conducive to positive mental health (Hughes and Gore, 1981), and on some indicators it is better to live alone than with those who are too critical or emotionally over-involved (Leff and Vaughan, 1985).

Brugha (1991) nevertheless sees social isolation as a predictive indicator of illness, and integration as an important objective for users. This correlates with Felce's (1996) finding that having a satisfying social life is among the most critical elements in quality of life studies and promotes insight into what is required. What requires development are opportunities for users to experience positive and life-enhancing interactions. This requires the creation of more inclusive communities with improved access to a range of environmentally sustainable vocational and cultural activities (Brandon, 1996).

How social inclusion is to be achieved remains a matter of some debate. The influential Sainsbury Report (1998), "Keys to Engagement," refers to work as being a key factor in promoting wellbeing. Leff et al. (1994) reported that following a five year follow up, service users who had been working demonstrated more significant levels of improvement in mental well-being than had been indicated previously. There are many complications and complexities concerning how to facilitate users' access to employment, with the Scandinavian model of gradual entry and a step-by-step approach likely to be particularly effective (Jarvela and Laukkanen, 2000).

In terms of UK policy development, the backdrop to the project is provided by New Labour's reform of the welfare state (DoH, 1998).

The modernisation programme is designed to tackle social exclusion (rather than poverty and inequality) and transform the welfare system around work (Clarke et al., 2000). It is indicative of what Tony Blair and Bill Clinton referred to as the 'third way'–how to balance the freedom of the market economy with a commitment to social justice (Jordan, 1998; Stepney, 2000). However, the emphasis on 'welfare to work' appears to be concerned with 'stemming the flow of people coming out of the workforce because of long term illness and disability, rather than the barriers that face people who have never been economically active' (Simons and Watson, 1999: 36). While the emphasis on jobs at all cost appears unreasonable, there are few resources currently available to help people with mental health problems obtain them anyway. Further, as Metteri notes there are gaps between social security, social policy and social work, such that 'social exclusion leaves the individual with hardly any freedom of choice with regard to his or her working life' (Metteri, 1999: 245).

Despite attempts to develop a wider range of community based support, non traditional day care 'without walls' and more vocationally related training, there remains no strategic framework within mental health services for facilitating inclusion (Sainsbury, 1998). The hope is that this modest research project will provide a model of what can be achieved by a green, land based approach to rehabilitation that will facilitate inclusion and influence wider service planning.

THE RATIONALE FOR ESTABLISHING A 'GREEN' LAND BASED PROJECT

American research tends to see therapeutic horticulture as a subject in its own right. Relf (1981) suggests that horticulture's powerful properties are helpful to mental health users and proposes that this should be tested at the level of randomised control trials. At present much of the evidence is more anecdotal in nature.

Horticulture can present a number of learning opportunities–motor skills can be developed via digging, the specific requirements of individual plants can be researched and various horticultural techniques acquired. Little can go badly wrong and there is usually a tangible end product. Moreover, it does not involve progressive linear learning. As a group activity it offers opportunities for social learning and interaction. With horticulture, participants have an opportunity to experience a safer world. They can be part of a group and apart from it simultaneously, whilst remaining in control and allowing for as much or as little social contact as is comfortable. Additionally, horticulture has a proven record in developing partnerships and enhancing access to other occupational domains (Davies, 1999).

The project was established, with support from various agencies including social services and health, on a horticultural site in Weston, the county town of North Somerset, in May 1999. North Somerset is an area of 120,000 pop. in southwest England, situated to the south of Bristol. It is characterised by pockets of high unemployment, with rates well above the average for the region. The local labour market is subject to seasonal fluctuations and is dependent on tourism and agriculture. The major areas of growth have been in the service sector where jobs are typically low paid and insecure.

Mental health users live in the shadow of the main tourist sites and may be perceived as an unwelcome sight for visitors. Consequently, they suffer discrimination and exclusion from mainstream resources. Social Services provision is characterised by crisis management allied to the psychiatric treatment of acute problems. The importance of work and occupational access had been recognised, but prior to the establishment of the project a network of occupational support services remained undeveloped.

RESEARCH METHODOLOGY

Evaluation of the project was carried out between September 1999 and July 2001. After discussion with key stakeholders it was decided to adapt a research methodology first used by Fuller (1992) and Badger (1998). This involved a mixed method approach, utilising a quasi-experimental design with hypothetical control and standardised psychological tests (HAD, 1983), followed by interviews with users, staff, and focus group discussion.

The choice of methodology reflected the need to balance a rigorous evaluation of the project's effectiveness in terms of outcomes alongside a wish to give meaning to participants' experience of the rehabilitation process (Cheetham et al., 1992). RCTs are seen as the gold standard in methodologies (Macdonald, 1997). However, this was not possible for practical and ethical reasons concerning the random allocation of service users and the establishment of an equivalent control group.

The experimental group (n = 10) comprised of nine white males and one white female who were all active cases from the local Social Services mental health team. Each participant volunteered and was accepted onto the project after consultation with their care manager. Appropriate approval was obtained from the ethics committee of the local Health Trust. A profile of each participant, detailing initial referral information and a summary of pre-test interview data, is summarised in Table 1.

A panel of experts were given diagnostic information on each participant at the beginning of the research process and asked to make predictions about the likely impact of the project 12 months ahead. The panel comprised of a clinical psychologist, an approved social worker, and a manager of rehabilitation services with an occupational therapy background. The panel was asked to make a professional judgement about each participant in the study concerning the following:

- their probable activity level during the first 12 months work on the project
- their likely attendance rate at the horticulture work sessions
- their potential suitability for some form of training/work preparation
- their potential suitability for inclusion in a social enterprise.

All three panelists combined their answers into one set of replies. A measure of effectiveness was obtained by comparing expert predictions with actual outcomes of the experimental group, and in this way the group, in effect, acted as its own control (Fuller, 1992).

A simple monitoring form was used by project staff to help measure hard and soft outcomes and 'distance travelled.' Hard outcomes are jobs, qualifications, attendance, etc., that can usually be quite easily quantified. However, more applicable to the project are soft outcomes associated with the more subtle changes in attitude and orientation to work and the development of key personal skills. The concept of 'distance travelled' involves a more holistic assessment based on a range of indicators concerning the overall impact of the project on participants.

FINDINGS FROM STANDARDISED PSYCHOLOGICAL TESTS

Following involvement in the project, pre-test and 12-month tests were carried out using standard instruments (HAD, 1983). It will be seen in Table 2 that participants were significantly less anxious and de-

TABLE 1. A profile of participants in the experimental group

Age and sex	Living circumstances	Diagnosis	Date of last admission to psychiatric hosp	Stated reason for involvement	Risks involved	Users view on work	Main self-reported occupation at outset	Most recent work
ONE 35 years Male	Alone in flat	Psychosis exacerbated by drug use	15.3.99	To grow veg and have somewhere to sit	Prison sentence For ABH 1987	Wants to be solicitor's clerk	Watching TV	Ecology project
TWO 35 years Male	Alone in flat	Paranoid Psychosis	7.12.98	To increase social contact	Violence to property 1993. Conviction for criminal damage	A good way of filling time	Family and friends	1994 Computer technician
THREE 42 years Male	Alone in flat	Psychotic Depression	14.11.96	To give me more to do	History of self harm and suicidal preoccupation	Would give me more to do	Doing voluntary work	Fishmonger 11 years ago
FOUR 32 years Male	Residential home	Schizophrenia	None	An alternative to college	Social isolation Psychological vulnerability	Would like to earn money	Fishing	1983/4 Y.T.S. scheme
FIVE 42 years Male	Alone in flat	Depression	July, 1994	To get back to employment	Many overdoses	I would jump at the chance of a normal life	Spending time with friends	In a factory as a power presser 1992
SIX 50 years Male	Bed and Breakfast	Depression and mild learning difficulties	None	To keep me active and keep my nose clean	Prison sentence For sexual Indecency	To know that the money you get is earned	Watching TV	Groundsman on golf course 1996
SEVEN 47 years Female	Alone in supported flat	Depression and memory loss via alcohol abuse	3.8.97	To gain more knowledge of horticulture	Self harm Overdoses	To give me self worth	Voluntary work	Store detective 1997
EIGHT 50 years Male	Lives with wife and teenage children	Brain damage and mild learning difficulties	None	To provide occupation	User very worried about family breakdown	Satisfaction in being occupied	Spending time with family	Factory cleaner 1985
NINE 35 years Male	Residential care	Paranoid illness and cerebral palsy	9.12.97	Occupation and to get a job	Self harm violence to others	Contributes to the community	Going to classes	Work in a supermarket 1991
TEN 50 years Male	Residential care	Alcohol abuse and depression	Jan 1999	To be occupied	Prison sentence for arson. Current probation order	To be physically and mentally active	Watching TV	Butchery Manager in supermarket 1995

TABLE 2. Changes in participants' scores in three psychological tests used to measure social fear, anxiety and depression at preliminary interviews and after 12 months

	Preliminary score	End score	Change
Participant One			
Social Fear	16	11	−5
Anxiety	11	0	−11
Depression	14	1	−13
Participant Two			
Social Fear	28	19	−9
Anxiety	9	9	0
Depression	8	4	−4
Participant Three			
Social Fear	41	26	−15
Anxiety	17	9	−8
Depression	15	9	−6
Participant Four			
Social Fear	9	14	+5
Anxiety	8	11	+3
Depression	2	2	Nil
Participant Five			
Social Fear	41	46	+5
Anxiety	20	15	−5
Depression	23	17	−5
Participant Six			
Social Fear	19	36	+17
Anxiety	13	16	+3
Depression	9	12	+3
Participant Seven			
Social Fear	11	16	+5
Anxiety	5	6	+1
Depression	5	10	+5
Participant Eight			
Social Fear	23	21	−2
Anxiety	10	7	−3
Depression	11	5	−6
Participant Nine			
Social Fear	26	24	−2
Anxiety	8	8	Nil
Depression	8	8	Nil
Participant Ten			
Social Fear	7	2	−5
Anxiety	8	4	−4
Depression	1	0	−1

pressed and were generally less affected by social fear in relation to a range of everyday social encounters.

Social Fear scores averaged 38 at initial interview but this reduced to 32 by the end of the 12 month study. It should be noted that the responses of four participants increased, one (participant six) by a significant margin.

Anxiety and Depression were both markedly less present at final interview. Some reduction in anxiety could be attributed to the fact that participants felt more comfortable with staff and researchers by the end of the study. This is less likely, however, to account for changing attitudes towards work and their generally positive comments about the project and its impact.

Overall, there would appear to be an association between project participation and positive changes in the psychological health of the group. The relationship appears strongest in the case of anxiety and depression, which reduced significantly by more than 25%, and weakest in relation to social fear, where the reduction was not statistically significant and actually increased in four participants.

PREDICTED AND ACTUAL OUTCOMES COMPARED

The following summarises the Expert Panel's predictions in response to the questions that they were asked and compares these against actual outcomes. The results for selected participants are grouped under three headings–(i) where outcomes were largely consistent with predictions, (ii) where outcomes were significantly better, and (iii) where outcomes were inconsistent.

Outcomes Consistent with Predictions

Participant Six: The panel said that without the project he would still be unemployed. His predicted attendance rate was 100%. The panel scored him as 100% ready for work preparation and 100% suitable for inclusion with a social firm.

The comments about his activity level would seem largely accurate. However, many of the comments about his different attitude to work and future prospects seem relevant. As a Schedule One offender (following a conviction as a 17-year-old boy), this man had begun to feel that his life was over. During the study he began to change his views on this and his concentration, commitment and energy were highly compatible with a return to paid employment. He had always been employed prior to a prison sentence in 1996, and with appropriate help there is no reason why he should not find work again. His actual attendance rate was 88%.

Outcomes Better Than Predictions

Participant Five: The panel predicted that without the Project he would continue with gardening. His predicted attendance rate was 50%. The panel suggested he was only 25% likely to be ready for work preparation but scored him at 75% in relation to potential participation in a social firm.

In reality some of his previous gardening has declined and would probably not have been maintained without the project due to conflict with family members. His actual attendance has been higher than predicted at 73%. He has shown considerable tenacity and despite his record of depression and minor overdosing, became a very enthusiastic participant.

The panel underestimated his work readiness, probably related to his high scores for depression and anxiety. His actual performance indicates that his presentation offers a restricted picture. His keyworker feels that his depression is more of an adjustment difficulty and that this could be addressed significantly within the project. The score in relation to membership of a social firm seems about right. He would benefit from being within a protected environment for some time given his record of ill health, but open paid employment would seem realistic with adequate supervision and support.

Participant Ten: The panel indicated that a detox programme might be considered and predicted that he might be involved in small amounts of gardening. His attendance rate was predicted at 75%. The panel scored him as 0% ready for work preparation and 25% likely to be suitable for inclusion within a social firm.

In fact this participant is doing a great deal of gardening. His mood is much improved and drink is currently not a problem for him. His attendance rate at 88% exceeded that predicted.

His involvement in the project has seen an enormous increase in his level of activity, and he is now much more motivated. Memory problems persist, and this leads to a query regarding his ability to work. In other respects his concentration, commitment, cheerfulness, and energy suggest that predictions about work preparation and a social firm are quite inaccurate. Much of this improvement he attributed to the project.

Outcomes Inconsistent and Variable

Participant Seven: The panel predicted that this woman would remain involved in activities around voluntary work, gardening and education classes. They predicted her attendance rate at 50% and suggested that she was 25% ready for work preparation and 50% suitable for inclusion within a social firm.

Predictions around her likely activity levels are largely accurate. She said that she feels the balance is about right. Her attendance rate at 80% is significantly higher that predicted. It demonstrates that she had the motivation to overcome her memory problems, and that motivation is generally a central factor within attendance. Were it not for a minor spinal disability her attendance might have been even higher.

The figure relating to her readiness for work preparation may be misleading. In fact, despite her active engagement in the project, she is not interested in paid employment. She would much rather concentrate on her voluntary work and adult education. Her actual score in relation to this and to participation within a social firm are likely to be nil, although she would be interested in a degree of therapeutic work to boost her personal spending money.

FINDINGS FROM INTERVIEWING EACH PARTICIPANT AND FOCUS GROUP DISCUSSION

These are discussed in terms of changes in attitude to work, changes in confidence, and the relationship between activity and mental health. The overall impact of the project or 'distance travelled' was evaluated during the focus group discussion.

Changes in Attitude to Work and the Future

These were relatively subtle. Participant one, following a short prison sentence and an associated severe depressive illness, had concluded that he might never have a job again. His involvement in the project led to a significant change in his attitude. Perhaps, he mused, his life may no longer be 'over' and his re-involvement in working activity meant that he might once again belong and be 'accepted' and 'trusted.' For participant six, work had telling repercussions for how he felt about himself, "it helps keep me occupied and keeps my nose clean." Later he made reference to working after the project ends "even if it is in a factory I might think

Christ, but it is a job." He sought an activity in which he could "put my whole body into it and get lost in it." Thus for him work had become a very serious matter, even though it was not without personal cost, as he was the participant who had recorded a significant increase in social fear.

Participants demonstrated that they wanted to work. National research has indicated that approximately half (49%) of long term mental health service users wanted help to find work (Hatfield et al., 1992). In fact this study found that 80% of the group wished to work. On closer questioning all said that they wanted to make some form of social contribution. However, they often lacked motivation and the self-belief to do so. Working on the Project helped beneficiaries in this area, and it was found that these factors were mutually reinforcing, i.e., gradual and tentative gains in self belief led to improved motivation. Over a period of 12 months, there were clear indications of participants contemplating paid or voluntary work in the future. This was noticeably stronger in participants two, three and six, whilst seven and eight remained more ambivalent. Without exception, however, this group of long-term service users wanted to move slowly towards this objective by degree. No one voted for a sudden change.

Changes in Confidence and How They Came About

There were noted changes in social interaction, especially amongst group members who had the most negative self-perception and the greatest difficulties in socialising. One respondent (participant seven) said that the project had helped her to "create something from nothing." She could make a difference and she felt more of a 'person.' Another, participant ten, said "you can get a bit stale if you don't meet people who have other interests." The project had given him a "reason for getting up and showered, I'm much less moody than I was . . . I feel I'm playing my part."

A more reticent participant (two) reported finding "eye contact a bit easier" and felt that he had achieved something. The shyest member of the group, participant four, who had a diagnosis of schizophrenia and features of an autistic spectrum disorder, began to communicate spontaneously. Subsequently, the gardening group helped him to communicate about his interests and what he was doing. In some way it seemed to help him to be clear about his identity and become more focussed. His mother and main carer confirmed that he had his most significant social contacts among other group members, who he seemed to regard as his friends.

The Relationship Between Activity and Mental Health

There was strong evidence that project based activity was conducive to improved mental health. Apart from participant four, who was fairly neutral, everyone else was clear that it had a positive impact on their mental health. This mirrors findings from other studies that activity is better than talk, although focussed counselling may enrich the experience of that activity (Sainsbury, 1998).

There was a high degree of unanimity epitomised by the view of participant two, "when I'm doing something I forget about my problems . . . it keeps your mind occupied and it helped me to sleep." Another, participant five, referred to a cognitive change– "activity helps you to concentrate." Participant eight described how boredom had "really got me down," and participant ten spoke of how activity within the project had helped him counteract his tendency to "go back into myself."

Focus Group Discussion–Considering the Overall Impact of the Project

A Focus group discussion took place after 12 months with 7 of the 10 participants from the experimental group at a local college and with staff separately. Participants four, five, and ten did not attend the focus group for various reasons (four could not tolerate any indoor group activity). The group discussion was facilitated by a staff member from the project and researcher, the latter in the role of participant observer. Two main themes were addressed:

- assessing the impact of the project on participants during the first 12 months
- identifying the hopes/concerns of participants regarding access to jobs and the likely problems or barriers they might face in the community.

Concerning the impact of the project, there were a number of positive responses elicited by the group. There was a consensus that 'teamwork' had been an important feature of project work that was greatly valued by everyone. Reference was made to the pleasure of working in the open (except of course when it rained), to 'fresh air' and the chance to 'exercise.' One participant spoke about 'not being hemmed in' and of being able to socialise in a more relaxed way. One participant said that he found it easier to relate to people in the project than in the mental health centre he had attended. He said that this was because "you could avoid someone without being rude, by just getting on with whatever you were doing." Others conferred with this with stories of previous encounters in institutional settings. Many relayed tales which contrasted their experience of cooperative team working on the project, where their contribution mattered, with repetitive menial tasks at a training centre or "dead-end jobs in the community." Some participants spoke of being labelled, let down and in some cases treated badly by 'the system,' whilst the perception of the project (even taking account of the grateful factor) seem to offer something qualitatively different.

More than one participant spoke of the project's horticulture site as being a safe and rewarding environment and, on prompting, it was clear that it was a less hostile world than the one many of them commonly experienced. The project created 'a positive social ambience' which arose from different sources: from within the group itself, from social interaction with other gardeners working on the site, and from working in a nurturing kind of way that modelled the 'green' environmental objectives of the project.

Concerning hopes and fears about the future and the prospects of work, this topic generated a variety of responses. However, whilst the group had a diversity of personal aspirations and activity interests, there was general agreement about the problems they faced in accessing them based on shared experience. The barriers identified included financial constraints, confidence, discrimination and medical limitations–after prompting it emerged that their perception of the latter had been shaped by sustained contact over a number of years with the psychiatric system and reinforced by medication. This criticism emerged much more strongly during the group discussion than the individual interviews.

Having established a broad consensus concerning the nature of the barriers they faced, a lively discussion ensued about how to address these factors. There was a belief that therapeutic earnings might assist with money shortages, a better option than open employment in the labour market. Five of the seven participants felt that their achievements on the project provided them with the confidence to go on, although it was acknowledged by some that they would need considerable encouragement to do so. The group wanted to be in a position to make "normal choices" that everyone makes about their lives. However, there was agreement that this did not amount to a 'licence for professional control.' What was needed was intensive one to one support, especially when embarking on a new activity.

In summary most participants said that they felt positive about the focus group discussion. It was too long for participant three, whilst seven felt it could have gone further. Participant three said that the discussion had become too heavy, and he had begun to hear voices. Some participants had suffered because smoking was not permitted in the college, but overall it proved to be a very useful experience.

Group Discussion with Project Staff

This took place after the focus group and attempted to gauge staff perceptions about the impact of the project both positive and negative. The group included two occupational therapists, a social worker, a psychiatric nurse, a gardening tutor and two healthcare assistants. They had discussed various matters within the project over a period of time, and this had involved other health and education staff and the Disablement Rehabilitation Officer.

The discussion was remarkable for the degree of enthusiasm generated within the project. There were tensions, however, on specific points. For instance, how far concerns about health and safety issues should apply to the selection of participants, the degree to which the project should concentrate on the development of a green infrastructure, as opposed to helping them to find educational and vocational outcomes within mainstream education and employment. Some felt that the project could become too biased towards horticulture. Others felt that if it moved too far from its land base then it would lose its clear identity.

Another subject that provoked discussion was the degree to which users should be helped to attend the project by being offered practical assistance, i.e., occasional lifts and telephone prompts among other measures. There was a dilemma. While the project was not a branch of the health service, many felt that significant allowances should be made to recognise the degree of mental distress participants experienced. Others talked more about commitment, responsibility and moving on. Sometimes this reflected the orientation of their agency, but not always. It became apparent that there was no entirely correct and consistent perspective within the staff group. However, it was agreed that compromise and balance was required, and that this had been significantly informed by the focus group.

DISCUSSION OF FINDINGS

As Badger (1998) and others have noted, caution is needed in attempting a detailed analysis when the sample is small and not representative of a wider population. Nonetheless this small-scale project evaluation has generated a considerable amount of data about mental health users. We identify some of the salient factors associated with achieving inclusion, for instance, changing attitudes to work, rebuilding confidence and self-esteem, and the importance of activity which reflects a 'green' environmentally sound agenda. The study has demonstrated that a group of service users, who were generally felt to have little capacity for change and significant limitations due to their psychiatric condition, have considerable potential for rehabilitation, provided the right blend of opportunity and support is available.

The Green Agenda

A possible synergy has emerged between meeting the vocational needs of mental health service users and the growing public concern for the environment. In the project participants' concern for and involvement in the latter not only brought dividends in terms of improved confidence and purpose, but provided a link with other local environmental initiatives. Fostering ecology and an 'alternative approach' may help participants to contribute actively as well as adjust to their local community. Deviating too far away from land-based activities as a central theme may run certain risks, as many workplaces and voluntary organisations are unlikely to be able to provide the sort of protective and nurturing environment which vulnerable participants require.

Comparing Hard Quantitative Outcomes with Soft Qualitative Data

Measuring hard outcomes, like jobs, qualifications, attendance rates, activity levels and so on, may appear to be a straightforward task, but care must be taken to assess changes in other related areas, such as reliance on welfare services, psychiatric symptoms and use of medication. Another problem with hard outcomes is that they may underscore the success of the project as a whole. In other words they do not offer a holistic view, and such measures may be an insufficient indicator of a participants' increased employability. Marginalised groups, such as mental health users, face multiple barriers and risks, and may be a long way from being able to obtain a recognised qualification or employment in the labour market (Pilgrim and Rogers, 1996). Hence, although hard outcome measures were used in the project evaluation, as part of the experimental design, they could not tell us the reasons why participants scored as they did or explain underlying patterns in the data.

Similarly, responses to the psychological tests provided useful baseline data about levels of anxiety, depression and social fear in the group, as well as a simple means for measuring how these changed over time. These data were important given the nature of each participants health status and the need to carefully monitor progress. However, it opened up other areas for consideration concerning what sort of environment participants found inclusive and what they found oppressive. Social fear remained an important barrier to inclusion for over a third of the group. The concept of work precipitated a fear amongst some participants of interacting with others and making new friends, together with the underlying fear of failing in any work related activity. In the majority of cases ongoing assessment and individual support helped participants to manage this satisfactorily.

The interviews gave researchers insight into some of the more subtle changes in a participant's life. Such data are sometimes referred to as 'soft outcomes' (for example, changes in attitude to work, confidence, personal skills), and this together with consideration of the 'distance travelled' by participants became an important part of the project evaluation (Dewson et al., 2000). This offered a different view of reality, compared with data from standardised test scores or hard outcome measures, giving meaning to how participants made sense of their experience. In addition, this had a practical pay off for staff in that it provided a better indication of the type of support and cluster of service interventions likely to be most effective.

Working with participants to record and monitor soft outcomes and distance travelled, and involving her/him in the process, can be a very empowering experience (Baistow, 1994). A project worker may be able to demonstrate to the participant that they have pre-existing skills and attributes of which they were unaware. In addition, it was found that when participants were made aware of the distance they had travelled it provided an enormous boost to their confidence.

The development and recognition of such skills is an important factor in many participants' long-term integration back into the labour market and is therefore critical to the process of social inclusion. There is strong evidence from the project and wider literature to suggest that participants are likely to be healthier and less dependent on care services if they can be helped to develop greater confidence and self belief, engage in purposeful activity and expand their range of social skills (Sainsbury, 1998).

Methodological Issues–Different Ways of Slicing the Reality Cake

The methodology utilised the concept of a hypothetical control rather than a control group. This overcame a number of logistical and ethical problems associated with RCTs viz. the random allocation of service users and establishing an equivalent control group, as neither was feasible within the resources available. The use of an expert panel proved illuminating and provided a useful baseline for evaluation as well as much contestation and debate.

The overly cautious prognosis, based upon the expert panel's predictions, and the genuine surprise on the part of project workers concerning progress made, are worthy of further comment. There appears to have been some instances where too much emphasis was placed on diagnosis. This is not to malign the panel, who provided a lot of valuable data. They had less information than they should ideally have had, but two points emerge—one relates to the degree to which diagnostic labels can be an overriding consideration within professional assessments. The other concerns the extent to which such an assessment may be limited and provisional (Acharyya, 1996).

It was found that no strong correlation existed between diagnosis and performance. Whilst anxiety and depression reduced, social fear actually increased for about a third of the experimental group. Many users who had internalised negative psychiatric labels performed far better than had been predicted by their diagnostic assessment. However, the reasons for this were unclear and went beyond the scope of an experimental approach. Here, the open-ended interviews enabled users to give accounts of their experience and identify the factors that had shaped their reality.

The data gathered during the two phases of the research derived from different epistemological positions (although the quasi-experimental design is not a common one). Thus rather than be tempted to try and conflate the data into one complete picture representing a single view of mental health users reality (oppressed, discriminated, and marginalised), it was felt that it represented two ways of slicing the reality cake (Silverman, 2000). Interpretation was thus informed by this dialectic: On the one hand, data derived from the quasi-experimental evaluation and standardised tests indicated how 'the system' diagnosed, managed, and 'objectively' measured service users potential. Whilst on the other, qualitative data provided insights into how participants responded to their situation, utilised the opportunities available through the project, and made sense of 'subjective' experience.

There is always a need in mixed method research involving interviews to establish the status of the data. In this instance to determine the extent to which participants gave one overriding meaning to their 'experience' of the project or different meanings depending on the context and whether they were speaking to staff, fellow participants, or researchers. This raises an important methodological issue about whether interviews point to the existence of some external reality and 'experience' or actively constructed 'narratives' which require analysis to give access to internal experience (Silverman, 2000; Holstein and Gubruim, 1995). Whilst the data could be analysed in ways that potentially support either position, the view adopted in this study is that the interviews enabled the 'subjective' meanings of participants to be explored and related to the more 'objective' quasi-experimental evaluation and standardised test results.

When the interview data were coded, it was found that various categories emerged: For example, 'push' factors derived from participants negative experience of the psychiatric system and 'pull' factors associated with positive views of the project (see also research by Miller and Glasner, 1997). This in turn could be said to reveal a tension between two parallel discourses: the care, control, and treatment discourse and the social inclusion discourse (Grove, 1998).

The qualitative interviews were supplemented with focus group discussion. This proved to be a revealing way of gaining further access to the process through which participants gave meaning to their experience (Bryman, 2001). The advantage of this was that the researchers had less control of the proceedings than the individual interviews, apart from setting the agenda and prompting from time to time. However, the discussion produced data that proved difficult to transcribe and analyse in terms of achieving a balance between content and process themes. And in the event it proved simpler to concentrate on the latter, using such headings as teamwork, activity, the environment and support.

It has been noted that a significant minority did not attend the focus group, suggesting that it is not suitable for every participant. There was also the problem of variable contributions as some participants were more comfortable with the group format and said a lot (one and six), whilst others were much more reticent. However, despite these problems the findings provided evidence that was largely consistent with the interview data and therefore contributed to the validity and reliability of the evaluation.

CONCLUSION

While currently something of a buzzword within the policy discourse of New Labour in Britain and other European governments (Jordan, 2000), the notion of social inclusion is a concept that is worth taking seriously. This study has demonstrated that it is participation, as part of a team, a sense of belonging and a wish to make a social contribution that has motivated participants rather than any magical properties associated with the labour market (Stepney et al., 1999). Current orthodoxy concerning paid work as a necessary step on the road to inclusion has been both supported and to some extent challenged by the responses of participants. It is clear that with improved accessibility and appropriate flexibility most of the participants would have welcomed some form of paid work. However, this could be hazardous and counterproductive without a great number of safeguards built in. A minority did not want it anyway.

At one level psychiatric labels can be inaccurate and self-limiting. Furthermore, the world of mental health services is a small one and users themselves are a heterogeneous group (Busfield, 1996). In the study participants varied in their willingness to use mental health services, and half the group had either declined or discontinued their involvement with mainstream rehabilitation services.

This study suggests that to maximise rehabilitation a project should become part of a wider strategy of inclusion or even linked to a social firm (Durie, 1998; see diagram in the Appendix). It has demonstrated the potential of horticulture as a catalyst and a context for inclusion in providing a range of incremental and connected opportunities. Social care services have often operated in relative isolation from education and training providers (Piling, 1991). As a consequence, there have been too many cul-de-sacs within vocational pathways that have lacked a connectedness with next step employment options and the real economy.

Participants are and will increasingly be central to the process of achieving inclusion. With appropriate intervention they will be able to recognise how their negative experiences of 'the system' may be used constructively to create positive employment opportunities that produce sustainable environmental outcomes.

A number of unknowns remain concerning our knowledge about 'what works' in promoting inclusion with mental health users. This study suggests that with improved service contexts and better blends of stimulation and support significantly more can be achieved (Leff et al., 1994). The research has demonstrated what is achievable at the local level when the principles of inclusion are taken as a starting point, and linked with a strong user-centred and evidence informed approach.

REFERENCES

Acharyya, S. (1996) 'Practising Cultural Psychiatry: The Doctor's Dilemma' in Heller, T. et al., (eds), *Mental Health Matters–A Reader*, Buckingham, Open University Press

Badger, D. (1998) *Researching the Effectiveness of a Small-scale Community Based Project for Sex Offenders* in Cheetham et al., *The Working of Social Work*, London, Jessica Kingsley

Baistow, K. (1994) 'Liberation and Regulation? Some Paradoxies of Empowerment,' *Critical Social Policy*

Bates, P. (1996) 'Lessons for Life,' *Health Service Journal*, 3 October 1996: 28

Brandon, D. (1996) *Normalising Professional Skills* in Heller et al., *Mental Health Matters–A Reader*, Buckingham, Open University Press

Brugha, T.S. (1991) *Support and Personal Relationships* in Bennett, D.H., and High, L. (eds.) *Community Psychiatry: The Principles*, Churchill, Livingstone

Bryman, A. (2001) *Social Research Methods*, Oxford, Oxford University Press

Busfield, J. (1996) *Professionally, The State and the Development of Mental Health Policy* in Heller et al., *Mental Health Matters–A Reader*, Buckingham, Open University Press

Cheetham, J., Fuller, R., McIvor, G. and Petch, A. (1992) *Evaluating Social Work Effectiveness*, Buckingham, Open University Press

Cheetham, J. and Kazi, M. (eds.) (1998) *The Working of Social Work*, London, Jessica Kingsley

Clarke, J., Gewirtz, S. and McLaughlin, E. (eds.) (2000) *New Managerialism, New Welfare?* London, Sage

Davies, J. (1999) *Towards a Happier Life, Therapeutic Horticulture–As a Means of Mental Health Rehabilitation, In a Life in the Day*, Vol 3, Issue 2, February 1999, Brighton, Pavillion

Department of Health (1998) *Modernising Social Services*, The Stationery Office, London

Dewson, S., Eccles, J., Tackey, N. and Jackson, A. (2000) Guide to Measuring Soft Outcomes and Distance Travelled, Institute for Employment Studies, Brighton

Durie, S. (1998) 'The Social Firm-An Idea Whose Time Has Come,' in *A Life in the Day*, Vol 2, Issue 3, August 1998

Felce, D. (1996) *Ways to measure quality of outcomes: An essential ingredient in quality assurance*, Tizard Learning Disability Review, 1(2):38-44

Fuller, R. (1992) *In Search of Prevention*, Aldershot, Avebury

Grove, B. (1998) *The Government's New Employment Agenda: Implications for Mental Health Service Managers*, Managing Community Care, Volume 6, Issue 5–October 1998

HAD, (1983) Hospital and Anxiety Scale (known as HAD), Zigmond As Snaith, RP, ACTA Psychiatric Scand 1983, 67 Social Fear Questionnaire, Author Unknown

Hatfield, B., Huxley, P. and Mohammed, F.H. (1992) 'Accommodation and Employment: A survey of circumstances and expressed needs of mental health service users in a northern town,' *Journal of Social Work*, 22: 68-73

Holstein, J. and Gubrium, J. (1995) *The Active Interview*, Thousand Oaks, CA: Sage

House, J.S., Umberson, D. and Landis, K.R. (1998) *Structures and Process of Social Support*, Annual Review of Sociology, 14, p293-318

Hughes, M. and Gore, W.R. (1981) *Living Alone and Social Integration and Mental Health*, American Journal of Sociology 87-1, p48-74

Jarvela, S. & Laukkanen, M. (2000) *Perspectives on Empowerment–Report on Employment Integra thematic work project*, Ministry of Labour, Finland

Jordan, B. (1998) *The New Politics of Welfare*, London, Sage

Jordan, B. (2000) *Tough Love: Implementing New Labour's Programme–Social Work and the 'Third Way,'* London, Sage

Leff, J. & Vaughan, C. (1985) *Expressed Emotion in Families*-New York, The Guildford Press

Leff, J., Thorncroft, G., Coshead, N., and Crawford, C. (1994) *The Taps Project* from Derham, T. 'Work related activity for people with long term Schizophrenia: A Review of the Literature,' British Journal of Occupational Therapy, 1997, 60 (6)

Macdonald, G. (1997) 'Social Work Research: The state we're in,' *Journal of Interprofessional Care*, Vol 11, No 1

Metteri, A. (1999) 'Researching Difficult Situations in Social Work' in Karvinen, S. et al., *Reconstructing Social Work Research*, SoPhi, University of Jyvaskyla Press, Finland

Miller, J. and Glasner, B. (1997) 'The "Inside" and the "Outside": Finding realities in interviews,' in Silverman, D. (ed) *Qualitative Research: Theory, Method and Practice*, London, Sage

Pilgrim, D. and Rogers, A. (1996) *Two Notions of Risk in Mental Health Debates, Britain in Moral Panic* in Heller et al., *Mental Health Matters–A Reader*, Buckingham, Open University Press

Pilling, S. (1991) *Rehabilitation and Community Care*, London, Routledge

Relf, D. (1981) 'Dynamics of Horticulture Therapy,' *Journal of Rehabilitation* 46: 147-150

Sainsbury (1998) *Keys to Engagement: Review of Care for People with Severe Mental Illness who are hard to engage with services*, London, The Sainsbury Centre for Mental Health

Silverman, D. (2000) *Doing Qualitative Research–a practical handbook*, London, Sage

Simons, K. and Watson, D. (1999) *New Directions? Day Services for People with Learning Disabilities in the 1990s. A Review of the Research*, The Centre for Evidence Based Social Services, University of Exeter

Stepney, P., Lynch, R., and Jordan, B. (1999) 'Poverty, Exclusion and New Labour,' *Critical Social Policy*, Vol 19, (1):109-127

Stepney, P. (2000) *An Overview of the Wider Policy Context* in Stepney, P. and Ford, D. (eds) *Social Work Models and Theories–A Framework for Practice*, Lyme Regis, Russell House Publishing

APPENDIX

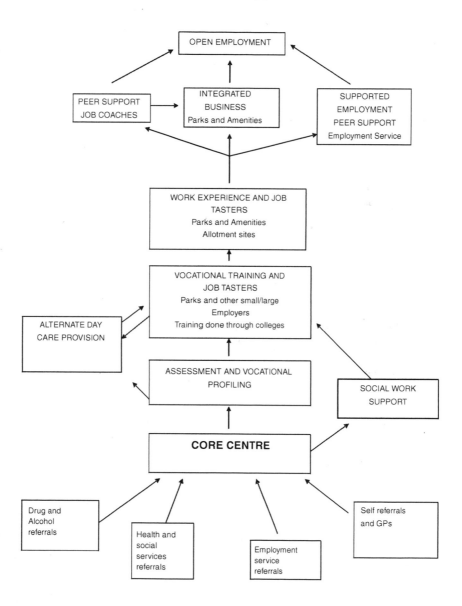

Social Vaccine for HIV Prevention:
A Study on Truck Drivers in South India

M. Ubaidullah, PhD

SUMMARY. Nearly everywhere that AIDS has been found, HIV infection is fast spreading. No one is known to have recovered from HIV infection. There is no vaccine to cure AIDS (Population Reports, 1989 and *The Hindu*, dated 9.3.2000). Until a cure or vaccine for HIV infection is found, the only way to prevent the spread of the disease is by changing people's behaviour through AIDS education programmes (Population Reports, 1986). Many national governments are using broadcast, print media, personal contact, counselling methods, etc., to educate people on AIDS and safer sex. Thus, the best vaccine is the 'Social Vaccine.' Social vaccine involves spreading education on how to protect oneself, hundred percent condom use, and changing sexual behaviour. In fact, the social vaccine was so successful in Thailand that the infection rate has come down by 50 per cent (*The Hindu*, dated 9.3.2000).

Truck drivers, prostitutes, and young adults are considered high risk groups for HIV/AIDS in India. An action research study was conducted in Chittoor District of Andhra Pradesh (India) among truck drivers. As part of this study, different strategies, namely mass media, personal con-

---

M. Ubaidullah is Associate Professor, Department of Population Studies, Sri Venkateswara University, Tirupati-517 502, Andhra Pradesh, India (E-mail: ubaidullahm@rediffmail.com).

[Haworth co-indexing entry note]: "Social Vaccine for HIV Prevention: A Study on Truck Drivers in South India." Ubaidullah, M. Co-published simultaneously in *Social Work in Health Care* (The Haworth Social Work Practice Press, an imprint of The Haworth Press, Inc.) Vol. 39, No. 3/4, 2004, pp. 399-414; and: *Social Work Visions from Around the Globe: Citizens, Methods, and Approaches* (ed: Anna Metteri et al.) The Haworth Social Work Practice Press, an imprint of The Haworth Press, Inc., 2004, pp. 399-414. Single or multiple copies of this article are available for a fee from The Haworth Document Delivery Service [1-800-HAWORTH, 9:00 a.m. - 5:00 p.m. (EST). E-mail address: docdelivery@haworthpress.com].

Digital Object Identifier: 10.1300/J010v39n03_11

tact, group discussion, folk media, and counselling, were adopted to provide AIDS education, to encourage increase in condom use for safer sex, and bring changes in their sexual behaviour. The strategies adopted in this study greatly enhanced the knowledge of the truck drivers on AIDS, changed their attitudes on sex, increased the use of condoms, and modified their sexual behaviour.

Thus, the social vaccine would help spread education on AIDS, bring changes in the sexual behaviour of the people, increase condom use, and thus help to prevent the AIDS scourge throughout the world. The social vaccine suggested in this study can also be extended to all the high risk group population for successful prevention of this dreadful disease in the world.*[Article copies available for a fee from The Haworth Document Delivery Service: 1-800-HAWORTH. E-mail address: <docdelivery@haworthpress.com> Website: <http://www.HaworthPress.com> © 2004 by The Haworth Press, Inc. All rights reserved.]*

KEYWORDS. AIDS, HIV education, India, truck drivers, prostitutes

INTRODUCTION

AIDS is found today nearly everywhere and HIV infection has been spreading fast. No one is known to have recovered from it so far. Of the 42 million people infected by HIV today in the world, 85 per cent live in Sub-Saharan Africa and the developing countries of Asia, which together account for less than 10 per cent of the global gross national product. While drugs and breast-milk substitutes have nearly eliminated mother-to-child transmission (MCT) of HIV in North America and Europe, people in the developing countries remain economically outside their reach. While antiretroviral drugs have dramatically prolonged both the duration and quality of life for most HIV positive people in North America and Europe, they too remain economically outside the reach of most HIV positive people in the developing countries (Sight and Life, 3/2000). Poverty and illiteracy go hand in hand in spreading HIV infection. Until a cure or vaccine for it is found, the only way to prevent the spread of the disease in the developing countries is by changing people's behaviour through AIDS education programmes (Population Reports, 1986). Many national governments are using the broadcast and print media, personal contact, counselling, and other methods to educate people on AIDS and safer sex. Thus, at present the best vaccine for HIV prevention is the 'Social Vaccine,' which involves spreading education on how to protect oneself against the infection, hundred per cent use of condoms, and changing sexual behaviour. In fact, the social vaccine has been so successful in Thailand that the infection rate has come down by 50 per cent (*The Hindu*, dated 09.03.2000).

REVIEW OF LITERATURE

The available literature pertaining to the topic has been reviewed and is presented here.

Unfortunately, India has become at present the AIDS capital of the world (Wainberg, 1999). It harbours four million people or roughly one out of every thousand citizens with HIV, which causes AIDS. A study commissioned by the National AIDS Control Organization (NACO) of India reported that the AIDS scenario was far more frightening than what global agencies had predicted long ago, that India was fertile ground for HIV infection, given the poor health care system, the virtual lack of public hygiene, and an uncomfortable literacy rate in the country (*The Hindu*, dated 15.4.1998).

In India, just within the recent one and a half decades, HIV infection has spread to all parts of the country. The epidemiological data indicate that the prevalence of HIV continues to increase and spread mostly through the heterosexual route, from urban to rural areas and from individuals practicing risk behaviours to the general population. The increasing trend of HIV infection and deaths through AIDS would in fact adversely affect not only individuals, households, and communities but also the bench marks of human development like infant survival, life expectancy, per capita income, school enrolment, health, loss of trained human resources and so on.

General awareness of the dangers of AIDS continues to be terribly low in India. It may come as a nasty revelation that HIV has spread so widely in India now that the cinema hall you are walking into may have ten people in the audience with this scourge. In every plane you take, there can be four positives, and in every college classroom there may be one such youth (Wainberg, 1999).

Now, AIDS is no more confined to prostitutes and drug addicts. There is no longer any such thing as a high risk group. HIV has certainly broken this barrier and spread to those hitherto considered safe, housewives and students for instance. And what is most painful is the fact that nine out of ten of the four million carriers of this fatal germ are below 45 years of age, the economically promising stratum in any society. Teen-agers and others must be enlightened on the gravity of the evil of AIDS, if they and the nation are to be saved.

India has one of the largest road networks in the world and an esti-mated 5 million long-distance lorry drivers. These men have to be away from their families for long durations and in unhealthy environments along the highways. They become easy prey to commercial sex workers. This fact has brought new dimensions to their lifestyle. Long-distance lorry drivers have become crucial in spreading sexually transmitted dis-eases (STDs) and HIV infection throughout the country in a short time. Knowledge of STDs including AIDS is found to be very poor among them (Rao, 1999). Creating awareness among them, prostitutes, and other vulnerable sections should be given top priority. If we educate 25 per cent of our drivers about HIV/AIDS, it will have a major impact on bringing down the number of fresh cases.

National AIDS Control Organisation has revealed that Andhra Pradesh, where the present study was conducted, has the dubious distinction of hav-ing the highest promiscuity among men and women and the second highest number of HIV positive persons in Indian states. Also, highest prevalence of sexually transmitted diseases (STDs) is recorded in A.P. The use of con-doms is proportionately very low. Consistent condom use even with non-regular partners in the state is only 25 per cent, whereas the all-India average is 32 per cent (*The Hindu*, dated 14-08-2003).

The Study

Narasimhulu (1999) conducted a study among the truck drivers in Chittoor District of Andhra Pradesh (India) and confirmed that their knowledge of HIV/AIDS was poor and that 40 per cent of the truck drivers were promiscuous. Pre-marital sex was reported to the extent of 53 per cent of the unmarried among them. On the basis of this study and the research experience of the author of this paper, an action research programme was launched in 1999 for the truck drivers of Chittoor Dis-trict for a period of one year (from December, 1999 to December, 2000). The programme was planned to inform the truck drivers about HIV/AIDS, the dangers associated with it, use of condoms for safer sex, and thus bring about changes in their sexual behaviour. As part of this study, different strategies were devised and adopted to provide them with the knowledge of HIV/AIDS, change their attitudes to sex, per-suade them to increase the use of condoms for safer sex, and bring about changes in their sexual behaviour. The programme is still on.

METHODS AND MATERIALS

Locale of the Study

The present study was conducted in the Chittoor District of Andhra Pradesh, which is in the south central region of India. This district is backward socially and economically.

Sample Size

The sample of respondents consisted of 300 truck drivers. To get at them for the study there were many problems which had to be overcome. First of all, their availability for a period of one long year was difficult, they being a highly mobile lot. As they were all alcoholic, they were not always sober. Despite these and other hurdles, earnest efforts were made to build up good rapport with them with the help of trained social workers, transport officials and their family members. Good hospitality too was extended to them. These rapport building strategies paid good dividends and helped to win the cooperation of the truck drivers for our study.

TOOLS DEVELOPED

In order to achieve the objectives of the study, a pilot study was conducted on a purposive basis among 30 truck drivers to find out their level of knowledge of HIV/AIDS, their attitudes to pre-marital and extra-marital sexuality, use of condoms, and their sexual behaviour. However, these 30 respondents of the pilot study did not form part of the sample of 300 chosen for the study. Based on the pilot study, three instruments were developed, namely (i) a knowledge test of HIV/AIDS, (ii) attitude scale on sexuality, and (iii) an interview schedule containing questions on the use of condoms for safer sex and sexual behaviour of the truck drivers. The details of the instruments developed and used in this study are given hereunder.

Knowledge Test

A knowledge test was constructed to assess the level of knowledge of the respondents regarding HIV/AIDS in terms of the symptoms of the disease, its dangers, modes of transmission, prevention techniques, diagnosis of the disease, etc. The test contains 20 questions. It was conducted twice, i.e., before the commencement of the educational programme (pre-test), and after its completion (post-test). The pre-test results helped the researcher to assess the level of knowledge of the truck drivers regarding HIV/AIDS and to plan suitable educational programmes on HIV/AIDS through films, counselling, group discussions, and the folk media. At the end of the study, the score differences between the pre- and post-survey results of the 300 respondents were statistically tested to find out the level of significance of the change occurred (increase/decrease in knowledge) through the four interventions, namely films, group discussions, folk media, and counselling.

Attitude Scale

An attitude *scale* was developed to find out and measure the attitudes of the truck drivers to HIV/AIDS, use of condoms, pre-marital and extra-marital sex, and to plan suitable educational programmes to bring about a change in their attitude towards all the issues already mentioned. This attitude scale contains 18 statements (9 positive and 9 negative). It is a three-point attitude scale. The minimum and maximum scores are 18 and 54, respectively. Accordingly, the attitude scale too was administered to the respondents twice (before the commencement of the education programme and immediately after its completion). The results of the attitude scale administered before the commencement of the educational programme helped the researcher to develop suitable interventions to bring about desirable changes in the respondents' *attitude towards* HIV/AIDS, use of condoms, and pre-marital and extra-marital sex. The score differences between the two surveys (before the commencement of the programme and after its completion) were tested to know the level of significant changes that occurred in terms of their attitude to AIDS, and the other issues closely connected with it.

Interview Schedule

An interview schedule was developed and administered to all 300 truck drivers well before the commencement of the educational programme to know whether they used condoms for safer sex whenever they participated in sex with sex workers and in their sexual behaviour. These data helped the researcher to assess the use of condoms by the truck drivers and the extent of their promiscuity. Based on the results, suitable educational programmes were planned to increase their use of condoms for safer sex and to change their sexual behaviour, particularly promiscuous behaviour. After the completion of the educational programme extended over a period of one year, the same interview schedule was once again administered to these 300 truck drivers. The score differences between the two surveys were statistically tested to find out the level of any significant change in the use of condoms for safer sex and change in their sexual behaviour.

Most of the questions used to measure the respondents' knowledge and attitudes were projective questions intended to infer the behaviour of the respondents. In fact, direct questions that might embarrass the respondents were avoided. In addition, little time was given to the respondents to answer the questions so that they would have no time for second thought. These precautions taken in the schedule enabled the respondents to give reliable responses. Further, in the pilot study, the schedule developed was also tested and retested on the same respondents to ascertain the genuiness of their responses. Thus, all precautions were taken to ensure that honest responses from the respondents could be elicited.

Conceptually, in the present investigation, the independent variables are communication variables like films, group discussion, folk media, and counselling. In fact, all these input variables for behavioural change among drivers were adopted for all the drivers, to reinforce the development of knowledge, provide credibility for the message and dramatise the situation. The dependent variables of this study are changes in the knowledge and attitudes of the respondents and regular use of condoms for safer sex.

DATA COLLECTION

The three instruments developed to elicit reliable data (knowledge test, attitude scale, and interview schedule) were administered twice to the sample respondents, first before the commencement of the educational programmes (pre-survey) and next after their completion (post-survey) to measure the impact of the educational programmes on the respondents.

Social Workers' Training and Roles

In the present study, five social workers were appointed, and they were trained for a period of one month well before the commencement of the programme. All the five were post-graduates in Social Work (Master of Social Work), and had a minimum of 5 years of experience in conducting programmes of this sort. They were taught thoroughly about HIV/AIDS, trained in the use of educational mechanisms to bring about attitudinal change regarding pre-marital and extra-marital sexual behaviour if any, use of condoms for safer sex among the respondents, rapport building, counselling techniques, etc., with the help of a team of doctors, psychologists, sociologists, and professors of Social Work and Population Studies through lectures, discussions, and films. The social workers who were involved in this programme performed multiple roles. Initially, they built up very good rapport with the truck drivers and their family members using counselling techniques. The programmes were conducted by them in "Telugu," the mother tongue of the truck drivers. Subsequently, they judiciously used the other educational strategies (films, group discussions, folk media, and counselling) to provide scientific knowledge to them about HIV/AIDS, the risk involved in pre-marital and extra-marital sex and thus sharpen their awareness. Further, the importance of using condoms to avoid the risk of STD/HIV infection was conveyed by means of films, group discussions, folk media and counselling. In fact, the skills of the social workers in building up rapport and communication with them eminently helped several truck drivers to increase their knowledge of HIV/AIDS, the need to change their risky sexual behaviour, and increase the use of condoms for safer sex. Whatever success this one-year long programme achieved was due to the committed efforts of the social workers in conducting the intervention programme. They deserve the thanks of all concerned.

PROGRAMME INTERVENTIONS

Based on the pre-survey results, the gaps in the truck drivers' knowledge of HIV/AIDS, their attitudes about it, their use of condoms, and sexual behaviour were identified and suitable educational programmes were drawn up. These programmes were conducted for a period of one year (from December, 1999 to December, 2000) to provide the respondents with correct knowledge about HIV/AIDS, to change their attitudes, increase the use of condoms and bring about changes in their sexual behaviour. The following methods/techniques were used for this purpose.

(1) Films, (2) Group Discussions, (3) Folk Media, and (4) Counselling

Films: Films on HIV/AIDS were shown to all the respondents once in every two months. Altogether, they were shown six times during the period of investigation. Before screening a film, the proposed date of screening was announced on the notice board of the transport offices well in advance. In addition, the drivers were informed about it in their houses by the social workers. Immediately after screening the films, the truck drivers were given an opportunity to seek clarification and clear their doubts, if any. Every time, a few among them used to ask questions which were answered by the social workers. Thus, the films provided them with essential knowledge about HIV/AIDS, its socio-economic aspects, its symptoms, diagnosis, prevention, treatment, etc.

Group Discussions: Once in two months, group discussions were arranged for the truck drivers with the help of trained social workers. The respondents were given an opportunity to discuss their sexual problems and get their doubts clarified on the use of condoms and other HIV/AIDS related issues. The place and date of the group discussion also was informed to all the respondents well in advance to enable them to be present and participate without fail.

Folk Media: India has a very high rate of illiteracy (35 per cent) and the vast majority of the population are from rural areas. But, there are several traditional and popular folkart forms among them. Therefore, folk media which have long been used as sources of entertainment as well as media to convey messages, and moral instruction programmes were arranged for the truck drivers with the help of folk artists to impress upon the rural audience, the drivers in particular, the mal-effects of HIV/AIDS, to bring about changes in their sexual behaviour and encourage them to use condoms for safer sex. In fact, this strategy has been used by the NACO of India successfully. The folk media messages on HIV/AIDS are well received in rural and semi-urban areas of India and the messages go home to them.

Counselling

The trained social workers used to meet the truck drivers at the transport offices and at their residences once a month and provide complete information to them on HIV/AIDS in terms of its symptoms, spread of the disease, prevention, dangers of promiscuity, etc., and counsel them to give up promiscuity in their own interest.

KNOWLEDGE

Knowledge is an important determinant of human behaviour. Hence, it is possible to predict the behaviour of people in direct ratio to their knowledge. As part of this study, as stated earlier, before the educational programme was commenced, a survey was carried out to identify the extent of knowledge of the truck drivers about the various aspects of HIV/AIDS in terms of the symptoms of the disease, its dangers, modes of transmission, diagnosis, prevention techniques, etc. The pre-survey helped to identify the gaps in the knowledge of truck drivers about HIV/AIDS and to plan suitable educational programmes to improve their knowledge. The pre-survey clearly showed that the knowledge of the truck drivers in this regard was poor as their educational level was very low, many of them being illiterate or semi-literate and only some of them having primary education (Mean Knowledge Score = 8.1).

Thereupon with the help of trained social workers, the truck drivers were exposed for one year to films, group discussions, folk media, and counselling and were helped to acquire sufficient knowledge of HIV/AIDS, etc. The next step was to assess whether the respondents had made any significant gain in their knowledge from the educational programme. After the educational programmes were conducted successfully using the various strategies already mentioned, a post-survey was conducted to assess the impact of the educational programme on the respondents regarding the knowledge they had gained about HIV/AIDS. The post-survey results clearly showed that there was a dramatic increase in the knowledge of the truck drivers. The post-test mean score was 16.4. The obtained 't' value of 13.53 was significant beyond the 0.01 level. Therefore, there was a quantum jump from the pre-survey (mean score: 8.1) to post-survey (mean score: 16.4) due to the knowledge provided to the truck drivers through the educational programme. Obviously, the educational programme greatly enhanced their knowledge of HIV/AIDS and made a positive impact on them, as Table 1 shows. Thus, it is worth replicating similar programmes in countries developed and developing alike, wherever a similar situation exists.

ATTITUDES

Attitudes denote what one feels or thinks about a particular topic or question. They are personal dispositions which impel individuals to react to objects or situations. Attitude is a most important element of human behaviour. "A knowledge of the attitude of an individual helps a great deal in predicting, other things being equal, how he will act in a given situation" (Roy et al., 1968). Attitudes are not inherited nor are they innate. But, in the course of experience, they may undergo a change. In the pres-

TABLE 1. Pre-Test and Post-Test Results of Knowledge Test on HIV/AIDS

Variable	Mean Scores		T-value
	Pre-test (N = 300)	Post-test (N = 300)	
Knowledge	8.1 ± 2.3	16.4 ± 10.9	13.53*

*Significant at 0.01 level.

ent study, before the commencement of the educational programme, an attitude scale was prepared and administered to the respondents to find out their attitude towards the use of condoms, AIDS, pre-marital sex and promiscuity.

The pre-survey results (attitudes) clearly showed a mean score of 19.0, which clearly indicated that the respondents had a positive attitude towards pre-marital sex, promiscuity, and a negative attitude towards the use of condoms, and HIV/AIDS. This was mostly due to a lack of knowledge and their ignorance largely because of illiteracy. Accordingly, suitable educational programmes were designed for the truck drivers, and they were provided with sufficient knowledge about AIDS, and AIDS-related issues such as general and particular dangers of pre-marital sex and promiscuity and the use of condoms. The purpose of the programme was to bring about desirable changes in their attitude to pre-marital sex, promiscuity, and the use of condoms. These programmes were conducted for a period of one year, and afterwards a post-survey was conducted to know whether there was any change in the attitude of the truck drivers on pre-marital sex, promiscuity, the use of condoms, AIDS and sexual behaviour. The post-test mean score was 43.3. The obtained 't' value of 15.15 was significant beyond the 0.01 level of probability. Compared with the pre-survey mean score (19.0), the post-test mean score (43.3) demonstrated that there was a sea-change in the attitudes of the truck drivers after their exposure to the educational programmes. They created in them negative attitude towards pre-marital sex and promiscuity, and a positive attitude towards the use of condoms (see Table 2).

USE OF CONDOMS

The use of condoms began to spread in rural India only during the last three or four decades, after the revitalisation of the family planning programme. Men need to know about contraceptive methods and un-

TABLE 2. Pre-Test and Post-Test Results of the Attitude Towards HIV/AIDS

Variable	Mean Scores		T-value
	Pre-test (N = 300)	Post-test (N = 300)	
Opinion	19.0 ± 11.31	43.3 ± 25.39	15.15*

*Significant at 0.01 level.

derstand the importance of condoms in preventing births and to get protection from STDs. Some men do not use condoms because of their fear that it comes in the way of sexual satisfaction for either partner or both. They like to have skin to skin touch during intercourse. Some are allergic to its use and some others do not like use it for one reason or the other or for no particular reason. Thus, many do not use condoms at the time of sex without minding the consequences of unprotected sex, especially with commercial sex workers. Those who engage in pre-marital or extra-marital sex do not like to use condoms because they wrongly believe that it delays ejaculation and does not give them enough sexual pleasure.

The survey data revealed that 120 truckers out of 300 were promiscuous/engaged in pre-marital sex. In the present study, before the educational programmes were started, an attempt was made through a survey to know how many truck drivers who were promiscuous or engaged in pre-marital sex were using condoms. The survey revealed that the use of condoms by them was very low for different reasons. Only 49 out of the 120 respondents who were promiscuous or engaged in pre-marital sex were using condoms and the remaining 71 did not. It means that only 41 per cent of the 120 truck drivers were using condoms and the remaining 59 per cent of the truckers were participating in unprotected sex.

The findings of the study demonstrated how grave the situation is regarding the spread of HIV infection from sex workers to truck drivers in the study area. They strengthen the fear that the conditions under which the truckers live and function in the rest of the country make them more liable to become victims of HIV infections on an unprecedented scale. Based on the startling findings, suitable educational programmes were designed and the messages to redeem the situation were passed on through educational films, group discussions, folk media, and counselling to see that every vulnerable truck driver used condoms for safer sex, without fail, wherever and whenever he participated in pre-marital or extra-marital sex. When the importance of condoms for safer sex was explained to the respondents by our social workers, a vast majority of those given to a promiscuous sex life could realise the necessity of using a condom during sex as a protective device. As a result, the post-test results clearly indicated that the use of condoms increases perceptively. The post-survey showed that 104 respondents were found using condoms whereas only 49 were using them before. It means that the majority of the promiscuous respondents who were not using condoms at the time of launch of the programme started using them to protect themselves from STDs. Thus, the educational programmes made an impact on the respondents, and significantly increased the use of condoms by the vulnerable truck drivers (see Table 3).

SEXUAL BEHAVIOUR

Sexual behaviour of people depends not only on physiological and psychological factors but also on their education, occupation, socio-economic and cultural background. Those who are better educated generally exercise restraint in matters of sex, pre-marital, or extra-marital. Those who are engaged in odd, occasional, and irregular jobs such as truck drivers are likely to engage in sex irrationally. In the social environment they live, not much importance is attached to privacy, or moral scruples which bind others who are more securely employed. Such people are more vulnerable to STDs and HIV infections than those engaged in other occupations. The vast majority of people who attend government clinics in the teaching hospitals of Andhra Pradesh are those who are engaged in odd jobs and who form the high risk group of the population.

Thus, it is clear from the data of this study that a good percentage (40 percent) of truck drivers among the respondents (120 out of 300) indiscriminately indulged with the sex workers in pre-marital and extra-marital sex. After conducting for a year the educational programmes specially designed to bring about a change in their sexual behaviour, a systematic post-survey was conducted by the social workers to find out whether the educational programmes had made any impact on the sexual behaviour of the truck drivers. Fortunately, there was a perceptible change, which was reflected in the post-test results. Counselling, group discussion, and exposure to the message through the folk media did bring down promiscuity and pre-marital sex to a significant level. The results indicated that only 57 (47.5 per cent) of the truck drivers continued with their old sex habits in spite of the concerted interventions on their behalf. This means

TABLE 3. Percentage Distribution of Respondents by Use of Condoms Before and After the Educational Programme

Variable	Mean Scores		Percent increase
	Pre-test (N = 120)	Post-test (N = 120)	
Use of condoms	49 (40.83%)	104 (86.67%)	45.84%

*Significant at 0.01 level.

that more than 50 per cent of the truck drivers (63) had given them up. The percentage of change was due to the impact of the education programmes on them. Thus, the educational strategies adopted in the present study are worth replicating in all places where such promiscuous sex behaviour has been extensively practiced by any occupational group in India and elsewhere (Table 4).

CONCLUSION

The information, education and communication (IEC) programmes experimentally tried by our team had a significant impact on the respondent truck drivers in terms of increasing their knowledge of HIV/AIDS. The study suggests that the current low level of knowledge among them of HIV/AIDS may be partly due to lack of understanding and their being unaware of the problem and its gravity. Their knowledge can be increased by means of suitable educational programmes. A good counselling programme would help them to understand the dangers of HIV/AIDS, its mode of transmission, and also how to prevent it by the proper precautions. Our IEC programmes enabled the respondent truck drivers to take well considered decisions and change their sexual behaviour. Those who are satisfied with this programme and benefited by it have even become extensive advocates for HIV/AIDS education. They are likely try to bring about changes for the better in the sexual behaviour of their friends and relatives who are vulnerable.

The present study, though difficult and time-consuming, is highly relevant. It provides valuable experience and insight into the complex problem. Other countries of the world, developing countries, and developed ones alike, wherever the HIV/AIDS infection is prevalent, would do well

TABLE 4. Percentage Distribution of Respondents by Promiscuity Before and After the Educational Programmes

Variable	Total Sample = 300			
	Pre-test (N = 120)		Post-test (N = 120)	
	No.	%	No.	%
Promiscuity	120	(40.0)	63	(52.5)

to conduct similar studies and devise suitable strategies, to arrest the menace. The success of the present study was possible because of our appropriate mix of four interventions, namely films, group discussions, folk media, and counselling, which together reinforced knowledge and gave credibility for the socially backward drivers for a learning situation. Any one of the interventions, however powerful in itself, could not have achieved the significant success that the combination of the four could achieve. Thus, this study demonstrates how an intelligent and successful combination of educational strategies can make a decisive impact on people and bring about a behavioural change. This is a valuable lesson for all social workers irrespective of the country in which they work.

Of late, in order to reduce the spread of STD/HIV among the general public and the truck drivers who form one of the high risk groups in India, a few innovative strategies have been initiated in Tamil Nadu and Andhra Pradesh States in India. They been very successful and worth replicating throughout the world. In Tamil Nadu, condoms are made available at all petrol pumps, particularly those on the highways that are invariably visited by truck drivers. The drivers can collect the required number of condoms or as many as they want free of cost. They are packed in a thick paper type valet, each containing three condoms. This programme in Tamil Nadu has been highly successful.

Some Non-Government Organisations (NGOs) working for the welfare of commercial sex workers in Andhra Pradesh, have taken up STD/HIV prevention programmes in a big way through Information, Education and Communication (IEC) Programmes. They, too, freely distribute condoms to those who require them. Trained social workers provide knowledge of STD/HIV and the need to use condoms for prevention of STD/HIV to the sex workers. Further, they distribute condoms to the sex workers at their places. As a result, 90 percent of the sex workers insist on their clients using condoms. Without it they do not permit them to have sex with them. Further, the social workers replenish sufficient number of condoms during their routine weekly visits to the sex workers. In case the sex workers fall short of condoms, they may telephone the NGO Office to deliver condoms immediately or they can even personally go to the NGO Office to collect them. This strategy has been highly successful.

REFERENCES

Narasimhulu (2001). Knowledge, Attitudes and Sexual Behaviour of Truck Drivers in Andhra Pradesh, Unpublished M.Phil. Thesis, S.V. University, Tirupati, Andhra Pradesh, India.

Population Reports (1986). Population Information Programme, Baltimore, The Johns Hopkins University.

Rao (1999). *AIDS Update*, AIDS Research and Control Centre, Mumbai, April-June, 1999.

Roy, P., and Koivlin, J. (1968). *Health Innovations and Family Planning: A Study in Eight Indian Villages*, Hyderabad, National Institute of Community Development.

Sight and Life Newsletter (2000), Sight and Life, P.O. Box 2116, 4002, Basel, Switzerland.

The Hindu, Daily Newspaper, (Dated 15-04-1998, 09-03-2000 & 14-08-2003), Andhra Edition, Chennai, Annasalai, India.

Wainberg (1999) in *The Hindu*, Daily Newspaper, Dated 07-01-99, Andhra Edition, Chennai, Annasalai, India.

FOCUSING ON THE UNIQUE LIFE-CYCLE: SOCIAL WORK KNOWLEDGE IN PROMOTING INDIVIDUAL LIFE CHANGES AND HUMAN RIGHTS

The Experience of Receiving a Diagnosis of Cystic Fibrosis After Age 20: Implications for Social Work

Eileen Widerman, PhD, MSW

SUMMARY. Using the phenomenological approach of Van Manen, this study explored the lived experience of receiving a diagnosis of cys-

Eileen Widerman is Assistant Professor, Temple University, School of Social Administration, 1301 Cecil B. Moore Avenue, Ritter Annex, 5th Floor, Philadelphia, PA 19122-6091 USA (Email: eileen.widerman@temple.edu)

The author wishes to thank Dr. Mary Bricker-Jenkins, Professor of Social Work at the School of Social Administration at Temple University, for her invaluable assistance in the conceptualizing, organizing, and writing of the manuscript.

[Haworth co-indexing entry note]: "The Experience of Receiving a Diagnosis of Cystic Fibrosis After Age 20: Implications for Social Work." Widerman, Eileen. Co-published simultaneously in *Social Work in Health Care* (The Haworth Social Work Practice Press, an imprint of The Haworth Press, Inc.) Vol. 39, No. 3/4, 2004, pp. 415-433; and: *Social Work Visions from Around the Globe: Citizens, Methods, and Approaches* (ed: Anna Metteri, et al.) The Haworth Social Work Practice Press, an imprint of The Haworth Press, Inc., 2004, pp. 415-433. Single or multiple copies of this article are available for a fee from The Haworth Document Delivery Service [1-800-HAWORTH, 9:00 a.m. - 5:00 p.m. (EST). E-mail address: docdelivery@haworthpress.com].

Digital Object Identifier: 10.1300/J010v39n03_12

tic fibrosis as an adult. Ten essential themes were generated from the stories of 36 participants: Awareness of Death, Change, Difference, Distraction, Family Indifference, Intrusion, Isolation, Normalizing, Time, and Uncertainty. Themes associated with gender, illness severity, and medical care were also developed. Although themes were similar to those in the chronic illness literature, late-diagnosis of CF was found to be a unique experience. Participants sought personal relationships with caregivers and educational materials targeted to their needs. Implications for social work are discussed. *[Article copies available for a fee from The Haworth Document Delivery Service: 1-800-HAWORTH. E-mail address: <docdelivery@haworth press.com> Website: <http://www.HaworthPress.com> © 2004 by The Haworth Press, Inc. All rights reserved.]*

KEYWORDS. Chronic illness, chronic illness themes, cystic fibrosis, cystic fibrosis adult diagnosis, new diagnosis

INTRODUCTION

Cystic Fibrosis (CF) is a chronic, progressive, genetic disease primarily affecting the lungs and pancreas. In 1999 the median age at diagnosis was six months and the median survival age was 29.1 years (CF Foundation, 2000). Because CF is usually diagnosed in young children, most treatment sites are located in pediatric facilities and patient education materials directed to parents and young children. However, some cases of CF are identified in adults. In 1999, 11.1% of individuals with CF in the US had been diagnosed at or over age 18, and 6.3% of all new diagnoses that year were confirmed in adults 18 years or older. In 1996, the mean age at which CF was identified in those over 18 was 27 years (Widerman, Millner, Sexauer, & Fiel, 2000).

Anecdotally, both caregivers and those affected say that receiving a diagnosis of CF as an adult is associated with unique experiences, issues, and needs. These arise from learning of an existing genetic disease during the early adult years and the accompanying necessities of beginning time-consuming treatment and re-evaluating life plans. Unfortunately, few published studies explore the phenomenon of receiving a diagnosis of CF as an adult. Professional caregivers, then, are without guidance in providing sensitive, comprehensive care, and those diagnosed as adults have little information to validate their experiences or answer their questions. This paper addresses these gaps. As part of a larger study exploring the lived experience of receiving a diagnosis of CF after age 20, this analysis focuses on (a) themes arising from this experience and (b) adults' self-expressed educational and support needs, interests, and preferences following a diagnosis of CF.

LITERATURE REVIEW

Late Diagnosis in CF

Over the years, several clinical case studies have described unusual presentations or unanticipated diagnoses of CF in adults (Drey et al., 1999; Gardiner & Cranley, 1989; Godby, 1985; Hellerstein, 1946; Fiel, 1988; Hunt & Geddes, 1984; vanBiezen, Overbrook, & Hevering, 1992; Vilar et al., 2000). The intent and contribution of these articles has been to alert physicians that CF can remain undiagnosed into the adult years and that men and women with undiagnosed CF can present with atypical symptoms. Reviewed as a body of literature, case study findings implicitly suggest that those diagnosed with CF as adults may differ medically from those diagnosed as children. More recent epidemiological and descriptive articles confirm differences. Milder pulmonary disease (Gan, Beus, Bakker, Lamers, & Heijerman, 1995; Hubert et al., 2000; McWilliams, Wilsher, & Kolbe, 2000; Widerman et al., 2000), less pancreatic insufficiency (Gan et al., 1995; Hubert et al., 2000; McCloskey, Redmond, Hill, & Elborn, 2000; McWilliams et al., 2000; Widerman et al., 2000), rarer CF mutations (Gan et al., 1995; McCloskey et al., 2000; Widerman et al., 2000), and longer life expectancy (Widerman et al., 2000) have been found to be associated with late diagnosis in CF. In addition, those diagnosed at or over age 18 in the US are more likely to be married, college educated, and working full-time than those diagnosed with CF during childhood (Widerman et al., 2000). Unfortunately, this research does not describe how receiving a diagnosis of CF as an adult or the characteristics associated with late diagnosis may affect individuals' experiences and psychosocial needs.

The Adult CF Literature

Common foci of research describing the psychosocial and medically-related characteristics of adults with CF, most of whom were diagnosed as children, include compliance/adherence (e.g., Abbott, Dodd, Gee, & Webb, 2001; Conway, Pond, Hamnett, & Watson, 1996;

Czajkowski & Koocher, 1987), psychological wellbeing (e.g., Anderson, Flume, & Hardy, 2001; Shepherd et al., 1990; Strauss & Wellisch, 1981), and quality-of-life (e.g., Congleton, Hodson, & Duncan-Skingle, 1996; Gee, Abbott, Conway, Etherington, & Webb, 2000). The findings of this research suggest that adults with CF demonstrate adequate-to-good overall functioning, that individuals' compliance is uneven, and that adults' gender and pulmonary function affect their perceived quality of life. One qualitative study explored the lived experience of ten men and women who grew up with CF and identified four descriptive themes: being different, don't call me terminal, a desire to be treated as an individual, and will power and faith (Tracy, 1997).

However, because this research does not include age-at-diagnosis as a variable, findings cannot be assumed to describe those diagnosed as adults. For example, the higher prevalence of pancreatic sufficiency among those diagnosed as adults could impact compliance (needing fewer doses of medication daily), self-image (achieving higher height and weight percentiles), and quality-of-life. But, the foci and the findings of this research were helpful in designing the study and suggesting areas for exploration.

THE EXPERIENCE OF CHRONIC ILLNESS

A substantial literature within the social sciences explores the chronic illness experience, both disease-specific and across diseases, including diagnoses occurring later in life. Three published overviews are helpful in understanding, evaluating, and summarizing this work. Thorne and Paterson (2000) conducted a metasynthesis of over 1000 articles on chronic illness written from an "insider" perspective between the years 1990 and 1998. They concluded that studies focusing on chronic illness as a generic phenomenon yield themes related to symptomatology (e.g., pain and suffering), adjustment patterns (e.g., changes in biographical course), and social contexts (e.g., stigma). Five contextual and mediating factors in illness experience were also identified: life stage, gender, social location, and ethnicity. Earlier, Conrad (1987) identified seven recurring themes that have both arisen from and been applied to chronic illness research activity: uncertainty; illness careers; stigma; biographical work and the reconstitution of self; managing medical regimens; information awareness and sharing; and family relations. Finally, Sidell (1997), reviewing chronic illness literature from a social work perspective, concluded that adjustment to chronic illness among non-geriatric adults is characterized by loss and grief, uncertainty, coping, and development issues. Additional themes, related to those described in the overview articles, have been also been described. Among these are self-pity (Charmaz, 1980), chronic sorrow (Eakes, 1993), frustration (Bertram, Kurland, Lydick, Locke, & Yawn, 2001), isolation (Bertram et al., 2001), and the concept of illness gains (Asbring, 2001; Petrie, Buick, Weinman, & Booth, 1999).

Thorne and Paterson (2000) point out that considering the specific attributes of diseases of interest can be helpful in evaluating and applying the many themes within the chronic illness literature. The attributes of CF differ from those of the diseases that, either individually or grouped, generated the themes reviewed in the literature above. Therefore, this study was conducted to better understand the CF late diagnosis experience and develop practice guidelines from that understanding. The findings within the generic and disease-specific chronic illness literature were helpful in developing the study design, suggesting areas for exploration, and informing qualitative data analysis.

METHOD

The absence of published work on the psychosocial aspects of late diagnosis in CF, as well as the exploratory and descriptive intent of this study, suggested the selection of a qualitative research method.[1] Specifically the interpretive phenomenological approach of Van Manen (1990) was chosen to guide data collection and analysis. This approach yields rich description and understanding through uncovering and interpretation of "essential themes" (p. 107). It differs in intent from the prevalent method within the chronic illness literature, grounded theory, which searches data for theoretical categories whose relationships are then analyzed to develop theory (Charmaz, 1990).

Sampling Plan

The population of interest was men and women living in the US who had received a diagnosis of CF at age 20 or older. Age 20 was chosen because the years 17-19 often involve leaving home, attending college, establishing relationships, etc., so that isolating the cognitive and emotional reactions specific to receiving a CF diagnosis during these years might have been difficult. Participants were recruited through notices placed in CF consumer newsletters, on a CF Listserv, and from flyers distributed to CF centers. A national sample of fifteen males and 21 females volunteered to participate.

The sampling plan assured diversity in gender and time-since-diagnosis (over/under three years). Gender differences in CF expression among those diagnosed as adults have been documented (Widerman, 2000) as has the potential for gender to influence illness experience (Thorne & Paterson, 2000). Sampling according to time-since-diagnosis assured the exploration of CF experiences at different points in the illness trajectory although in different individuals.

The Interview Process

Twenty telephone and 16 face-to-face interviews, ranging in length from 45 minutes to over two hours, generated the data for the study. Participants provided CF and demographic data (e.g., perceived illness severity, educational attainment, age, marital status, etc.). A semi-structured interview guide was developed to promote an efficient organization of the data to be collected. Questions encouraged participants to talk about experiences related to their late diagnosis of CF (e.g., Describe a "typical" day in your life. How, if at all, did your life change after your diagnosis? Describe your relationship with your doctor). Reading and re-reading initial interviews uncovered issues and experiences for further exploration in remaining interviews.

Data Analysis

In keeping with the approach of Van Manen (1990), data analysis began with an in-depth consideration of each individual's story and its accompanying case notes. Case notes included the researcher's reflections, insights, and tentative interpretations following each of the interviews. Words, phrases, and interpretations that appeared essential to the phenomenon of late diagnosis for each individual were highlighted and named as individual themes.

To determine the extent to which these analyses were successfully capturing individuals' experiences, each of ten participants, selected to mirror the diversity of the sample, was mailed a list of the themes developed from her story and asked to comment on their relevance. Nine responded, and all indicated that the themes captured the experiences and feelings they recalled relating during their interviews.

The themes were then assembled, read, and re-read, along with field notes. Field notes were recordings of the researcher's questions, notations, reactions, etc., across cases, during the entire research process. Similar individual themes were grouped together, retaining the language and descriptive experiences of each. Data reduction involved eliminating repetitions within these groups to highlight the essential qualities of the described experiences, generating cross-case themes. These were named by using the language of the participants (e.g., "Difference"), by summarizing similar narrative content (e.g., "Uncertainty"), or interpreting common participant experiences (e.g., "Distraction").

Next, cases were grouped according to gender and self-perceived illness severity in order to search for themes associated with each of these characteristics. Themes were also developed from participants' stated educational and care needs, as well as from their descriptions of their experiences interacting with medical professionals.

The themes generated from the analysis of the individual stories were shared and discussed with a CF activist who was diagnosed with CF as an adult, a CF newsletter editor who frequently interacts with readers who were diagnosed as adults, and three experienced qualitative health researchers. All indicated that the themes were consistent with their understandings of the experiences and issues related to receiving a diagnosis of CF as an adult.

Participants

Participants' ages ranged from 20-69, with a mean age of 28 (26 for males and 29 for females). Time-since-diagnosis ranged from four months to 29 years. Approximately half of those interviewed were married, raising children, and engaged in professional occupations; three-quarters attended or completed college; and almost a third worked full-time outside of the home.

Most participants' diagnoses were the first known in their families and were confirmed as the result of pulmonary complaints. Half self-assessed their current illness severity as mild, 39% as moderate, and 11% as severe. Many respondents received care in pediatric settings reflecting the scarcity of adult CF programs at the time (1996), particularly in rural areas.

FINDINGS

Themes

Cross-Case Themes

Table 1 lists the ten inter-related cross-case themes that were generated from the stories of the 36 men and women interviewed and that describe their experience of receiving a diagnosis of CF as an adult. These themes are presented in alphabetical order because each is essential to understanding the late diagnosis experience.

Awareness of Death. Participants said that, upon diagnosis, they became aware of the probability of a shortened life span and responded with fear. A married mother of two recalled, "I thought I was going to die . . . I really thought my days were numbered." A male in his late 20s commented, "I started to pick out shrouds." Their fear was in part prompted by the often-outdated educational materials they consulted shortly after their diagnoses. A woman explained, "I immediately went to the library the next day and looked up CF. And everything said you were going to die by the time you were 16. And here I was 40, and I was like, you know, this is it!" Fortunately, for most, this immediate fear subsided as they learned more about CF, began treatment, and developed coping strategies. However, the awareness of a shortened life span remained persistent although not constant. One woman said, "Depend-

TABLE 1. Cross-Case Themes Describing Experiences Related to Adult Diagnosis of CF

Theme	Description
Awareness of Death	Aware of probable or possible short life span
Change	Lifestyle and self-view must accommodate CF
Difference	Unlike "normals" and others with CF
Distraction	CF competing with typical life stage demands for attention
Family Indifference	Birth families not accepting of CF nor supportive
Intrusion	Effect of CF on daily life and future plans
Isolation	Shrinking social circles and loneliness
Normalizing	Desire to maintain pre-diagnosis life style
Time	Sense of time altered; future "shrinks"
Uncertainty	Long and short-term future not predictable

ing on the day. I can go days and not think about it. Then I get a call, or someone will ask me about it." Another woman said, "I flip-flop between denial and self-consciousness."

Change. Once diagnosed with CF, men and women were confronted with new information about themselves, information affecting their self-view, their futures, and their daily functioning. One woman recalled, "I was amazed at how life can change so quickly. One day you think everything's fine and the next day you think it's all over." Most had to re-evaluate plans, careers, and lifestyle choices. A woman diagnosed in her mid 20s had been unhappy in her marriage. She thought, "OK, if I'm going to have a shortened life span, then I better get my act into gear and make the changes I need to make." She filed for divorce within a month of receiving her diagnosis. More than one participant changed careers. Others moved to be nearer to a CF center.

Almost all reported that CF brought positive changes as well as troubling ones. As one woman explained, "CF brings gifts with it." Because of their diagnoses, many began valuing time and relationships differently, respecting the fragility of health, and developing a sense of purpose. A young man reflected, "I was speeding through life. I enjoy life now."

Difference. Participants repeatedly used the word "different" to describe themselves and their stories reflected an overwhelming sense of difference. First, they felt different from adults with CF who were diagnosed as infants or children. Commenting on a friend diagnosed at age six, one woman related, "He grew up with [CF]. He was comfortable with it. It was like a little blanket. To me it wasn't. It was threatening." Another woman mused, "[Those diagnosed as children] have all their decisions to make . . . Do I get married, have kids, go to college? . . . I didn't get to make those decisions." Their sense of difference was often heightened, and occasionally defined, by physicians who were said to have stressed the rarity of late diagnosis or individuals' atypical symptoms. One woman said she was told, "You're not a normal CF person anyway, because you weren't diagnosed until this age." A man in his early 20s was reassured, "You're going to live to 30 or 40 or 50." Although many experienced their difference as distancing themselves from others, they also drew upon their perceived difference to enable them to construct and maintain an optimistic outlook: As long as they were different from those diagnosed as children, they could believe that their prognoses and their lives would also be different.

Participants also felt different from those with other diseases. One woman commented, "Diagnosis as an adult is different than a diagnosis of cancer. You didn't just get it. You've always had it. You've been sick and didn't know it." A number commented that, unlike those with AIDS or lung cancer, they "didn't do anything" to "cause" CF and viewed themselves as "innocents" or "victims." A man reflected, "Hey, I didn't give myself cystic fibrosis . . . My parents were carriers."

Finally, participants felt different from those they termed "normal," for all of the reasons that chronic illness can change lives–symptoms, appearance, treatment demands, dependency, shortened life expectancy, etc. Another man mused, "I have an uncertain future. What's important to me is different than what is important to others."

Distraction. Most participants were diagnosed in their late twenties when important life events, many common to the early adult years, were also occurring. The urgency of these events distracted them from thinking about having CF. A 35-year-old man explained,

> In that first year we were having a family crisis. It just so happens that my father was diagnosed with cancer in January . . . I was diagnosed a month after him. So, um, there were a lot of other things going on in the household that took away some of the dramatics . . . We were dealing with other issues.

In this man's case, he and his family were absorbed in caring for his father, in anticipating his father's death, and in supporting each other. He kept clinic appointments, but he said he did not reflect on the meaning of having CF until months after his father died. Another man was struggling with sexual identity issues when he was diagnosed. "Well, I was very preoccupied with coming out, so that was the thing even bigger on my mind than my CF diagnosis." Other participants were distracted by the demands of college, career, or children. Dealing with life events and dealing with a new diagnosis, simultaneously, with equal energy, was impossible. The phenomena of distraction was adaptive. While distractions relegated CF to the periphery of awareness, they afforded men and women time to "ease into" the reality of their late diagnoses.

Family Indifference. Most participants said that at and before their diagnoses, their birth families showed little interest in their health and were rarely helpful or supportive. A young college student recalled that her first thought at diagnosis was, "Thank God . . . someone is saying it's not in your head. Because that's what my parents were saying. 'It's all in your head. You're making this up . . . It's just a nervous cough.'" Over and over again individuals said that their parents ignored or minimized symptoms and accused them of malingering or of seeking attention. Participants were angry, sad, and confused by their families' reactions and lack of help or support. One woman said, ". . . my first thought when I was finally diagnosed was that I wished my mother were still alive to finally know that it really was something!" Another indicated she was sure her family will "feel bad" after she dies, but went on to say, "I want involvement now, not when I'm dead."

Intrusion. CF was seen as an intrusion into lives already planned without awareness of CF. One man related, "I was building my life. We had been married for three years. We were preparing to build our home. We were getting along successfully financially speaking . . . We saw life optimistically ahead of us." Rather suddenly, he learned that the sinus problems he had suffered throughout childhood were actually symptoms of CF. He was advised by his physician to consider a less stressful career and move to a warmer area of the country. He had to begin a time-consuming regime of self-care and treatment. He was resentful that CF would affect the flow of his daily life as well as his future planning. Others also saw the necessary self-care and physician appointments as intrusive. A young woman remarked, ". . . maybe because I wasn't brought up on medicines, on physiotherapy, with a viewpoint towards illness. Being constantly aware you have this monkey on your back."

Isolation. Participants reported that they minimized their socialization and consequently felt isolated because of the time involved in CF self-care, from embarrassment related to CF symptoms (primarily coughing), and/or from the effects of the disease (e.g., fatigue, shortness-of-breath). Because they felt "different" from other adults with CF, they did not actively participate in CF patient list-servs. The emotional, and often physical, indifference of families further contributed to their sense of isolation.

Normalization. The men and women interviewed did everything possible to maintain their pre-diagnosis routines of work, church, parenting, etc., and to pursue plans made pre-diagnosis. At an average age-of-diagnosis of 28, participants had existing obligations (particularly children and expenses) that required them to maintain a high level of daily activity. But pursuing a normal life was not just a response to established demands, it was a way of "proving" to themselves and others that they were indeed different, that CF would not define who they were and how they lived their lives. Men and women repeatedly expressed that they really had not changed upon diagnosis, a label had simply been applied to them. "I was so used to [my symptoms] that whatever they called it, it was still the same," was a young woman's comment. A man explained, "I'm the same guy as the day before I found out."

Time. Participants reported that, following diagnosis, their sense of time changed and their conception of "future" became more restricted. Even though many thought they would live a relatively long life given their already older age and their mild symptoms, almost all said that they lived "day to day" nonetheless. Participants also said they had difficulty finding the time necessary to care for themselves given busy lives. One woman sighed, "There's not enough hours in the day."

Uncertainty. Participants were uncertain about what lay ahead, how CF would affect them, and how long they would live. One woman ruefully commented, "I've learned not to let [CF] rule me and take over my life. Ha Ha. But it's hard to make plans, buy tickets, because I never know if I'm going to be sick."

Data analysis also identified themes that were not descriptive across cases, but were strongly related to gender or to illness severity.

Gender Related Themes

Difficulty of Parenthood. Mothers repeatedly said that the physical and self-care demands of CF made taking care of their children difficult. A number said that if they had known they had CF they would not have had children. None indicated plans to have additional children. One woman described how she was raising her children "from the couch." Others said they were "cheating" their children, because they could not play games with them, volunteer for school functions, or be sure they would live to see them graduate or get married. As indicated, few had families willing to help them. None of the men who were adoptive or step-parents were primary caregivers nor did they identify their parental role as difficult.

Devastated by Sterility. Almost 100% of men with CF are sterile. The men interviewed were devastated by sterility. In some cases sterility was more disturbing than the shortened life span associated with CF. A 32-year-old married man recalled, "The actual CF part wasn't bad. I dealt with that part really well. But still the infertility thing made me feel like less than a human, less of what I am." Another man interviewed over 30 years after his diagnosis said, "It's the worst of the worst [news] ... for a man to find out that he can't father children." Although CF can affect fertility in women, none of the women interviewed expressed concern they could not have children or might have difficulty conceiving and/or carrying a baby to term.

Fear of Rejection. Three men in the study offered that they were homosexual, and all feared that their CF symptoms (malnutrition, frequent pneumonia) and treatment (antibiotics) could be mistaken for the symptoms and treatment of AIDS. One explained, " . . . with the sickness I have they are immediately going to think about AIDS . . . So, when I think it's going to become an issue with that person . . . I'll look them in the eye and say, 'Look, I have this and it's not a big deal . . .' And that's when you don't hear from them anymore." No women in the study self-identified as lesbian or bisexual, and no females indicated they were concerned that others might think they had AIDS/HIV.

Themes Related to Illness Severity

Probability of an Early Death. Participants who described themselves as moderately or seriously ill said that they were acutely aware of the probability of an early death, which they found depressing. Because they experienced ongoing symptoms, were frequently hospitalized, etc., these men and women were constantly aware of CF. Some were receiving or considering disability. A 26-year-old man acknowledged, "I guess I'm always getting worse. That's a simple fact, though. You know, no matter how much I do, the bottom line is you're getting worse." Another man related, "I'm not looking forward to retirement, because I don't know if I'll even make it that far." A woman in her 40s explained, " . . . when you do get bad, and you are looking at a transplant, it's another world. It's someplace I never thought I'd be."

Self-Pity/Wanting Sympathy. Moderately or seriously ill participants admitted feeling self-pity and wanting sympathy, particularly from family members and caregivers. They said they tried so hard to meet their obligations, lead "normal" lives, and take care of themselves. Yet their struggles seemed, to them, rarely understood or appreciated. One woman said, "Once in a while, I'd like someone to feel sorry for me." Participants said they envied and resented the concern of the public for CF "poster children." But, because CF is not outwardly apparent in most adults, participants felt their families, friends, and coworkers underestimated its impact.

Importance of Exercise. Those describing themselves as mildly ill were believers in the importance of exercise and described their routines in great detail. Determining and maintaining a challenging activity level were consciously employed not only as a means of improving health status, but also to reassure themselves that they were not "getting worse." For example, one man ran three miles every day. As long as he could run those three miles he had "evidence" that his CF was not progressing. Despite the lack of supporting research and their physicians' skepticism, those who espoused exercise were convinced that vigorous activity can stop, or even reverse, the progression of CF.

In addition to cross-case, gender-related, and CF severity-related themes, data analysis revealed themes describing participants' experiences with medical caregivers and preferences related to their medical care.

Themes Related to Interactions with Medical Caregivers

Personal Relationships. Participants expressed that they wanted to feel that their physicians knew them and cared about them. One woman said, "I tell you, I don't care how good the doctor is. If you don't feel safe or you don't like them, you won't want to go back." Another woman explained, "If I get sick between visits I want to feel that [my doctors] care and are interested. It is very important to me."

The prevalent clinic approach to CF treatment can seem more like being processed than being cared for to an adult never before treated for a chronic disease. One man responded to a trial visit to a CF center which offered adult care within a pediatric setting. "These CF factories, factories, they see 10, 20, 30 CF kids a day. They just bring them in and turn them out." He opted instead to receive his care from a pulmonologist in private practice in his community. A woman commented that at her CF center she felt "pushed aside and brushed through like cattle."

Craving CF Information. Participants expressed frustration that they were either given no information on CF at the time of their diagnosis or were provided with cartoons directed to a pediatric audience. Few adult-focused materials were available and nothing for those diagnosed as adults. "It seems there is not enough information for me to research on my own out there. I want to know about adult stuff," said one man. A woman wanted directions on how to do chest percussion; she was given was a booklet with illustrations of an infant.

Participants were not particularly interested in biomedical descriptions of CF, or even in instructions on self-care. One man explained, "We need more on everyday stuff." A woman lamented that her CF education involved "technical things" and "nothing about what life would be like." Participants wanted information on longevity, treatment options, and research directions, information that would help them construct hope. "I want to know . . . how not to think I am going to die soon so often," wrote a young man. Also, seeing themselves in educational materials helped participants accept having CF. A man diagnosed in his thirties recalled, "We started hitting the books and getting all the information we could about CF. And, um, every single thing about it pertained to me, except in a very mild extent."

Insurance Worries. Many participants felt they had to continue working full-time so as not to lose medical coverage. Or, they felt "trapped" in unsatisfying jobs because they feared their pre-existing condition would prevent them from being covered if they were to move. Others struggled to meet medical co-payments or to afford uncovered prescriptions. Some fought with managed care organizations who refused specialized CF center care, rejected requests for newer models of medical equipment, or denied home care as an option.

DISCUSSION

Each of the ten across-case themes generated from participants' stories describes an essential and important aspect of their individual and collective lived experience of receiving a diagnosis of CF after age 20. But, to understand the breath and depth of their experiences, the themes must be appreciated as an interrelated cluster, each affecting and affected by the others. For instance, individuals' needs to *change* their lifestyles to accommodate CF resulted in their experiencing CF as an *intrusion* which affected the *time* they had available to devote to socialization, resulting in *isolation*. The themes, then, cumulatively and synergistically impacted how the phenomenon was experienced and integrated by any one individual. The stories of the participants also reflected the ways that gender and illness severity mediated and differentiated their experience, giving rise to additional themes.

Thorne and Paterson pointed out that the study of individual diseases yields "a range of experiential features . . . that cannot be captured by a generic orientation to the phenomenon" (2000, p. 8). The contribution of this study has been to describe these as they relate to late-diagnosis in CF. Nine themes, not similarly named or articulated in Conrad's (1987) or Sidell's (1997) overviews of the chronic illness literature, were identified: Difference, Distraction, Family Indifference, Intrusion, Change, Awareness of Death, and Normalization. While these could be conceptualized as similar to or subsumed by themes in these overview articles (e.g., developmental issues or biographical work), there are differences.

For instance, the theme related to family that emerged from this study was very different from the "family relations" themes identified in other research. The family theme in this study reflected indifference and withdrawal. In other studies it described either the effect of chronic disease on families or how families cope with the stresses of caregiving. The findings of this study also demonstrate that disease experiences may vary, even within the same disease. Only two of Tracy's (1997) themes describing the life experience of adults diagnosed with CF as children emerged in this study: difference and wanting to be treated like an individual.

This study was qualitative, descriptive, and exploratory. The cross-case, gender-related, and severity-related themes describe the experiences of the 36 participants and cannot be generalized nor assumed to represent the phenomenon of late diagnosis of CF as it may be experienced by others. Nonetheless, the participants' stories illuminate the heretofore understudied phenomenon of late-diagnosis in CF and suggest foci for exploring other chronic diseases. Additional research is recommended to affirm and "fine tune" the themes generated, assess how men and women experience an adult diagnosis of CF over time, and discover how adults' CF experience and needs are influenced by their age-at-diagnosis.

IMPLICATIONS FOR SOCIAL WORK

The cross-case and other themes identified in this study reflect that those who receive a diagnosis of CF as adults are as concerned about and affected by psychosocial issues as they are bio-medical ones, rendering the social work role on CF teams important and essential. The findings of this study suggest that to meet the diverse and complex needs of those late-diagnosed with CF social workers must (a) reach out to these patients and (b) help colleagues appreciate and respond to the ways in which these patients differ from those diagnosed as children. To do so, social workers must, as Sidell (1997) encouraged, function outside the confines of the medical perspective of the clinic setting and adopt a more client-centered approach.

Most adults who attend CF Centers were diagnosed as children and are familiar with the disease, with clinic routines, and with the roles of team members. Brown, Krieg, and Belluck (1995) recommend that CF team social workers help these patients deal with the cumulative effects of a chronic illness and mobilize coping abilities. Given the findings of this study, however, it is apparent that those late-diagnosed have additional needs and issues.

CF social workers must reach out to the late-diagnosed patients in their clinic populations and make sure they are comfortable and familiar with the clinic setting and the services available to them. In working with these individuals, social workers should draw upon the themes discovered in this study to guide their assessments, anticipate patients' needs, suggest foci for exploration, and to better understand the impact of receiving a late-diagnosis of CF.

However, because CF social workers carry large caseloads, multiple responsibilities, and are engaged in a field that is emotionally exhausting (Coady, Kent, & Davis, 1990), establishing a helping, ongoing relationship with every late-diagnosed man or woman with CF, although ideal, may not be possible. Therefore, to assure that late-diagnosed adults within CF center populations receive comprehensive, integrated, and personalized care, social workers on CF teams should work closely with their professional colleagues, especially physicians, to help them understand the impact of late diagnosis and the challenges that these patients face over time. In addition, social workers should examine their CF Center routines and patient/provider interactional styles from the perspective of those diagnosed as adults and suggest ways in which the CF team can personalize the care they provide. In particular, CF social workers should join with their medical colleagues to locate, or create, educational materials that include content on late-diagnosis and are responsive to issues identified in this study.

NOTE

1. This study was approved by the author's university Institutional Review Board. Individuals' rights as research participants were explained to them, and steps were taken throughout the study to protect their confidentiality and to promote their physical and psychological comfort.

REFERENCES

Abbott, J., Dodd, M., Gee, L., & Webb, K. (2001). Ways of coping with cystic fibrosis: Implications for treatment adherence. *Disability Rehabilitation*, 23, 315-324.
Anderson, D.L., Flume, P.A., & Hardy, K.K. (2001). Psychological functioning of adults with cystic fibrosis. *Chest*, 119, 1079-1074.

Asbring, P. (2001). Chronic illness—a disruption in life: Identity transformation among women with chronic fatigue syndrome and fibromyalgia. *Journal of Advanced Nursing*, 34, 312-319.

Bertram, S., Kurland, M., Lydick, E., Locke, G.R. 3rd, & Yawn, B.P. (2001). The patient's perspective of irritable bowel syndrome. *Journal of Family Practice*, 50, 521-525.

Brown, D.G., Krieg, K., & Belluck, F. (1995). A model for group intervention with the chronically ill: Cystic fibrosis and the family. *Social Work in Health Care*, 21, 81-94.

Charmaz, K. (1990). 'Discovering' chronic illness: Using grounded theory. *Social Science and Medicine*, 30, 1161-1172.

Charmaz, K. (1980). The social construction of self-pity in the chronically ill. *Symbolic Interaction*, 3, 123-145.

Coady, C.A., Kent, V.D. & Davis, P.W. (1990). Burnout among social workers working with cystic fibrosis. *Health and Social Work*, 15, 116-124.

Congleton, J., Hodson, M.E., & Duncan-Skingle, F. (1997). Quality of life in adults with cystic fibrosis. *Thorax*, 52, 397.

Conrad, P. (1987). The experience of illness. In: J.A. Roth & P. Conrad, (Eds.), *The experience and management of chronic illness* (pp. 1-32). Greenwich, CT: JAI Press.

Conway, S.P., Pond, M.N., Hamnett, T., & Watson, A. (1996). Compliance with treatment in adult patients with cystic fibrosis. *Thorax*, 51, 29-33.

Cystic Fibrosis Foundation. (2000). Patient registry 1999 annual data report. Bethesda, MD: Cystic Fibrosis Foundation.

Czajkowski, D., & Koocher, G. (1987). Medical compliance and coping with cystic fibrosis. *Journal of Child Psychology and Psychiatry*, 28, 311-319.

Drey, X., Zinzindohohoue, F., Cuillerier, E., Cugnenc, P.H., Barbier, J.P., & Harteau, P. (1999) Acute pancreatitis revealing cystic fibrosis in an adult. *Gastroenterologie Clinique et Biologique*, 8-9, 974-977.

Eakes, G.G. (1993). Chronic sorrow: A response to living with cancer. *Oncology Nursing Forum*, 20, 1327-1334.

Fiel, S. (1988). Cystic fibrosis in an adult. *Emergency Medicine*, 20, 109-111,114,121.

Gan, K.H., Geus, W.P., Bakker, W., Lamers, C.B., & Heijerman, H.G. (1995). Genetic and clinical features of patients with cystic fibrosis diagnosed after the age of 16 years. *Thorax*, 50, 1301-4.

Gardiner, K., & Cranley, B. (1989). Acute presentation of cystic fibrosis in an adult. *Postgraduate Medical Journal*, 65, 471-472.

Gee, L., Abbott, J., Conway, S.P., Etherington, C., & Webb, A.K. (2000). Development of a disease specific health related quality of life measure for adults and adolescents with cystic fibrosis. *Thorax*, 55, 946-954.

Godbey, J. (1985). Cystic fibrosis in adults. *Journal of the Mississippi State Medical Association*, 26, 161-163.

Hellerstein, H. (1946). Cystic fibrosis of the pancreas in an adult. *Ohio Medical Journal*, 42, 616-617.

Hubert, D., Rivocal, V., Desmazes-Dufeu, N., Lacronique, J., Maurer, C., Richaud-Thiriez, B., & Dusser, D. (2000). Characteristics and specificities of cystic fibrosis in adults: Evolutive disease of childhood or recently diagnosed disease? *Revue des Maladies Respiratoires*, 17, 749-757.

Hunt, B., & Geddes, D. (1984). Newly diagnosed cystic fibrosis in middle and later life. *Thorax*, 40, 23-26.

McCloskey, M., Redmond, A.O., Hill, A., & Elborn, J.S. (2000). Clinical features associated with a delayed diagnosis of cystic fibrosis. *Respiration*, 67, 402-407.

McWilliams, T.J., Wilsher, M.L., & Kolbe, J. (2000). Cystic fibrosis diagnosed in adult patients. *New Zealand Medical Journal*, 113, 6-8.

Petrie, K.J., Buiick, D.L., Weinman, J., & Booth, R.J. (1999). Positive effects of illness reported by myocardial infaction and breast cancer patients. *Journal of Psychosomatic Research*, 47, 537-43.

Shepherd, S., Howell, M., Harwood, I., Granger, L., Hofstetter, C., Molguard, C., & Kaplan, R. (1990). A comparative study of the psychosocial assets of adults with cystic fibrosis and their healthy peers. *Chest*, 97, 1310-1316.

Sidell, N.L. (1997). Adult adjustment to chronic illness: A review of the literature. *Health and Social Work*, 22, 5-11.

Strauss, G., & Wellisch, D. (1981). Psychosocial adaptation in older cystic fibrosis patients. *Journal of Chronic Disease*, 34, 141-146.

Thorne, S., & Paterson, B. (2000). Shifting images of chronic illness. *Image the Journal of Nursing Scholarship*, 30, 173-178.

Tracy, J. (1997). Growing up with chronic illness: The experience of growing up with cystic fibrosis. *Holistic Nursing Practice*, 12, 27-35.

vanBiezen, P., Overbrook, S., & Hevering, C. (1992). Cystic fibrosis in a 70 year-old woman. *Thorax*, 47, 202-203.

Van Manen, M. (1990). *Researching lived experience: Human science for an action sensitive pedagogy*. Albany: SUNY Press.

Vilar, M.E., Najib, N.M., Chowdhry, I., Basssett, C.W., Silverman, B.A,. Giusti, R.J., Rosa, U.W., & Schneider, A.T. (2000) Allergic bronchopulmonary aspergillosis as presenting sign of cystic fibrosis in an elderly man. *Annals of Allergy, Asthma, & Immunology*, 85, 70-73.

Widerman, E., Millner, L., Sexauer, W., & Fiel, S. (2000). Health status and sociodemographic characteristics of adults receiving a cystic fibrosis diagnosis after age 18 years. *Chest*, 118, 427-433.

What Social Workers Can Do About Violence: Learnings from the Lives of 37 Men

Dorothy Van Soest, DSW

SUMMARY. Descriptive results of a study of the lives of 37 men who were executed for capital murder reveal the complex and multi-varied problem of violence at individual, institutional, and societal levels. The role of social workers is discussed in relation to prevention of violent crime rather than focusing on punishment. The study provides support for an anti-death penalty policy stance by the social work profession. *[Article copies available for a fee from The Haworth Document Delivery Service: 1-800-HAWORTH. E-mail address: <docdelivery@haworthpress.com> Website: <http://www.HaworthPress.com> © 2004 by The Haworth Press, Inc. All rights reserved.]*

KEYWORDS. Capital punishment, anti-death penalty, prevention of violent crime, multi-level nature of violence

---

Dorothy Van Soest is Dean and Professor, School of Social Work, University of Washington, 4101 15th Avenue N.E., Seattle, WA 98105-6299 USA (E-mail: dorothyv@u.washington.edu).

This paper was presented at the Third International Conference on Social Work in Health and Mental Health, July 1-5, 2001, Tampere, Finland.

[Haworth co-indexing entry note]: "What Social Workers Can Do About Violence: Learnings from the Lives of 37 Men." Van Soest, Dorothy. Co-published simultaneously in *Social Work in Health Care* (The Haworth Social Work Practice Press, an imprint of The Haworth Press, Inc.) Vol. 39, No. 3/4, 2004, pp. 435-453; and: *Social Work Visions from Around the Globe: Citizens, Methods, and Approaches* (ed: Anna Metteri et al.) The Haworth Social Work Practice Press, an imprint of The Haworth Press, Inc., 2004, pp. 435-453. Single or multiple copies of this article are available for a fee from The Haworth Document Delivery Service [1-800-HAWORTH, 9:00 a.m. - 5:00 p.m. (EST). E-mail address: docdelivery@haworthpress.com].

http://www.haworthpress.com/web/SWHC
© 2004 by The Haworth Press, Inc. All rights reserved.
Digital Object Identifier: 10.1300/J010v39n03_13

435

INTRODUCTION

Capital punishment, more than any other public issue, has given rise to considerable differences of opinion within U.S. society. Although the Supreme Court struck down the death penalty as unconstitutional in 1972, several states subsequently passed new laws that the Supreme Court ruled as constitutional in 1976. Executions across the country were resumed in 1977. By 1998, death penalty laws existed in 38 states and under federal and military law. In reality, the death penalty has been found to be administered in the U.S. today much the same way as it was in 1972 (Amnesty International, 1998). In relying on the death penalty, the U.S. is out of step with much of the world; 108 countries and territories have reduced or eliminated the death penalty, and only 87 still use it (Amnesty International, 1998). While the pace of executions increases, pressures are again mounting to abolish the death penalty. Undoubtedly, this public issue will continue to be debated with legislative and legal actions changing with political climates over time.

The debate is fueled by fears of the U.S. public, instilled by heinous violent crimes that capture media attention. The response is often a tendency to look for a quick fix and, thus, deterrence through harsh punishment has become a preferred prevention strategy in spite of evidence of its lack of success (Bailey & Peterson, 1994). A collective attitude of zero tolerance toward youth has also developed in recent years. This is reflected in a transformation of many educational and criminal justice systems toward punishment and away from prevention and rehabilitation and calls for applying the death penalty at younger ages.

This article is based on the premise that social work as a profession has a responsibility to challenge capital punishment as a practice that is in opposition to its fundamental values and ethics. Descriptive results of a study that aimed to understand personal and environmental factors in the lives of men who murdered and who were subsequently executed are presented. The study investigated the lives of 37 men who were executed for capital murder by the state of Texas in 1997, with a focus on those who committed crimes characterized by extreme rage, violence, and lack of remorse. The article first presents the conceptual framework upon which the study is grounded and describes the research methodology. Descriptive results are then presented and discussed. The goal of the article is to promote informed discussion related to the death penalty and to support prevention as an alternative.

CONCEPTUAL FRAMEWORK

The study of 37 men is based on a belief that part of the answer to violent crime prevention is to understand the route that those who have committed violent crimes have traveled. Violence was broadly defined as any act or situation that injures the health and well-being of others, including direct attacks on a person's physical or psychological integrity and destructive actions that do not necessarily involve a direct relationship between the victims and the institution or persons responsible for the harm (Van Soest & Bryant, 1995). The study is grounded in the notion that risk factors for violence are multi-level in nature at individual, institutional, and structural/cultural levels and that the levels are inseparable from each other and form an intractable cycle of violence (Van Soest, 1997; Van Soest & Bryant, 1995).

At the individual level of violence are individually oriented harmful actions against persons or property. This is the level that is most often considered and quickly condemned. Violence at this level is the most visible and easiest to assess, since it usually involves direct actions and means and immediate consequences. When politicians talk about the problem of violence, they are talking about this level of crime, murder, rape, battery, robbery, assault, etc. The capital crimes committed by the men in the current study belong at the individual level of violence, as do many of the risk factors they experienced at different stages of their lives. These include violent actions against the murderers by others, often when they were children (e.g., physical and sexual abuse, physical and emotional neglect, parental and peer rejection); harmful actions by the murderers against others (e.g., bullying, sexual assault, domestic violence); and harmful actions by the murderers against themselves (e.g., suicide attempts, substance abuse).

Violence at the individual level, however, is only the tip of the iceberg. An institutional level of violence is submerged from view so that its forms are almost completely invisible. Violence at this level includes harmful actions carried out by social institutions and their agents that obstruct the spontaneous unfolding of human potential. Institutional violence occurs in prisons, juvenile detention facilities, governmental bodies, corporations, the military, and–the institution with which social workers work most often–the family. The institutional level is equally as important to our understanding of violence and how to prevent it as knowing that it occurs at the individual level; as Gilligan (1996) points out, human violent action "is also, unavoidably, familial, societal, and institutional" (p. 7). Thus, the study of 37 men investigated risk factors for violence such as interventions and access to formal and informal helping systems at the institutional level. Risk factors at this level can involve either harmful actions (e.g., physical abuse, inappropriate, and punitive punishment in school) or a failure to intervene at different developmental stages (e.g., lack of child protective services, failure to provide special education).

The third level of violence is a firmly embedded foundation containing the normative/ideological roots of violence that under gird and give rise to the other levels. Any microcosm of individual and institutional levels of violence can only be understood fully when it is "seen as part of the macrocosm, the culture and history of violence, in which it occurs" (Gilligan, 1996, p. 15). It is at the structural/cultural level where normative and ideological roots of violence reside in the form of a comprehensive worldview that reveals itself in beliefs about race and gender superiority, an easy acceptance of the threat or use of violence as a form of social control (e.g., murder by lethal injection used to enforce the death penalty), an appropriate solution to problems (e.g., police force, war), and a form of entertainment (violence in television, film, and videogames). Conventional values at this level include ideas about male behavior and how boys should be socialized to become men. The impact of male socialization, not only on what children are exposed to but how they handle risk and stress, may be a significant contextual risk factor (Canada, 1995; Garbarino, 1999; Levant et al., 1992; Scher, 1980; Sones Feinberg, 1996). Thus, the study explored questions about the men who were executed for capital murder related to socialization processes coupled with childhood victimization.

Violence was conceptualized as being of three distinct types, each of which occurs at the individual, institutional, and cultural levels. The violence of omission involves not providing help to people in need or danger; e.g., failing to address issues of domestic violence or not providing help for students with learning disabilities. Repressive violence includes infractions of civil, political, economic, and social rights of individuals or groups; e.g., murder and physical assault, differential punishment for a person who is a member of a marginalized population compared with the punishment conferred on a person of the dominant group. Alienating violence deprives people of higher rights, such as the right to emotional, cultural, or intellectual growth; e.g., denigrating another person's cultural identity.

THE STUDY QUESTIONS

This study investigated lifelong personal and environmental factors influencing men executed for capital murder. In the first phase of the study, the following questions were explored: How did the men get from birth to committing a violent crime that resulted in their execution? How do their stories vary depending on the nature of the murder committed? What constellation of risk factors did they experience at individual, institutional, and societal/cultural levels?

RESEARCH METHODOLOGY

A two-tiered qualitative multifactor research design was used to examine the lives of 37 men who were executed in Texas in 1997. Using a purposive sampling technique based on the best opportunity to learn, cases of inmates executed in a single year in a single state were selected. Since the resumption of the death penalty in the United States in the late 1970s, Texas has accounted for more than one-third of all executions (Graczyk, 1999) and Texas led the nation in the number of executions in 1997. The state of Texas and the year 1997 were thus selected, which resulted in the sample of 37 men who include all those executed by Texas in that year. The sample was selected for several reasons: The 37 men represent 50% of the total number of people executed in the United States in 1997 (n = 74) and 25.6% of the total number executed by Texas from 1977 to 1997 (n = 144); the number and variety of those executed in a one-year time frame in one state provide an opportunity to look for themes among a substantial and diverse population within a manageable geographic area; and the accessibility of data.

Data Collection

There were two levels of data collection. The first level included public information such as reports introduced and testimony given at trial for each of the 37 men (both state and defense evidence), appeal documents, and information related to psychiatric, psychological, neurologic, medical, social service, welfare, school, probation, police, prison, and military records. In addition, web searches yielded media reports in newspapers and television shows related to the crimes, executions, and the lives of the men in the study. The second level of data collection included prison packets for each of the 37 men, containing their social and criminal histories. A Social Summary is completed by nonprofessional staff at the Texas Department of Criminal Justice (TDCJ) Unit Administration and Treating Departments within two weeks of an inmate's assignment to death row. These summaries provided information related to family, marriage, and children and inmate's statement about the nature of his familial relationships; physical and mental health history; educational, employment, and military histories; and involvement with the criminal justice system. The prison packets also included a FBI report that includes a list of all arrests, charges, and date and type of disposition for each arrest. Prison packets are kept in files at the TDCJ in Huntsville, Texas. In order to obtain the packets, a Request for Permission to Conduct Research in the TDCJ was submitted and permission obtained.

The range of available documents enabled the research team to practice triangulation, that is, to examine a single phenomenon from more than one vantage point (Schwandt, 1997). Several types of triangulation identified by Denzin (1978) were incorporated to enhance the rigor of the study. The first was data triangulation, which is defined as the use of more than one data source. While the two levels of data collection relied solely on available records and media reports, the data within the records were triangulated since the documents were collected from different sources representing various viewpoints, such as witnesses for the defense and prosecution. This proved to be invaluable, as the sources of the documents tended to present a different perspective in order to substantiate their own agendas. Observer triangulation was achieved by having multiple readers and coders for each data file.

Data Analysis

The unit of analysis used in this study was predominantly demographics and events. After a through reading of the cases and the pertinent literature, 93 variables were identified and a codebook developed. The frequency of each variable was then counted based upon the presence-absence of particular content (Berelson, 1952); for example, the presence or absence of a criminal history was noted rather than counting the often-conflicting number of arrests.

Problems with reliability and validity in content analysis usually "grow out of the ambiguity of word meanings or the ambiguity of category definitions or other coding rules" (Weber, 1985, p. 15). In this study these concerns were addressed by establishing a definition for each variable. One case was selected for testing the coding by all four members of the research team in order to obtain an interrater reliability. The first measure of interrater reliability was calculated at 72%. According to Rubin and Babbie (1997), an 80% rating is preferred with 70% agreement considered acceptable. In order to increase the interrater reliability, the definition for each variable was further refined and it was decided that two different coders would rate every case. Subsequent interrater reliabilities increased to 90%. In order to assist with data management and data reduction, as well as produce descriptive statistics, the data were coded in a format that allowed data entry into SPSS.

Based on their criminal histories and facts of the capital murder(s), each of the 37 men was assigned one of two possible criminal categories based on severity of violence and presence or absence of remorse. Category 1 includes particularly heinous criminal histories characterized by rage, intense violence, lack of remorse, and sadism (e.g., victim-degrading, getting pleasure from inflicting pain); Category 2 includes both a more murky representation of serious violence but without the horrendous, victim-degrading quality of the first category and with evidence of some sense of conscience or remorse and criminal histories characterized mostly by property crimes without intentional harm to people (e.g., one murderer panicked during a robbery and shot the victim while attempting to flee). Three reviewers independently ranked each of the 37 men by qualitatively analyzing the facts of the crime and the criminal history data in each case file. In the few cases where there was a disparity in rankings, the reviewers discussed their rationale and consensus was reached through further analysis. Twenty-three of the men were determined to be in Category 1 and 14 in Category 2. Cases in the two categories were compared to discern any differences between the most serious violent criminal profiles and the others.

RESULTS

Descriptive Results

The men in the study include 22 Caucasians (59.5%), 13 African Americans (35.1%), and 2 Latinos (5.4%). Table 1 shows that the demographic characteristics of the 37 men executed in Texas are similar to all those who were executed in the U.S. (n = 74) and to all prisoners under sentence of death in the United States (n = 3,335) in 1997. Virtually all of those sentenced to death are male and a disproportionate number are Black or Hispanic. This racial disparity is consistent with the overall picture of who has been on death row at any given time since the revival of the death penalty in the mid-1970s: About half of those on death row at any given time have been black (U.S. General Accounting Office, 1990). While Table 1 does not show the demographics related to the

TABLE 1. Demographic Characteristics of Prisoners Under Sentence of Death in the U.S. and Those Executed in 1997

Characteristic	Prisoners under sentence of death in 1997			Prisoners executed in 1997		
	U.S.*		U.S.*		Texas	
	n = 3,335		n = 74		n = 37	
	n	%	n	%	N	%
Gender						
Male	3,291	98.7	74	100	37	100
Female	43	1.3				
Race						
White	1,878	56.3	45	60.8	22	59.5
Black	594	42.2	27	36.5	13	35.1
Other	53	1.6	2	2.7	2	5.4
Hispanic Origin						
Hispanic	307	9.2	2	2.7	2	5.4
Non-Hispanic	3,028	90.8	72	97.3	35	94.6

* Source: U.S. Department of Justice (Dec. 1998). Capital punishment 1997. Bureau of Justice Statistics: Bulletin.

murder victims, a U.S. General Accounting Office (1990) report of empirical studies on racism and the death penalty showed that if the murder victim is white, the killer is treated much more severely than if the victim is Black. Almost all death sentences in the U.S. (82%) involve white victims, and the report concluded that our criminal justice system essentially reserves the death penalty for murderers (regardless of their race) who kill white victims. Just ten years ago, it was a fact that no white person had ever received the death penalty for killing a black person in this country. However, now the statistics show that of all the white murderers (n = 178) executed between 1977 and 1995, only three had been convicted of killing a victim of color (U.S. Department of Justice, 1997). This racial disparity is true of the murders in this study as well, with most of the murder victims having been white.

In Table 2, characteristics of the men who committed the most heinous category of crimes (n = 23) are compared with those of the men who committed less heinous crimes (n = 14). The men who committed the most heinous crimes were more likely to be white, to have used multiple weapons, and to have sexually assaulted their victims, while the men who committed less heinous crimes were more likely to have murdered in the course of committing a robbery. Those who committed the most heinous crimes were more likely to have experienced the following risk factors: poverty; victims of childhood physical, sexual, and emotional abuse; victims of childhood physical/emotional neglect; post-traumatic stress disorder; alcohol abuse and alcohol/drug abuse

TABLE 2. Characteristics of Sample by Category

Characteristic	Total n = 37		Heinous Crimes n = 23		Less Heinous Crimes n = 14	
	N	%	n	%	n	%
Race						
White*	22	59.5	16	69.6	6	42.9
Black	13	35.1	6	26.1	7	50.0
Other	2	5.4	1	4.3	1	7.1
Nature of Capital Crime						
Involved robbery	22	59.5	11	47.8	11	78.6
Involved sexual assault*	16	43.2	15	65.2	1	7.1
Used multiple weapons*	13	35.1	11	47.8	2	14.3
Socioeconomic Status						
Low/poverty*	14	37.8	11	47.8	3	21.4
Other	23	62.2	12	52.2	11	78.6
Attachment Variables						
Change in primary care-taker in first 5 years	13	35.1	8	34.8	5	35.7
Temporary separation	7	18.9	4	17.4	3	21.4
Loss of significant person	21	56.8	14	60.9	7	50.5
Violence Victimization						
Physical abuse*	20	54.0	15	65.2	5	35.7
Sexual abuse*	8	21.6	8	34.7	0	0
Emotional abuse*	9	21.6	6	26.1	2	14.3
Physical/emotional neglect*	6	16.2	6	26.1	0	0
Perpetrator of Violence						
Sexual abuse*	14	37.8	12	52.2	2	14.3
Physical abuse	15	43.2	10	43.5	6	42.9
Domestic violence*	10	27.0	8	34.8	2	14.3
Trauma Variables						
Witnessed domestic violence	8	21.6	5	21.7	3	21.4
Medical trauma	6	16.2	5	21.7	1	7.1
Victim of violence (extra familial)	9	24.3	6	26.1	3	21.4
PTSD*	10	27.0	8	34.7	2	14.2
Physical & Mental Health						
Chronic health problems	7	18.9	5	21.7	2	14.3
Alcohol abuse*	29	78.3	20	87.0	9	64.3
Substance abuse*	33	89.2	20	87.0	13	92.8
History of selling drugs	10	27.0	6	26.1	4	28.6
History of suicide attempts	9	24.3	6	26.1	3	21.4
Hospitalized-mental illness	9	24.3	6	26.1	3	21.4
Hospitalized-drug-related	10	27.0	5	21.7	5	35.7
Hallucinations*	5	13.5	4	17.4	1	7.1
Brain dysfunction*	10	29.7	8	34.8	3	21.4
Family History						
Family alcohol/drugs*	16	45.9	13	56.5	4	28.6
Mental illness in family	3	8.1	2	8.7	1	7.1
Criminal behavior of family member	13	35.1	6	26.1	7	50.0
Parental incarceration*	4	10.8	4	17.4	0	0
Educational History						
Illiterate	7	18.9	5	21.7	2	14.3
Dropped out of H.S.	31	83.8	19	82.6	12	85.7
Special education classes	6	16.2	4	17.4	2	14.3
Mental retardation*	8	21.6	7	30.4	1	7.1
School behavior problems**	14	37.8	7	30.4	7	50.0
Bullied peers**	5	10.8	1	4.3	3	21.4
Employment History						
Unskilled labor	24	67.6	15	65.2	10	71.4
History of erratic employment	27	73.0	18	78.3	9	64.3
Served in military	10	27.0	7	30.4	3	21.4
Criminal History						
Juvenile criminal history**	32	86.5	18	78.3	14	100
Adult criminal history**	35	94.6	21	91.3	14	100

* Variables related to most heinous crimes
** Variables related to less heinous crimes

both by themselves and by family members; hallucinations and organic brain dysfunction; parental incarceration; and mental retardation. They were also more likely to have been perpetrators of sexual abuse and domestic violence. The men who committed less heinous crimes, on the other hand, were more likely to have bullied their peers, and men who bullied their peers were more likely to have profiles that include being Black, a high school dropout, and having a juvenile criminal history and attachment disruptions with significant people in their lives.

Both categories of men had high rates of substance abuse. Twenty to thirty percent of the 37 men were reported to have exhibited first signs of trouble including alcohol, drugs, and school behavior problems by age 11. By age 15, over 60% were reported to have alcohol and drug problems, and over 70% exhibited school behavior problems or other signs of trouble. However, there were differences between the two groups of men related to ages of onset of risk variables. Substance abuse manifested itself at a younger age in the men who committed the most heinous crimes. The mean age for onset of alcohol abuse was 12.6 years for men in Category 1 compared with 14.3 years for men in Category 2 and the mean age for onset of drug abuse for men in Category 1 was 13.9 compared with 16 for men in Category 2. On the other hand, men who committed the most heinous crimes, when compared with those who committed less heinous crimes, were older at onset of school behavior problems (mean = 14 years of age compared with mean = 12.8), first report of trouble (mean = 14.6 compared with mean = 13.4), and first criminal offense (mean = 18.8 compared with mean = 15.6).

DISCUSSION

The most striking portrayal that emerges of the men in this study is the prevalence of violence in many of their lives. This was often true beginning at a young age, when many of them were victimized by multiple forms of violence, and continued to be true to the end, when they committed the violence of murder and their lives were ultimately ended by the State. Violence seems to be a particularly predominant theme in the lives of the men who committed the most heinous crimes. Preliminary results suggest that, of the men for whom there is evidence of childhood sexual abuse and emotional or physical neglect, all of them were among the group that committed the most heinous crimes. Of 20 men for whom there is evidence of childhood physical abuse, 15 went on to commit the most heinous crimes. Boys who were victims of sexual abuse seem to grow into men who are sexual abuse perpetrators, which supports the poignant observation that "violence, like charity, begins at home" (Gilligan, 1996, p. 5) as well as the age-old adage that violence breeds violence.

Yet, not all victims of childhood abuse grow up to commit heinous crimes. Violence is "more complicated, ambiguous and, most of all, tragic, than is commonly realized or acknowledged" (Gilligan, 1996, p. 5). Preliminary results of this study suggest that multiple risk factors, operating in clusters at particular stages of the life cycle, may culminate in what may seem to be a senseless act of violence but which, when understood within the context of life circumstances, becomes not only eminently rational but perhaps also even predictable. Several risk factors related to the lives of the men who committed the most heinous crimes are suggested by the data. Several of them are consistent with the risk factors identified by Loeber and Farrington (1997) as being associated with serious and violent juvenile offenders.

More in-depth data need to be collected and analyzed to understand trauma experiences associated with combinations of neglect, abuse, and other indicators. Of particular relevance for further study and analysis is Lewis et al.'s (1997) finding of reported conditions that might be associated with remorseless murder, such as being able to block out physical pain and experiencing trance-like states in adulthood. For some of the executed murderers in this study, the level of abuse they experienced was similar to the kind described by Lewis et al. (1997) as "torture." Lack of remorse may be related to the self-protective mechanism of "shutting down" when faced with such life-threatening situations. This may result in loss of any memory of the pain or fear and denial of reality that may lead to an inability to feel pain for self or others as an adult. Studies of dissociative identity disorders among murderers suggest a linkage between the traumatizing experience of childhood victimization and a kind of "shutting down" that manifests itself in the development of one or more personalities, absence of memory of the trauma, or minimizing or denying any pain (Carlisle, 1991; Coons, 1991; Lewis et al., 1997). The role of male socialization, as a factor in shutting out feelings of pain, needs to be investigated further as well (Canada, 1995; Garbarino, 1999; Gilligan, 1996).

Another interesting finding is the age at onset of first sign of troubled behavior. By age 15, a very high percentage (over 60%) of all of the men had been identified as having some kind of problem. The significance of the developmental stage between ages 11 and 15 and the importance of identifying risk factors and implementing effective interventions has been well documented (Loeber & Farrington, 1997; Loeber & Stouthamer-Loeber, 1986). Results of the current study also suggest differences in both the kinds of problems manifested and the age of onset for the men who committed the most heinous compared with those who committed less heinous crimes. Men who committed the less heinous crimes may have exhibited more overt and detectable behavioral problems (such as school behavior problems or arrests) at a younger age, while those who committed the most heinous crimes may have more quietly withdrawn through the use of alcohol or drugs at a younger age. While alcohol and drug abuse seems to have been rampant among all the men, results suggest that men who committed the most heinous crimes began using alcohol and drugs at younger ages, which may be reflective of trying to cope with other risk factors.

Other differences between the two categories of men merit serious attention. The men who committed the most heinous crimes were more likely to be victims of sexual abuse, and men who were sexually abused were more likely to have profiles that included being Caucasian, experiences of childhood victimizations that included both abuse and neglect, and a range of health and mental health problems. On the other hand, the men who committed less heinous crimes were more likely to have bullied their peers, and men who bullied their peers were more likely to have profiles that include being Black, a high school dropout, and having a juvenile criminal history and attachment disruptions with significant people in their lives. These two profiles seem to show that Black men were executed by the state of Texas in 1997 for less heinous crimes than those committed by white men. While this is a serious charge, it is consistent with the history of the death penalty in the U.S. that shows that it has been applied in a racist manner (Amnesty International, 1998, p. 109).

The two profiles also suggest different behavioral manifestations during childhood that would predictably give rise to different interventions. Within a societal and institutional context characterized by racism and an emphasis on controlling behavior, it seems reasonable to speculate that boys with profiles similar to the first one might not be identified as having problems or whose problems might be overlooked or excused. In fact, there is almost no evidence of interventions by institutions such as child protective services, mental health agencies, schools, or churches when this group of men were children. At the institutional level, the type of violence most prevalent seems to have been the violence of omission, a failure to help or to intervene. The family as an institution, in the lives of these boys, was often the perpetrator of violence against them.

It further seems reasonable to speculate that boys with the second profile tend to elicit more negative interventions that could be characterized more as a criminalization response than a helping response. In fact, a recent study sponsored by the U.S. Justice Department found that Black and Hispanic youths are treated more severely than white teenagers charged with comparable crimes at every step of the juvenile justice system (Poe-Yamagata & Jones, 2000). This includes adjudicating Black youth as adults at an astoundingly higher rate than white youth and administering the death penalty. Currently, there are 29 people on death row in Texas who were younger than 18 at the time of the crime, and 23 of them (79%) are minorities (11 African Americans and 12 Latinos) (Death Penalty Information Center, 2000). Results of this study are seen to illustrate how violence at the individual level is dealt with differentially by institutions based on hidden criteria grounded in the structural/cultural level of beliefs based on an ideology of race superiority.

What seems to be clear from the preliminary findings is that a complex of multiple events, environmental conditions, socialization influences, and individual characteristics may converge in powerful constellations, resulting in a violent outcome. Children can usually handle one stressor in their lives, even if it is chronic. But when negative conditions pile up, the rate of maladjustment is multiplied (Capaldi & Patterson, 1991; Sameroff et al., 1993). This study of the lives of 37 executed men suggests complex and multi-varied problems at the individual, institutional, and societal levels. At the individual level were the acts of violence the men committed against others and against themselves. Life stories portray histories of multiple types of violence against them as children at both individual and institutional levels. A too frequent pattern of physical and sexual abuse was found within the family as an institution. At the institutional level, the most frequent type of violence outside the family institution seems to have been the violence of omission, a failure to detect and to help. For the boys of color, interventions by the juvenile justice system can be suspected as possibly including the other two types of violence: repression and alienation. The differential application of both interventions and the death penalty itself illustrates the structural level of violence with its hierarchical ordering of people.

LIMITATIONS OF THE STUDY

One limitation of the study is that the cases chosen reflect a selection bias since whether a person receives a sentence of life in prison or the death sentence is based upon many biases of the legal system (Farr, 1997; International Commission of Jurists, 1997), and men who were not executed were not included in the study. However, representativeness was not a goal since emphasis of the study was on what the particular cases could teach us rather than generalizing to the prison population of those who commit murder.

Another limitation was the lack of depth of information available in the case records. Some records were incomplete and sometimes superficial. For example, the social summary completed in prison was compiled using a form that captured only quick, short answers. Rarely were the inmates' own words used. Additional questions and probes were either not utilized and/or not recorded. Without in-depth description, resorting to particularistic categories and variables became necessary.

IMPLICATIONS FOR SOCIAL WORK PRACTICE AND POLICY

While the results of this study are preliminary and descriptive, they suggest a chain of multiple risk factors and events that, when linked together in complex configurations, can create people who commit dangerous and violent acts. The study has implications for social work practice related to prevention and intervention programs at each stage of the life cycle. When people look at someone who has committed a particularly heinous crime, they see the finished product at the end of a lengthy developmental process. Lonnie Athens (1992), in a book about his theory building research on how people who engage in dangerous, violent crimes are created, writes:

> When people look at a dangerous violent criminal at the beginning of his developmental process rather than at the very end of it, they will see, perhaps unexpectedly, that the dangerous violent criminal began as a relatively benign human being for whom they would probably have more sympathy than antipathy. Perhaps more importantly, people will conclude that the creation of dangerous violent criminals is largely preventable, as is much of the human carnage, which follows in the wake of their birth. Therefore, if society fails to take any significant steps to stop the process behind

the creation of dangerous violent criminals, it tacitly becomes an accomplice in creating them. (p. 6)

The life stories of the 37 men in this study point to the need to focus on prevention activities at the front end rather than the death penalty at the end of a series of violent events that have culminated in the act of murder. Social workers are uniquely situated to promote and engage in interventions that could break the chain of events leading to violent crime at any of several links. The first links related to prevention occur during the prenatal stage of the life cycle, followed by infancy and early childhood. Social workers should promote pre-natal and early infancy programs for parents at the earliest point possible. What is striking about the stories of the 37 men in this study is the apparent lack of interventions by helping professionals, not only at infancy but at all stages of the life cycle.

School social workers are in a particularly key position to intervene at all levels of the educational system. By exploring the prevalence of behaviors and risk factors that could be identified during the early school years, they can recommend ways to assess the nature and severity of problems at a younger age, before a child reaches adolescence, and recommend community-based interventions. The high rate of alcohol and drug abuse found in this study suggests that social workers need to be aware of the use of alcohol or other drugs at a young age as a way to self-medicate symptoms of underlying problems such as physical or sexual abuse, neglect, or psychiatric symptoms. It also points to the need for chemical dependency treatment at younger ages.

During adolescence, individualized intervention approaches are needed that differentiate teenage boys by risk profile. The current investigation suggests varied life histories and risk factors related to the race/ethnicity of the men in the study and raises questions that social workers need to conscientiously address. What role does racism play in the type of intervention selected and the outcome? Do boys who are labeled as troublemakers eventually believe that they *are* troublemakers and continue to put themselves in risky situations (like robbing a store)? On the other hand, do boys who are quiet sufferers of abuse attempt suicide, use drugs and alcohol to numb their pain, and eventually explode in a violent and deadly rage? Some of the questions raised by the current study seem counter to the conventional idea that boys who act out and bully others are those most at risk. Recent incidents of youth violence, such as that committed by the Columbine High School killers, cast similar doubt on such conventional wisdom.

450 Social Work Visions from Around the Globe: Citizens, Methods, and Approaches

The current study provides support for an anti-death penalty policy stance by the social work profession based on two arguments. The first is that some child victims grow up to victimize and, in such cases, capital punishment can be seen as the final victimization and failure of society. While most people who were victims of violence as children do not commit dangerous crimes, all of the men in this study who committed the most heinous crimes were wounded child victims who grew up to victimize in horrendous ways. With increased knowledge about the etiology of particularly heinous crimes, social workers can shift the debate to include calls for more effective prevention programs and resources. Social workers should clearly take the second position in Garbarino's (1999) articulation of two sides of the debate:

> On one side stands a simple moralism that says if kids can kill, kids should die (or at least serve long prison terms), as if they were adults. On the other side stands an impulse to understand and, if understanding is possible, to rescue the troubled and hurt child from inside the killer. (p. 21)

The second argument in support of a professional anti-death penalty stance is related to evidence of racism and classism in the system. In the current study the men who committed less heinous crimes, and were more likely to be Black, received the same penalty (death) as the men who committed the most heinous crimes, who were more likely to be White and of lower socioeconomic status. This finding is consistent with studies that reveal that the likelihood of receiving a death sentence is several times higher if the defendant is Black (Amnesty International, 1998). As U.S. Supreme Court Justice Blackmun contended in 1994: "race continues to play a major role in determining who shall live and who shall die" (cited in Amnesty International, 1998, p. 108).

Social workers as individuals and through their professional organizations can work to eliminate capital punishment and play a role in expanding the public debate to include discussion about the need for more focused and effective violence prevention policies and programs. They can support calls for a moratorium on the death penalty. Professional social work organizations can adopt anti-death penalty policies. Social workers can also do mitigation work at the penalty phase of capital trials after a jury has found the accused guilty of a murder under aggravating circumstances. During this phase of trial, the jury can hear any mitigating evidence that would justify a life sentence rather than execution. Social workers are well qualified to become part of the defense team by investigating the life history of the person found guilty and helping to explain the relationship of that evidence to the offense. Finally, it is important to consider how to move social workers back into the corrections system where they can influence reform and work to shift the focus from punishment to rehabilitation and healing (Casarjian, 1995).

CONCLUSIONS

This study of the lives of 37 executed men shows how complex and multi-varied the problems of violence are at the individual, institutional, and societal levels. The preliminary study results demonstrate this with documentation of physical and sexual abuse at the individual and institutional levels and racism at the structural/cultural level. By examining the root causes of violent crime, we are not suggesting that violent behavior should go unpunished. The need for this caveat is clearly articulated by Garbarino (1999):

> Sometimes as I listen to people talk about violent youth, I doubt that they really want to understand the dangers that our boys face and to make sense of how their violent acts flow from their experiences in our society. Sometimes it seems that few people really care about hurt little boys who have grown up to be violent teenagers, except as potential threats to the community. It is as if we want to forget how they got to be kids who kill in the first place. We are willing to incarcerate them but not to understand them. Perhaps we feel that understanding them is unnecessary because punishment is the only issue, or perhaps we feel that an attempt to understand them is dangerous because it might excuse their actions. (p. 20)

Rather than look for excuses or justifications for violent behavior, what is being suggested is that punishment should not be our sole response to violent crime. It makes more sense to prevent someone from committing violent crime than it does to further violence on a state level through use of the death penalty after the fact. Social workers have a unique understanding that they bring to their work with children, adolescents, and adults in schools and agencies. We need to bring that unique understanding to criminal justice issues as well.

REFERENCES

Amnesty International (1998). *United States of America: Rights for all*. London: Amnesty International Publications.

Athens, L. (1992). *The creation of dangerous violent criminals*. Urbana and Chicago: University of Illinois Press.

Bailey, W.C. & Peterson, R.D. (1994). Murder, capital punishment, and deterrence: A review of the evidence and an examination of police killings. *Journal of Social Issues, 50* (2), 53-75.

Berelson, B. (1952). *Content analysis in communication research*. NY: Hafner Publishing Co.

Canada, G. (1995). *Fist, stick, knife, gun: A personal history of violence in America*. Boston: Beacon Press.

Capaldi, D.M., & Patterson, G.R. (1991). Relation of parental transitions to boys' adjustment problems: I. A linear hypothesis. II. Mothers at risk for transitions and unskilled parenting. *Developmental Psychology, 27*, 489-504.

Carlisle, A.L. (1991). Dissociation & violent criminal behavior. *Journal Contemporary Criminal Justice, 4*, 273-285.

Casarjian, R. (1995). *Houses of healing: A prisoner's guide to inner power and freedom*. Boston, MA: Lionheart Press.

Coons, P.M. (1991). Iatrogenesis and malingering of multiple personality disorder in the forensic evaluation of homicide defendants. *Psychiatric Clinician North America, 14*, 757-768.

Death Penalty Information Center (2000, November 10). *Facts about the death penalty*. www.deathpenaltyinfo.org

Denzin, N.K. (1978). *The research act: A theoretical introduction to sociological methods* (2nd Ed.). New York: McGraw-Hill.

Farr, K.A. (1997). Aggravating and differentiating factors in the cases of white and minority women on death row. *Crime & Delinquency, 43*(3), 260-278.

Garbarino, J. (1999). *Lost boys: Why our sons turn violent and how we can save them*. New York: The Free Press.

Gilligan, J. (1996). *Violence: Reflections on a national epidemic*. New York: Vintage Books.

Graczyk, M. (1999, August 2). State set to execute 6 killers as it closes in on 1997 record. *Houston Chronicle*, pp. 9A, 19A.

International Commission of Jurists. (1997). Administration of the death penalty in the United States. *Human Rights Quarterly, 19*, 165-213.

Levant, R.F., Hirsch, L.S., Celentano, F., Cozza, T.M., Hill, S., MacEachern, M., Marty, N., & Schendker, J. (1992). The male role: An investigation of contemporary norms. *Journal of Mental Health Counseling, 14*, 325-337.

Lewis, D.O., Yeager, C.A., Swica, Y., Pincus, J.H., & Lewis, M. (1997). Objective documentation of child abuse and dissociation in 12 murderers with dissociative identity disorder. *American Journal of Psychiatry, 154* (12), 1703-1710.

Loeber, R. & Farrington, D.P., eds. (1997). *Never too early, never too late: Risk factors and successful interventions for serious and violent juvenile offenders.* Final report of the Study Group on Serious and Violent Juvenile Offenders (grant number 95-JD-FX-0018). Washington, DC: U.S. Department of Justice, Office of Justice Programs, Office of Juvenile Justice and Delinquency Prevention.

Poe-Yamagata, E. & Jones, M. (2000). *And justice for some.* Washington, D.C.: Building Blocks for Youth. <www.buildingblocksforyouth.org/justiceforsome/jfs.html>

Rubin, A. & Babbie, E. (1997). *Research methods for social work* (3rd ed.). Pacific Grove, CA: Brooks/Cole Publishing Company.

Sameroff, A.J., Seifer, R., Baldwin, A., & Baldwin, C. (1993). Stability of intelligence from preschool to adolescence: The influence of social and family risk factors. *Child Development, 64,* 80-97.

Scher, M. (1980). Men and intimacy. *Counseling and Values, 25,* 62-68.

Schwandt, T.A. (1997). *Qualitative inquiry: A dictionary of terms.* Thousand Oaks, CA: Sage.

Sones Feinberg, L. (1996). *Teaching: Innocent fun or sadistic malice?* Far Hills, N.J.: New Horizon Press.

U.S. Department of Justice (1997, December). *Capital punishment 1996,* Bureau of Justice Statistics Bulletin NCJ-167031, Washington, DC.

U.S. General Accounting Office (1990). *Death penalty sentencing: Research indicates pattern of racial disparities, 5,* Washington, DC: GAO.

Van Soest, D. (1997). *The global crisis of violence: Common problems, universal causes, shared solutions.* Washington, DC: NASW Press.

Van Soest, D. & Bryant, S. (1995). Violence reconceptualized for social work: The urban dilemma. *Social Work, 40,* 549-557.

Index

Elderly
participation and citizenship of,
user experiences in Finland,
181-207
advocates for, 198-201
study of
active disengagement in,
197-198
activity of friends or relatives
in, 189-191
advocates in, 198-201
contacting in, 194
cooperation in, 194-195
data from, 186-188
demanding in, 195-197
described, 191-192
disagreement with, 192-193
discussion of, 201-203
dissatisfactory initiation in,
192-193
historical background of,
188-193
method in, 186-188
need for help in, 188-189
negotiation in, 194-195
participation in, 193-198
passive disengagement in,
193-194
personal initiative in,
188-189
in social service system in
Finland, citizenship of,
184-186
EMDR. *See* Eye movement
desensitization reprocessing
(EMDR)
Emotion(s), of HIV seropositive wives
of men with HIV/AIDS,
40-41
Empowerment, in postmodern social
work, 351-352
Ephross, P.H., 293
Ervast, S-A, 151
Escape, as coping mechanism, 34

Ethical issues, in working with
culturally diverse patients
and their families, 249-262.
See also Cultural diversity,
cultural and ethical issues in
working with patients and
their families
"Ethnic discrimination and psychic
illness," 239
Ethnicity
effects on health of minority ethnic
women in Britain, 11-27. *See
also* Health, ethnicity,
gender, and social class
effects on, of minority ethnic
women in Britain
health and, 15-19
Ethnographic assessment, in
postmodern social work,
349-350
Exercise, importance of, adult
diagnosis of cystic fibrosis
and, 427-428
Eye movement desensitization
reprocessing (EMDR), 265

Falck, H.S., 292
Falkov, A., 314, 321
Families for Children with Cancer, 109
Family(ies)
of children with cancer, long-term
psychosocial effects of,
129-149. *See also* Cancer,
diagnosis of, long-term
psychosocial effects on
children and their families
culturally diverse, cultural and
ethical issues in working
with, 249-262. *See also*
Cultural diversity, cultural
and ethical issues in working
with patients and their
families

in, 249-262. *See also*
Culturagram, in promoting
cultural competent practice in
health care settings
in study of health care services of
Canadian urban Aboriginal
persons, 174
Health Departments, in Ukraine,
101-102
Health maintenance organizations
(HMOs), 303
Health Trust, 380,381t
Health-related issues, for families
caring for disabled children at
home in Ukraine, 89-105. *See
also* Ukraine, disabled
children in; Ukraine, families
of disabled children in
Heffernan, S., 131
Herbert, M., 165,290
Herman, J., 268
Hidden Children Hard Words, 322
Higgs, P., 185
HIV. *See* HIV/AIDS; Human
immunodeficiency virus
(HIV)
HIV seropositive wives, of men with
HIV/AIDS, psychosocial
problems and coping patterns
of, 29-47. *See also*
HIV/AIDS, HIV seropositive
wives of men with,
psychosocial problems and
coping patterns of
HIV seropositivity, described, 30
HIV/AIDS
HIV seropositive wives of men with
caregiving by, 39-40
children of, 36-37
coping patterns of, 41
disclosure and social support
stigma, 38-39
emotions of, 40-41
marital relationship of, 37-38

psychosocial problems and
coping patterns of, 29-47
study of
discussion of, 41-44
finances in, 35-36
findings in, 35-41
method in, 33-34
recommendations related
to, 44-45
sample characteristics in,
34-35
quality of life of, 40
receiving by, 39-40
research related to, 31-33
prevention of
attitudes in, 408-409,409t
condoms in, 409-411,410t,412t
counseling in, 407
films in, 406-407
folk media in, 407
group discussions in, 407
knowledge in, 407-408
literature review of, 401-402
programme interventions in,
406-407
sexual behavior in, 411-412,
413t
social vaccine in
introduction to, 400-401
study on truck drivers in
South India,
399-414
social workers in, roles of,
405-406
study of
attitude scale, 404
data collection, 405-406
described, 402
interview schedule, 404-405
knowledge test in, 403-404
locale of, 403
materials in, 403
methods in, 403
sample size in, 403
tools developed in, 403-405

BOOK ORDER FORM!

Order a copy of this book with this form or online at:
http://www.haworthpress.com/store/product.asp?sku=5245

Social Work Visions from Around the Globe
Citizens, Methods, and Approaches

_____ in softbound at $39.95 (ISBN: 0-7890-2367-9)
_____ in hardbound at $69.95 (ISBN: 0-7890-2366-0)

COST OF BOOKS _____

POSTAGE & HANDLING _____
US: $4.00 for first book & $1.50
for each additional book
Outside US: $5.00 for first book
& $2.00 for each additional book.

SUBTOTAL _____
In Canada: add 7% GST. _____

STATE TAX _____
CA, IL, IN, MN, NJ, NY, OH & SD residents
please add appropriate local sales tax.

FINAL TOTAL _____
If paying in Canadian funds, convert
using the current exchange rate.
UNESCO coupons welcome.

❑ BILL ME LATER:
Bill-me option is good on US/Canada/
Mexico orders only; not good to jobbers,
wholesalers, or subscription agencies.

❑ Signature _____

❑ Payment Enclosed: $ _____

❑ PLEASE CHARGE TO MY CREDIT CARD:

❑ Visa ❑ MasterCard ❑ AmEx ❑ Discover
❑ Diner's Club ❑ Eurocard ❑ JCB

Account # _____

Exp Date _____

Signature _____
(Prices in US dollars and subject to change without notice.)

PLEASE PRINT ALL INFORMATION OR ATTACH YOUR BUSINESS CARD

Name

Address

City   State/Province   Zip/Postal Code

Country

Tel   Fax

E-Mail

May we use your e-mail address for confirmations and other types of information? ❑ Yes ❑ No We appreciate receiving
your e-mail address. Haworth would like to e-mail special discount offers to you, as a preferred customer.
We will never share, rent, or exchange your e-mail address. We regard such actions as an invasion of your privacy.

Order From Your **Local Bookstore** or Directly From
The Haworth Press, Inc. 10 Alice Street, Binghamton, New York 13904-1580 • USA
Call Our toll-free number (1-800-429-6784) / Outside US/Canada: (607) 722-5857
Fax: 1-800-895-0582 / Outside US/Canada: (607) 771-0012
E-mail your order to us: orders@haworthpress.com

For orders outside US and Canada, you may wish to order through your local
sales representative, distributor, or bookseller.
For information, see http://haworthpress.com/distributors

(Discounts are available for individual orders in US and Canada only, not booksellers/distributors.)

Please photocopy this form for your personal use.
www.HaworthPress.com

BOF05

DATE DUE

AG 29 02			

Please remember that this is a library book,
and that it belongs only temporarily to each
person who uses it. Be considerate. Do
not write in this, or any, library book.